Carcinogens and Related Substances

Carcinogens and Related Substances

Analytical Chemistry for Toxicological Research

MALCOLM C. BOWMAN

Division of Chemistry
National Center for Toxicological Research
Food and Drug Administration
Jefferson, Arkansas

MARCEL DEKKER, INC.   New York and Basel

Library of Congress Cataloging in Publication Data

Bowman, Malcolm C   [Date]
    Carcinogens and related substances.

    Includes bibliographical references and indexes.
    1. Carcinogenicity testing. 2. Carcinogens--
Analysis. 3. Chemistry, Analytic. I. Title.
RC268.65.B68   616.9'94'071   79-20476
ISBN 0-8247-6885-X

This volume was written by Malcolm C. Bowman in his private
capacity. No official support or endorsement by the Food and
Drug Administration is intended or should be inferred.

MARCEL DEKKER, INC.
270 Madison Avenue, New York, New York 10016

Current printing (last digit):
10 9 8 7 6 5 4 3 2 1

PRINTED IN THE UNITED STATES OF AMERICA

PREFACE

Mankind is currently being exposed to thousands of chemicals and
many new ones are being introduced each year. Since only a few
of these substances have been adequately tested, serious questions
have arisen concerning possible adverse effects on human health that
could result from the presence of such agents in the environment.
Public awareness of the problem and recommendations by environmental
scientists resulted in the establishment of the National Center for
Toxicological Research (NCTR) in 1971. The major objective of this
new national resource was to study the biological effects of potentially toxic or hazardous chemicals with emphasis on carcinogenesis
(cancer), teratogenesis (birth defects), and mutagenesis (inherited
defects) as determined by long-term, low-dose bioassays with large
numbers of test animals. The author has been concerned with the
analytical chemical requirements for valid and safe toxicological
experiments at NCTR since its inception.

Analytical chemical control of test substances should begin
when the chemical enters the laboratory and end only after its safe
disposal. The purpose of this book is to outline and discuss some
of the important principles, problems, and pitfalls encountered in
the chemistry of toxicological testing and to provide analytical
methodology in sufficient detail to enable a trained chemist to
perform many of the assays that may be required.

Although the book may be most useful to researchers in the fields
of chemistry, biochemistry, pharmacology, toxicology, and biology, it
is hoped that all scientists and laymen alike who are concerned with
toxicological research will find its contents to be of interest.

Malcolm C. Bowman

iii

CONTENTS

Carcinogens and
Related Substances

1

ANALYTICAL CHEMICAL REQUIREMENTS FOR TOXICOLOGICAL RESEARCH:
AN OVERVIEW

I   INTRODUCTION

The chemical industry has undergone vast expansion during the
past few decades. Of the 3,500,000 chemicals currently known, about
25,000 are now being produced in significant amounts in the United
States; new industrial chemicals are being added to the list at a
rate of about 700 annually [1]. Although the introduction of new
chemicals through the years has made an important contribution to
our quality of life, we must be assured that such substances can be
used safely and do not pollute the environment. It is estimated that
of all the chemicals now on the market, only about 6000 have been
tested for carcinogenic effects [2,3] and that about 1000 of these
have been found to produce tumors in animals [4]. An excellent compendium of potential industrial carcinogens and mutagens was recently
prepared by Fishbein [5].

Public awareness coupled with recommendations from the scientific
community concerning the need for safety evaluations of potentially
hazardous environmental chemicals was voiced in 1969 by recommendations of the Pesticide Advisory Committee to the Secretary of the
Department of Health, Education, and Welfare. This committee concluded that inadequacies existed in the safety evaluation of chemicals and that tests for carcinogenicity, teratogenicity, and mutagenicity merited immediate and urgent attention. The committee
further recommended the initiation of a major national effort to
correct these deficiencies.

In January 1971, President Nixon announced the establishment of
the National Center for Toxicological Research (NCTR) located on a
500-acre site between Little Rock and Pine Bluff, Arkansas. This
new national resource, although administered by the Food and Drug
Administration (FDA), is also a joint research venture with the
Environmental Protection Agency (EPA). The primary mission of the
NCTR is to conduct research pertaining to the biological effects of
potentially toxic chemical substances found in the environment with
emphasis in the following areas: (1) determination of adverse health
effects resulting from long-term, low-level exposure to chemical
toxicants, (2) determination of basic biological processes involving
chemical toxicants in animals to provide better extrapolation of data
from laboratory animals to humans, (3) development of improved meth-
odologies and test protocols for evaluation of the safety of chemical
toxicants, and (4) development of data that will facilitate the extrapolation of toxicological data from laboratory animals to humans.
Although these objectives are directed toward three broad research
categories consisting of carcinogenesis (cancer), teratogenesis
(birth defects), and mutagenesis (inherited defects), a wide variety
of explicit research programs exists within each category.

No toxicological test can be accomplished with assurance of
validity or safety without extensive analytical chemical tests becoming an integral part of the protocol. In the pages that follow,
the author, who has been responsible for the development of analytical chemical methods at the NCTR since its inception, will describe
some of the important principles concerning the chemistry of toxicological research, some problems encountered, and some of the
detailed chemical procedures employed, modified, and/or developed.

II   GOOD LABORATORY PRACTICES

Although researchers have long recognized the need for guidelines that will ensure the integrity of toxicological tests, the
standardization of good laboratory practices (GLPs) is still in its
infancy. Currently, the only published Federal documents on the

subject are the proposed regulations of the U. S. Department of Health, Education, and Welfare--FDA for nonclinical laboratory studies [6]. The finalized version of these regulations is expected to appear in 1979; however, it is not available at the present time. Problems encountered by the author during the past 5 years underline the need for standardized chemical control in toxicological tests. However, at best, the finest formal GLPs can only emphasize general principles of control; details of problems concerning individual test substances can be resolved only by utilizing the competency and judgment of the researcher.

The control of a test substance begins when it enters the laboratory and ends only after its safe disposal. Salient elements of the GLPs as they are related to the chemistry of a toxicological test have been previously discussed by the author [7,8]. Some of these elements that are of primary concern are

1. Identity, purity, chemical properties, and stability of the chemical
2. Handling and storage of the substance
3. Analysis of bioassay supplies for essential ingredients and deleterious substances
4. Homogeneity, stability, and proper concentration of test substance in the dosage form
5. Safety surveillance of personnel and work areas
6. Safe disposal of the chemical and contaminated experimental material

It should be noted at this point that none of these factors can be evaluated without adequate analytical methodology for the analysis of the substances in various substrates. Since there is no general agreement on the "threshold" level at which most carcinogens cause cancer or at which other substances produce damage, the analyst must strive for the ultimate sensitivity allowed by the state of the art.

III   PROPERTIES, IDENTITY, PURITY, AND STABILITY
OF THE CHEMICAL

Some of the analytical techniques that are generally accepted
and currently used at our laboratory for determining the properties,
identity, purity, and/or stability of test substances are listed as
follows:

Spectrophotometry (ultraviolet, visible, and infrared)

Spectrophotofluorimetry

Melting point

Boiling point

Solubility determinations

Thin-layer chromatography

High-pressure liquid chromatography

Atomic absorption spectrometry

Emission spectrometry

Derivatization techniques

Elemental analysis

Mass spectrometry

Nuclear magnetic resonance spectrometry

Solvent partitioning behavior

Vacuum volatiles

Recrystallization

Zone refinement

Gas-liquid chromatography (with various specific and nonspecific
    detectors)

The chemical nature of the test substance is the primary factor
governing the selection of appropriate techniques and, in practice,
only a limited number of the methods listed are actually used for an
individual test substance. For example, before initiating long-term,
low-dose studies with 2-acetylaminofluorene (2-AAF) in mice, our
primary analytical standard of the chemical was subjected to analysis.
(Note: 2-AAF which produces bladder tumors in mice is used as a
positive standard in bioassays.) It was found that our primary
standard of 2-AAF yielded identical melting points, spectrophoto-

fluorescent excitation and emission spectra, and temperature-
programmed gas chromatograms (containing no extraneous responses) by
using flame ionization detection both before and after recrystallization from methanol-water [9]. These data, coupled with a mass spectrum which gave the proper molecular weight and fragmentation pattern,
were considered sufficient evidence of identity and purity. The primary standard was then used as the basis for purity assays of kilogram
amounts of 2-AAF required for animal studies; specifically, spectrophotofluorescence, temperature-programmed gas chromatography, and
vacuum volatile determinations.

The initial batch (10 kg) of 2-AAF, acquired in 1972 for our
animal studies, was found to be about 85-90% pure and the impurities
were attributed to volatile materials which probably remained from a
recrystallization process. After the entire batch was dried at 135°C
overnight a purity of 99.6% was obtained. A decision was then made
that the purity and amount of test substance was adequate. In 1974
it was found that our supply of 2-AAF was inadequate for continued
testing and we attempted to purchase an additional 10-kg amount from
the original supplier. When we received the new shipment (June 1974)
it was assayed and found to contain 16.2% of 2-AAF. The manufacturer
was notified that the chemical was unsatisfactory and agreed to purify
the batch. In August 1974, a sample of the purified substance was
received and assayed at 1.68% purity. Had this low purity gone un-
detected, the entire long-term toxicity study may have been lost
without recognition of the loss, and worse, erroneous data may have
been generated. At this point, negotiations were started with a
different vendor, and in December 1974 their product was received,
assayed, and found to be 99.4% pure. This whole series of events
occurred before the existence of GLPs and provides an illustration
of the need for them. Current GLPs do in fact recommend that sufficient test substance consistent with stability and the needs of the
experiment is acquired, and that the identity, purity, and quality
of each batch of material should be determined [6].

No rigid rules can be cited concerning purity specifications
for test chemicals and each case must be separately assessed by the

researcher. It is suggested, however, with chemicals found to have
purities near 100%, that further assays should be directed toward
trace analyses for specific impurities. Candidate compounds for such
tests might include chemicals used in the synthesis and possible by-
products of the reaction or purification. An experienced toxicologist
can usually identify potential problems that could arise from the
presence of such contaminants. For example, in purity assays of
2,4,5-trichlorophenoxyacetic acid (2,4,5-T), trace assays should also
be conducted for the reaction by-product 2,3,7,8-tetrachlorodibenzo-
p-dioxin at the parts-per-billion (ppb) level (ng/g) because of its
extremely high biological activity.

Another example of the importance of identity and purity control
is given in a study of diethylstilbestrol (DES) carried out at our
laboratory [10]. This study shows (see Table 1.1) the relative stability of trans DES in 95% ethyl alcohol as contrasted to the isomerization of trans to cis DES in chloroform (Table 1.2). It is
known that the extent of chemical isomerization is governed by various
conditions (e.g., temperature, type of solvent, and light) and that
the trans isomer is the most active biologically. Therefore, it is
important not only to assay for the chemical per se but to be prepared to determine the isomeric ratio of the cis and trans forms.

Stability testing of the pure chemical becomes a fairly simple
matter if a good analytical method is available and a schedule of
reanalysis is instituted. This idea is contained in the GLPs which
state that periodic testing for purity, quality, and strength should
be undertaken. In actual practice, most pure chemicals are stable if
stored in a sealed light-tight container under ambient conditions.
Nevertheless, the stability of test chemicals must be determined on
an individual basis prior to the initiation of toxicological studies.

Information concerning the chemical and physicochemical properties of each test substance is essential for its analysis, control,
and use. Some of the properties of practical interest, in addition
to those previously listed, are (1) volatility, (2) acidic, basic,
or neutral properties, and (3) solubility and stability in a variety

Table 1.1. Isomeric content of DES in 95% ethyl alcohol after standing at ambient temperature for various periods of time.

	Percent isomeric content of DES at concentration indicated					
Hours after preparation	10 ppm		300 ppm		1000 ppm	
	cis	trans	cis	trans	cis	trans
0[a]	0	100	0	100	0	100
24	1.0	99.0	1.2	98.8	1.1	98.9
96	1.6	98.4	1.5	98.5	--	--
120	0.5	99.5	2.2	97.8	--	--
144	0.5	99.5	2.1	97.9	3.3	96.7

Source: King et al. [10].

[a]No detectable isomerization had occurred after 5 hr.

Table 1.2. Isomeric content of DES in chloroform after standing at ambient temperature for various periods of time.

	Percent isomeric content of DES at concentration indicated			
Hours after preparation	10 ppm		300 ppm	
	cis	trans	cis	trans
0	0	100	0	100
0.35	6.7	93.3	--	--
0.60	--	--	6.2	93.8
0.85	7.1	92.9	--	--
1.05	--	--	7.7	92.3
1.40	10.0	90.0	--	--
2.00	--	--	10.1	89.9
2.70	10.7	89.3	--	--
4.00	14.4	85.6	13.1	86.9
10.6	15.7	84.3	--	--
11.0	--	--	14.7	85.3
28.0	17.7	82.3	17.5	82.5
51.5	17.8	82.2	18.0	82.0

Source: King et al. [10].

of solvents (especially water). These properties and the practical
manner in which they are related to animal studies are discussed
throughout this book.

IV   HANDLING AND STORAGE OF THE TEST SUBSTANCE

Some of the most sophisticated guidelines for handling hazardous
substances are those described for radioactive materials [11]. Extensive thought has also been given to hazards involved in handling pathological organisms [12,13]. More recently, increased awareness of the
potential for injury by carcinogens, mutagens, teratogens, and other
toxic substances has stimulated interest in general rules for handling
and storage of these chemicals [14-16]. It is recommended that such
chemicals should be handled as if they were radioisotopes without the
requirement for radiation shielding. For example, in our laboratory
all chemicals known to be hazardous are held in a glove box equipped
with a high-efficiency particulate air (HEPA) filter (which retains
99.7% of particles of diameter 0.3 μm or more) and kept under reduced
pressure (0.5 in. of water) during operation. Weighings, dissolutions,
and preparation of formulations are performed in the glove box. The
preparations which are removed contain no higher concentrations than
those allowed under the guidelines of the Occupational Safety and
Health Administration (OSHA) [16].

The conditions under which test compounds are stored are dictated
by the stability of the chemical. Of course, storage of all chemicals
at liquid nitrogen temperature (-196°C) would be highly desirable.
However, where larger amounts of chemicals are required, this is
almost always impractical. In our laboratory, chemicals that are
under current study (e.g., 2-AAF, benzidine dihydrochloride, 4-amino-
biphenyl hydrochloride) which are required in large amounts and were
found to be stable, are stored in sealed containers under ambient
conditions in a locked room under the control of the Safety Officer.
Those chemicals requiring only a few grams for large-scale tests
(e.g., DES, estradiol) are stored in a freezer (-15°C). It is a
policy at our laboratory to reserve a few grams of each test substance

in a freezer repository to serve as a reference standard in the event
that questions might arise in the future concerning the integrity of
the chemical. This reference standard also allows the monitoring of
stability of bulk chemicals stored under other conditions or in
dosage forms.

V   HOMOGENEITY, STABILITY, AND PROPER CONCENTRATION OF TEST SUBSTANCE IN THE DOSAGE FORM

A broad spectrum of techniques of varying complexity has been
described for administering measured doses of chemicals to test animals; these techniques are briefly discussed in Chapter 3. However,
many of the techniques are not amenable to bioassays involving thousands of animals since a convenient means of administering the proper
dose must be employed. Thus far, in large-scale bioassays with mice
at the NCTR, the test chemical has been spiked either into the drinking water or the diet (animal feed).

The GLPs are fairly specific in their recommendations for the
provision of a pure compound and for its analysis and control. However, when it comes to actual handling of a test substance in an
experiment, the recommendations must be vague.

In practice, in our laboratory when chemicals are administered
in the drinking water, a concentrated stock solution is made with
the aid of sonication, filtered to exclude any possible undissolved
microparticles, assayed, and diluted to the proper dose concentrations. These dilutions are also assayed for correct dose levels.
Once a true solution is achieved, homogeneity can be assumed. Obviously the drinking water is the medium of choice because it generally
eliminates laborious assays, provides for rapid availability of the
analytical information, and results in a marked reduction in the cost
of analysis. Factors that determine whether dosed drinking water may
be used are the solubility and stability of the chemical in water and
the amount of the chemical required to produce the desired biological
response. For example, with 2-AAF and 3,3'-dichlorobenzidine dihydrochloride solubilities of 6 and 30 ppm in water at $25 \pm 2°C$ were insufficient to administer the desired dosage in drinking water; therefore,

they were fed in the diet. On the other hand, benzidine dihydrochloride and 4-aminobiphenyl hydrochloride were soluble at 61,700
and 4140 ppm and stable in water; therefore, they were administered
in the drinking water.

The development of suitable methodology and monitoring of dosage
concentrations in drinking water is relatively simple as compared to
that in the diet. Many of the carcinogens of interest were found to
fluoresce and methods for determining the hydrochloride salts and
free amines of benzidine, 4-aminobiphenyl, 3,3'-dimethylbenzidine,
3,3'-dimethoxybenzidine, and 2-naphthylamine were developed [17,18].
In our studies with 4-aminobiphenyl hydrochloride, a sample of the
dosage solution was simply diluted with aqueous HCl (pH 2) to about
1 µg/ml and its fluorescence (excitation and emission maxima, 260
and 382 nm, respectively) compared directly with that of a standard
solution [18]. The procedure is simple and rapid; many samples can
be prepared, analyzed, and used in the animal tests on the same day.

The stability of the test substance administered in drinking
water must be established under simulated test conditions (animals
absent) prior to the initiation of animal studies. For example, the
stability of 4-aminobiphenyl hydrochloride in water and aqueous HCl
(0.01 N, pH 2) under such test conditions is illustrated in Table 1.3
[18]. These studies included the highest and lowest anticipated dose
levels, and they were continued for 16 days, which was more than twice
as long as the solutions would normally be used. Aqueous HCl was the
medium of choice because the test substance was unstable in water
alone.

The certification of proper dose levels in the diet is a more
complex problem and usually centers around the necessity for an extensive cleanup prior to analysis. This is illustrated in our assay for
DES at low ppb levels which requires extraction, a three-step cleanup
consisting of a Sephadex LH-20 column, liquid-liquid partitioning,
and a silica gel column, followed by derivatization to pentafluoro-
propionyl-DES and subsequent analysis by electron-capture gas chromatography [10]. Assays of four samples (in duplicate) plus appropriate
controls and spiked samples require about 5 work days for completion.

Table 1.3. Stability of aqueous solutions of 4-aminobiphenyl
hydrochloride for 16 days.

Sampling intervals (days)	Concentration (ppm) of 4-aminobiphenyl·HCl solutions indicated[a]			
	1.0 ppm[b]	100 ppm[b]	1.0 ppm[c]	100 ppm[c]
0	0.989 ± 0.003	98.9 ± 0.35	1.01 ± 0.001	93.8 ± 0.00
1	0.973 ± 0.012	99.2 ± 0.42	0.781 ± 0.001	79.3 ± 0.02
2	0.968 ± 0.005	97.9 ± 0.90	0.649 ± 0.019	73.5 ± 0.17
4	0.976 ± 0.021	98.6 ± 1.00	0.459 ± 0.020	60.4 ± 2.30
8	0.950 ± 0.001	98.3 ± 0.31	0.365 ± 0.023	62.4 ± 0.66
16	0.936 ± 0.002	98.9 ± 0.50	0.282 ± 0.011	57.4 ± 1.10

Source: Holder et al. [18].

[a]Mean and standard error from triplicate assays.

[b]Aqueous HCl solution (0.01 N, pH 2); samples adjusted for control.

[c]Deionized water solution; samples adjusted for control.

Generally, where chemicals of low volatility and high thermal
stability are administered in the diet, alcoholic solutions containing
the proper amounts of test substances are sprayed onto the animal feed
while it is being agitated in a V-type solid processor operated at
elevated temperature and under reduced pressure. Results from chemical assays of multiple samples, taken from the batch, which are essentially identical and correspond to the theoretical dose are evidence
of homogeneity and stability during the mixing process. For example,
multiple assays of production batches (45 kg) of feed spiked with 0,
25, and 12,800 ppb of estradiol, which represent a control and the
lowest and highest levels of the chemical to be administered in large-
scale studies with mice, were carried out for a 43-day period and
indicated that homogeneity of mixing had been achieved and that the
chemical was essentially stable at these levels when stored in a
sealed stainless steel container at ambient temperature. Homogeneity
and stability of DES in the diet at levels as low as 2.5 ppb have also
been demonstrated.

From the chemist's point of view, drinking water is obviously the medium of choice because it generally eliminates long and tedious assays, provides for rapid availability of analytical information, and results in a marked reduction in cost of analysis.

VI   SAFETY SURVEILLANCE OF PERSONNEL AND WORK AREAS

The amount of effort expended in surveillance of personnel and work areas is determined by the relative hazard of the chemical entering the experiment. In the case of clearly hazardous materials, e.g., carcinogens, every effort must be made to assure that zero exposure is attained and that analytical chemical methods are available for monitoring extremely low, e.g., ppb or even parts per trillion (ppt, pg/g), levels of the substance. Since our laboratory is currently involved in animal studies with benzidine, which is a known carcinogen in humans [19], the surveillance approaches that we use with this compound are described below for the purpose of illustration. It should be emphasized that the general concept and techniques used for surveillance with various test chemicals remain essentially unchanged; however, the analytical chemical methodology employed for the detection and measurement of traces of the substances may be expected to vary widely.

Before surveillance for traces of benzidine dihydrochloride could be initiated it was necessary to develop suitable methodology; spectrophotofluorescence (SPF) was found to provide a relatively simple, rapid, and specific means of performing the assays [17]. At the onset of animal tests with benzidine dihydrochloride, routine monitoring of human urine, air, and work areas was also initiated to detect any accidental exposure of personnel.

Periodic analysis of the urine is a convenient means of determining human exposure to a chemical. Benzidine is known to be partially metabolized; however, no method for routine analysis of the metabolites is available. Nevertheless, it is believed that a sufficient amount of the parent compound is excreted through the urine to signal exposure if a sensitive analytical procedure is employed.

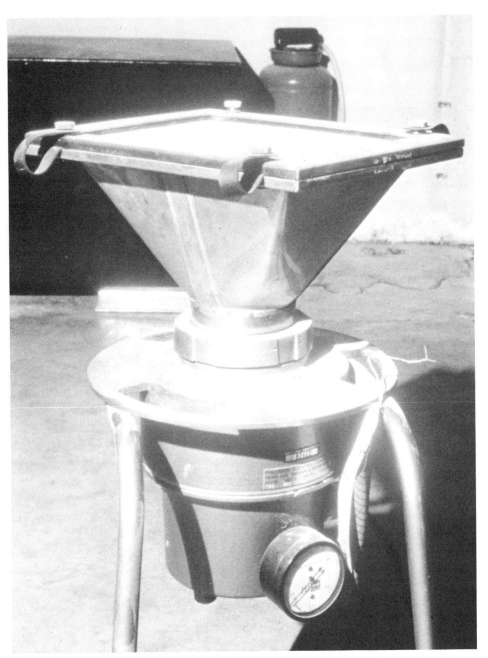

Figure 1.1. A High Volume Air Sampler equipped with a fiberglass HEPA filter for monitoring airborne particulate matter in work areas.

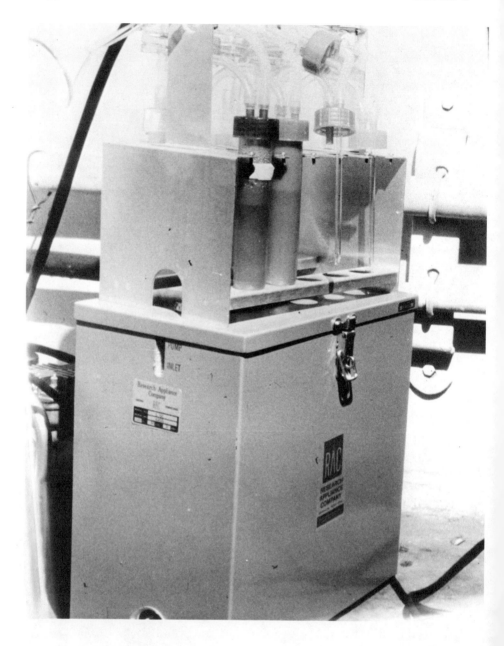

Figure 1.2. A portable Gas Collecting Sampler equipped with scribbers for monitoring vapors in work areas.

Therefore, our surveillance of personnel in these experiments is based on determining parent benzidine in urine. The minimum amount of benzidine detectable in urine (based on twice SPF background) is about 10 ppb; recoveries from samples spiked with 20 ppb are about 90%.

Any airborne particulate matter that might be present in the work areas is collected by using the High Volume Air System (No. 63084, Precision Scientific Co., Chicago, Ill.) shown in Figure 1.1. The apparatus is equipped with a fiberglass HEPA filter and operated continuously with a flow rate of about 2000 liters/min during the work day; the filter is removed weekly for chemical analysis and replaced by a new one. The smallest amount of benzidine that can be measured and confirmed in air by SPF analysis of the weekly filter samples is about 4 parts per trillion (ppt), based on twice SPF background.

It is recognized that any vapors of benzidine dihydrochloride or its free amine would probably not be retained by a HEPA filter. Therefore, the portable Gas Collecting Sampler (No. 2333-A, Research Appliance Co., Gibsonia, Pa.) shown in Figure 1.2, which is equipped with gas scrubbers (aqueous HCl is used for the amines), is also operated continuously in the work areas. The sensitivity obtained by using the air scrubbing device is several decades less than that of the particulate method because of the smaller volume of air sampled (ca. 2 liters/min); nevertheless, data obtained by using the apparatus are required for the efficient monitoring of a work area. Thus far, no residues of particulate benzidine or its vapor have been detected in the air from our work areas.

The monitoring of work areas (cages, floors, benches, apparatus, etc.) suspected of being contaminated with benzidine of its hydrochloride salt is accomplished by using kits consisting of a cotton applicator and a 5-ml culture tube equipped with a screw cap and containing exactly 2 ml of aqueous HCl (pH 2). The applicator is moistened with the aqueous acid and used to swab a specific area (ca. 100 cm^2); then the applicator is vigorously stirred in the acid solution after each of several subsequent swabbings of the same area.

The tube and contents are then centrifuged to remove any suspended
material and the supernatant is analyzed directly or after appropriate
dilution. Areas contaminated with as little as 0.3 µg of the benzidine salt are readily detected and the identity of the chemical is
confirmed by its characteristic excitation and emission maxima. The
efficiency of decontaminating areas where spills have occurred has
been confirmed by using this test.

Surveillance for other compounds or mixtures is performed in a
similar manner except that different solutions may be used in the air
scrubbing device and in the kit used for monitoring work surfaces.
Analytical procedures superior to the SPF method described for benzidine, because they are more sensitive, specific, and amenable to the
analysis of test substances and metabolites in admixture, are described in Chapter 4. However, such sophisticated procedures require
more time to perform the analysis.

VII   SAFE DISPOSAL OF THE CHEMICAL AND CONTAMINATED
EXPERIMENTAL MATERIAL

The decontamination of large volumes of wastewater, generated
in a toxicological research facility such as the NCTR, is one of the
most formidable problems. When all of our programs become operational, volumes of about 500,000 gallons will be discharged daily,
and contamination with several test substances will be the rule
rather than the exception. Indeed, the task of removing a single
contaminant is no small problem. Initially, when we were confronted
with the task of cleaning up wastewater containing only residues of
2-AAF, several means that were tested included millipore filtration,
organic solvent extraction, hydrolysis, distillation, and adsorption
on granular carbon and nonionic polymeric resin (XAD-2). Of these
methods, only adsorption was of use because it removed all detectable
residues (<0.2 ppb) and had the potential to accommodate large volumes of wastewater. A clean-up procedure based on a tandem arrangement of granular carbon and XAD-2 resin adsorbers was developed and
a pilot-scale system (up to 60,000 gallons) was evaluated [20]. This
system, which is described in detail in Chapter 5, is now used to

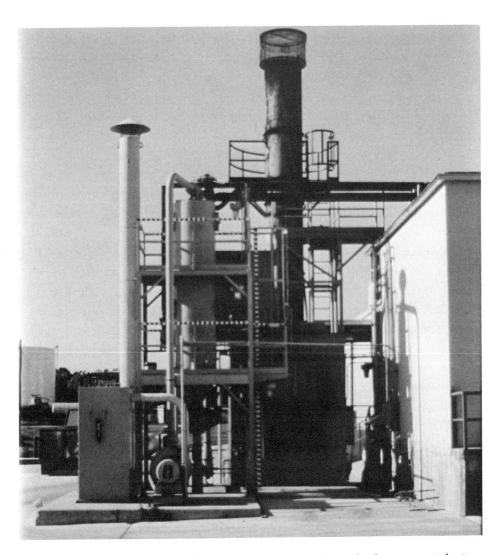

Figure 1.3. A two-chamber incinerator (secondary chamber operated at 850°C or higher) for disposal of contaminated experimental material.

decontaminate water from our most hazardous experiments. Current plans call for the scaling-up of the present system to accommodate all of the effluent from the facility. The system has potential for broad applicability as evidenced by the fact that all of the compounds evaluated thus far are retained by the adsorbers. Analytical procedures for use in determining residues of individual test substances in wastewater, human urine, air, and samples from work areas are presented in Chapter 3; a procedure for assaying mixtures of the substances is described in Chapter 4.

All highly contaminated waters, e.g., unused dosage forms and stock solutions, are subjected to a preliminary purification by percolating them through a 100-cm column made of plastic pipe [10 cm inside diameter (i.d.)] and filled with granular carbon (1.5 kg). When 164 liters of aqueous benzidine dihydrochloride (200 ppm, 32.8 g) were percolated through the column, the effluent contained no detectable residue (<1 ppb). Washing the column with an additional 132 liters of distilled water failed to elute any benzidine. This column was found adequate to purify all of the discarded highly contaminated water produced during a 1-week period. At the end of each week the plastic column was destroyed by incineration and a new one prepared. It should be noted that this column cannot be used for solutions containing organic solvents.

All contaminated solid waste, such as spent carbon adsorbers from the wastewater cleanup system, bedding, carcasses, diet, cardboard feeder boxes, clothing, and apparatus, are burned in a two-chamber incinerator with the secondary chamber maintained at about 850°C or higher (Figure 1.3). Liquid waste, whether organic or aqueous, may be atomized into the incinerator for disposal. Provision must also be made for the sampling and analysis of the exhaust gases from the incinerator stack to provide assurance that no test substance or harmful thermal degradation products are being discharged into the environment.

VIII   SUMMARY

The efficient control of chemicals during a nonclinical laboratory study is of the utmost importance from three main points of view:
(1) integrity of the experiment, (2) safety of personnel, and (3)
protection of the environment. While the general principles involved
in chemical control may be set forth in formal GLPs, detailed problems concerning individual test substances can only be resolved by
utilizing the competency and judgment of the researcher who is cog-
nizant with adequate analytical chemical methods.

The integrity of an experiment requires knowledge of the identity,
purity, and stability of the test substance, as well as its chemical
properties and a knowledge of its proper handling and storage. Tests
must also be performed to ensure the presence of essential ingredients
and the absence of deleterious substances in the bioassay system.
Assurance of homogeneity, stability, and proper concentration of the
chemical in the dosage form is also of primary importance.

The development and use of adequate analytical chemical procedures for determining the test agent in human samples, air, clothing,
and on work surfaces is necessary for the initiation of surveillance
procedures to assure safety of personnel from exposure to the test
substances.

The environment must be protected from exposure to the test substances by using adequate disposal techniques for the chemical and all
contaminated materials. This usually involves development of wastewater cleanup systems and continuous monitoring of the effluent to
prevent discharge of hazardous substances. Incineration is the most
useful method for disposal of solids and highly contaminated liquids;
however, the gases from the incinerator stack must also be monitored
to prevent contamination of the environment.

REFERENCES

1. National Cancer Institute. 4th Annual Collaborative Conference, Carcinogenesis Program, Orlando, Fl., February 22-26 (1976).

2. Anonymous. The spector of cancer. *Environ. Sci. Technol. 9,* 116 (1975).

3. B. Toth. Synthetic and naturally occuring hydrazines as possible causative agents. *Cancer Res. 35,* 3693 (1975).

4. World Health Organization. Prevention of cancer. WHO Tech. Report Ser. No. 276, Geneva, Switzerland, 1964.

5. L. Fishbein. Potential industrial carcinogens and mutagens. No. EPA 560/5-77-005, Office of Toxic Substances, *U. S. Environmental Protection Agency,* Washington, D.C.

6. *Federal Register.* Nonclinical laboratory studies: Proposed regulations for good laboratory practices. *41,* 51206-51230 (November 19, 1976).

7. M. C. Bowman. Control of test substances. *Clin. Toxicol.* in press (1979).

8. M. C. Bowman. Trace analysis: A requirement for toxicological research with carcinogens and hazardous substances. *J. Ass. Offic. Anal. Chem. 61,* 1253-1262 (1978).

9. M. C. Bowman and J. R. King. Analysis of 2-acetylaminofluorene: Residues in laboratory chow and microbiological media. *Biochem. Med. 9,* 390-401 (1974).

10. J. R. King, C. R. Nony, and M. C. Bowman. Trace analysis of diethylstilbestrol (DES) in animal chow by parallel high-speed liquid chromatography, gas chromatography and radioassays. *J. Chromatogr. Sci. 15,* 14-21 (1977).

11. U. S. Nuclear Regulatory Commission. *Code of Federal Regulations, Title 10,* Chapt. 1, Parts 30-35.

12. *National Institutes of Health Biohazards Safety Guide.* DHEW, PHS, NIH, 1974.

13. *Laboratory Safety at the Center for Disease Control.* DHEW, PHS, Publ. No. CDC 75-8118, 1974.

14. *National Cancer Institute Safety Standards for Research Involving Chemical Carcinogens.* DHEW Publ. No. (NIH) 75-900, June 2, 1975.

15. *Carcinogens, Control Procedures for the Safe Handling and Use of Cancer-causing Substances in the Workplace.* U. S. Dept. of Labor, OSHA Publ. No. 2204, January, 1975.

16. *General Industry Standards and Interpretations* Vol. 1, Part 1910, Subpart Z, Toxic and hazardous substances. U. S. Dept. of Labor, OSHA, October, 1972, pp. 642.14-642.111.

17. M. C. Bowman, J. R. King, and C. L. Holder. Benzidine and congeners: Analytical chemical properties and trace analysis in five substrates. *Int. J. Environ. Anal. Chem. 4,* 205-223 (1976).

18. C. L. Holder, J. R. King, and M. C. Bowman. 4-Aminobiphenyl, 2-naphthylamine, and analogs: Analytical properties and trace analysis of five substrates. *J. Toxicol. Environ. Health 2,* 111-129 (1976).

19. T. J. Haley. Benzidine revisited: A review of the literature and problems associated with the use of benzidine and its congeners. *Clin. Toxicol. 8,* 13-42 (1975).

20. C. R. Nony, E. J. Treglown, and M. C. Bowman. Removal of trace levels of 2-acetylaminofluorene (2-AAF) from wastewater. *Sci. Total Environ. 4,* 155-163 (1975).

2

THE BIOASSAY SUPPLIES: ANALYSIS FOR ESSENTIAL
AND/OR DELETERIOUS SUBSTANCES

I INTRODUCTION AND GENERAL SPECIFICATIONS

The basic components of a simple bioassay system for mice are
illustrated in Figure 2.1. The system consists of (1) a transparent
polycarbonate cage containing hardwood chips which are used as bedding, (2) a glass bottle (ca. 400 ml) for drinking water which is
equipped with a rubber stopper and a stainless steel "sipper tube"
containing a stainless steel ball to serve as a valve, (3) a wire
cage cover which supports the water bottle in an inclined position,
(4) a feeder constructed of stainless steel, and (5) a filter bonnet
that covers the top of the cage. The diet, contained in a cardboard
box, is inverted and inserted into the top of the stainless steel
feeder.

The presence of excessive amounts of aflatoxins, pesticides,
heavy metals, minerals, vitamins, and other substances in the untreated animal diet used in bioassays could bias the results obtained
with the test chemical. Also, in some instances, a deficiency of
certain nutrients, minerals, and vitamins could also exhibit a biological effect. Therefore, all animal feed (diet) used in toxicological studies should be subjected to analysis for a series of
essential and/or deleterious substances, and only those lots that
meet the desired specifications should be accepted for use in animal
studies. However, the preparation of a comprehensive list of all
such substances together with rigid tolerances and analytical procedures that would apply to various animal bioassay systems would be
an almost insurmountable task. Nevertheless, in order to minimize

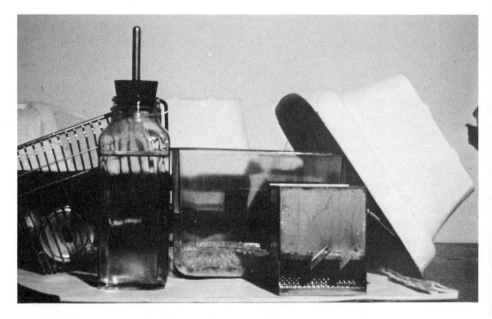

Figure 2.1. A simple bioassay system for
toxicological tests with mice.

adverse effects from the diet, a panel of scientists [1] at the
National Center for Toxicological Research (NCTR) has proposed the
tentative specifications presented in Table 2.1 for use in accepting
or rejecting the animal feed slated for bioassays with mice. It
should be emphasized that Table 2.1 is only a guideline; substances
for assay are likely to be added or deleted and their tolerances
changed as additional data are collected concerning their effects.
It should be noted the levels of selenium, vitamins A and B_1, and
fat and protein must be within specified ranges; calcium, copper,
and zinc must be present in at least the amount specified. Levels
of heavy metals, aflatoxins, and pesticide-related compounds must
not exceed the amounts indicated. The specifications for deleterious
substances are based upon current knowledge concerning minimum amounts
of each substance required to produce a biological response; it should
be recognized, however, that little is known concerning the additive

Table 2.1. Tentative specifications for essential and deleterious
substances in chow used for bioassays with mice

Substance	Specifications[a]
Aflatoxins (B_1, B_2, G_1, G_2)	5 ppb, max.
Estrogenic activity	5 ppb equivalents of DES, max.
Arsenic	1.0 ppm, max.
Cadmium	250 ppb, max.
Calcium	0.75%, min.
Copper	8.0 ppm, min.
Lead	1.5 ppm, max.
Mercury	200 ppb, max.
Selenium	0.05 ppm, min.; 0.65 ppm, max.
Zinc	75 ppm, min.
Dieldrin	20 ppb, max.
Heptachlor	20 ppb, max.
Lindane	100 ppb, max.
Malathion	5 ppm, max.
Polychlorinated biphenyls	50 ppb, max.
Total DDT-related substances	100 ppb, max.
Vitamin A	15 IU/g, min.; 75 IU/g, max.
Vitamin B_1	0.075 mg/g, min.; 0.125 mg/g, max.
Total fat	4.3%, min.; 6.7%, max.
Total protein	21.0%, min.; 28.0%, max.

[a]Abbreviations: ppm, parts per million; ppb, parts per billion;
max., maximum; min., minimum; IU, international units; DES, diethylstilbestrol.

Table 2.2. Tentative specifications for deleterious substances
in cardboard and animal bedding

	Specifications[a]	
Substance	Cardboard	Bedding
Pentachlorophenol	2.0 ppm, max.	2.0 ppm, max.
Polychlorinated biphenyls	10.0 ppm, max.	10.0 ppm, max.
Total DDT-related substances	1.0 ppm, max.	--
Dieldrin	0.1 ppm, max.	--
Heptachlor	0.1 ppm, max.	--
Lindane	0.1 ppm, max.	--
Malathion	5.0 ppm, max.	--
Total organochlorine pesticides	--	1.0 ppm, max.
Total organophosphorus pesticides	--	5.0 ppm, max.
Moisture	--	8%, max.

[a]Abbreviations as for Table 2.1.

effects of the substances as well as their interactions with the
test chemical or with each other.

Other materials introduced into large-scale bioassays with mice
include feeder boxes constructed of cardboard (used to dispense feed
into the stainless steel feeders) and the animal's bedding (hardwood
chips). Since these materials could also contain deleterious substances, they must be tested prior to use. Tentative specifications
for the cardboard and bedding are presented in Table 2.2.

The drinking water is another possible means of introducing
deleterious substances into the bioassay system. However, the author
is not aware of any current specifications governing the treatment of
water slated for use in bioassays or analytical parameters for its
acceptance or rejection. It is suggested that the filtration of tap
water, followed by deionization, subsequent percolation through
activated carbon, and finally distillation from glass, will provide
potable water for the animals that is of sufficiently high quality.
Periodic assays of the potable water supply is recommended for

possible contaminants such as total organochlorine pesticides and related substances, total organophosphorus pesticides, arsenic, cadmium, selenium, lead, mercury, iron, nickel, beryllium, chromium, copper, and chloroform. In the absence of specifications governing permissible levels of various substances in potable water, the researcher must independently assess the possibility of adverse effects. Since a mouse may consume about twice as much water as diet, a fairly safe conclusion might be that twice the residue of a substance found in the water added to that found in the diet should not exceed the specification for the diet. Those substances found in potable water that are not mentioned in the specifications for the diet must be assessed individually, based on any biological effects reported in the literature.

The adequate control of microorganisms in the bioassay system is an essential part of long-term experiments. Although the details of microbiological control are beyond the scope of this book, it should be pointed out that measures taken to achieve a specific-pathogen-free environment (e.g., autoclaving the diet) could bias the chemical quality of the bioassay system. Therefore, chemical tests must be designed to provide assurance that such sterilization techniques do not result in a deficiency of essential ingredients or the addition of deleterious substances.

The chemical analysis of all bioassay supplies for all of the essential and deleterious substances previously discussed is expensive and requires a wide variety of analytical procedures of varying complexity; nevertheless, such assays are necessary to provide assurance of a valid toxicological test. Descriptions of most of these procedures in sufficient detail to allow a trained chemist to perform the assays are presented in the remaining pages of this chapter. Although the assay for estrogenic activity is not a chemical procedure, details are included as a convenience to the analyst. In the procedures that follow, all solvents are pesticide grade and all chemicals are CP (chemically pure) grade unless otherwise specified. Extreme care must be taken to ensure that all glassware and apparatus

are free of any traces of substances that might interfere with the
analysis.

II   ANALYSIS OF THE DIET

A. Aflatoxins

1. *General Description of Method*

This method which determines traces of aflatoxins B_1, B_2, G_1, and G_2
in animal feed [2] is based on a modification of procedures previously
reported [3-6]. Aflatoxins are extracted with methanol [4], cleaned
up by solvent partitioning, separated and estimated by using a two-
dimensional thin-layer chromatography system [5], and confirmed by
treatment with trifluoroacetic acid on the TLC plate [6]. Formulas
of the four aflatoxins are presented in Figure 2.2.

2. *Extraction and Cleanup Procedure*

Extract 50 g of the feed sample with 150 ml of methanol for 2 min at
high speed in a Waring blender. Centrifuge a 35-ml portion of the
extract at 1000 revolutions per minute (rpm) for 3 min then transfer

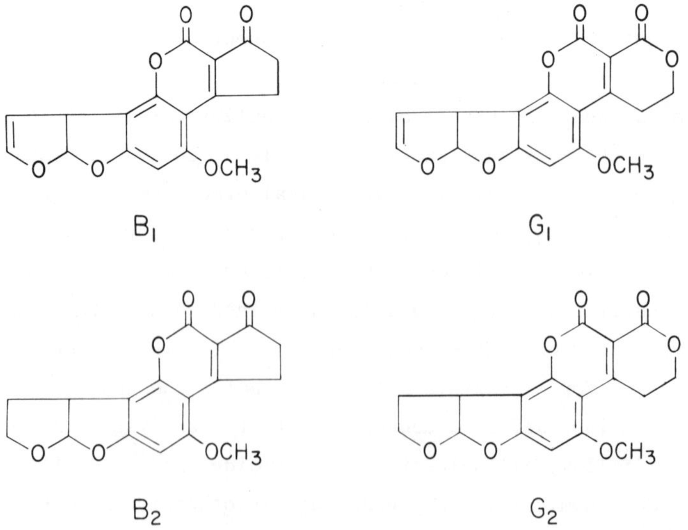

Figure 2.2. Formulas of aflatoxins B_1, B_2, G_1, and G_2.

20 ml of the clear extract to a separatory funnel containing 40 ml
of aqueous ammonium sulfate (20%) and 30 ml of hexane. Shake the
contents for about 1 min; transfer the bottom layer (aqueous) to a
second separatory funnel and discard the hexane layer. Extract the
aqueous layer with two additional 30-ml portions of hexane. After
the last extraction, drain the aqueous layer into a separatory
funnel containing 5 ml of dichloromethane, and discard the hexane..
Shake the contents for about 30 sec, allow the layers to separate,
and carefully drain the dichloromethane layer (bottom) into a 50-ml
round-bottom flask containing a boiling bead. Evaporate the contents
just to dryness by using water pump vacuum and a 60°C water bath.

   3. Thin-layer Chromatographic Analysis

Add 100 µl of benzene-acetonitrile [98:2, volume/volume (v/v)] to
the flask containing the dry extract and gently swirl the flask to
dissolve the residue. Spot 10 µl of the solution in the right corner
of a TLC plate (Brinkman MN-Silica Gel-GHR, 20 x 20 cm, used as received) and first develop the plate with diethyl ether-methanol-water
(90:4.5:1.5). Turn the TLC plate on its right side and develop it a
second time with chloroform-acetone (90:10). Use a long-wave ultraviolet lamp (360 nm) to view the four aflatoxins which emit a bluish
fluorescence. With both of the TLC solvent systems, R_f (retention
factor) values for B_1, B_2, G_1, and G_2 are about 0.60, 0.55, 0.50, and
0.48, respectively; however, the second development (chloroform-
acetone) is much more efficient in separating the aflatoxins from
interferences in the feed. A sample of the feed spiked with known
amounts of the four aflatoxins is also carried through the procedure
to provide a semiquantitative estimation of the residues in the sample
of unknown aflatoxin content.

   4. Confirmatory Test for Aflatoxins B_1 and G_1

Divide a TLC layer into two halves by scratching a vertical line.
On one side spot two equivalent portions of sample extract thought
to contain 0.2-2 ng of B_1 and G_1. Superimpose an equal amount of
aflatoxin standard of B_1 and G_1 on one of the spots of extract and
also spot separately the same amount of B_1 and G_1 standard. Cover

the unused half of the plate with cardboard then superimpose 2 μl of a benzene-trifluoroacetic acid (TFA) mixture (1:1, v/v) on each of the three spots; allow 5 min for the TFA to react. Spot the same pattern of three spots on the other half of the plate substituting standards of aflatoxin B_2 and G_2; do not superimpose TFA. Dry the plate for 10 min by using cool air from an air blower, then develop the plate by using benzene-ethyl alcohol-water (46:35:19). Allow the plate to dry in the dark and examine it under ultraviolet light (360 nm).

The derivative of aflatoxin B_1 will appear as a blue fluorescent spot (R_f 0.18-0.3) while the derivative of G_1 is a green fluorescent spot (R_f 0.15-0.25). The TFA reacts completely with B_1 and G_1 while B_2 and G_2 are not affected. The formation of derivatives in the sample with the same R_f value of the derivatized standards confirms the presence of B_1 and G_1. Examination of the plate under short-wave ultraviolet light often reveals spurious spots in the area of afla-toxin G_1 and G_2. Spray the plate with aqueous nitric acid (25%); the fluorescence of all four aflatoxins and the derivatives of B_1 and G_1 changes from blue or green to yellow. This also provides additional confirmation of identity.

B. Estrogenic Activity (Bioassay) [7]

1. *General Description of Method*

Three groups of female mice are fed diets as follows: (1) a negative control, (2) a positive control (DES added), and (3) the diet for analysis. After 7 days, comparisons are made of the ratios of mean uterine weight to terminal body weight of each group.

2. *Preparation of Rations for Use in Bioassays*

a. *Negative control*   This ration, which is for use in establishing baseline uterine weights, is prepared by extracting a control diet (similar in nutrient content to the rations to be assayed) with diethyl ether for at least 2 hr. The crude fat content is then adjusted to the same level as the rations to be assayed. The source of added fat may be refined cottonseed oil, corn oil, or soybean oil

b. *Positive control*   This ration is prepared in the same manner as the negative control except that the fat added back to the ration after extraction with diethyl ether contains an appropriate amount of DES to provide a concentration of 5 ppb in the final ration mixture. Ether or acetone is used to dissolve the DES prior to adding it to the fat in order to provide a more uniform distribution of the hormone throughout the ration.

c. *The diet for assay*   The ration being assayed for estrogenic activity is fed in the same physical form as the two control rations. Purified fat may be added to test rations of low crude fat content to increase palatability.

   3. The Bioassay

Groups of 15 prepuberal female mice 14-17 days old (6-12 g body weight) are assigned to the positive and negative control rations and to samples of the diet to be assayed for estrogenic activity. The mice are assigned to groups in a manner that results in a near equal mean body weight and the groups are randomly assigned to the various rations (and controls) for assay. The mice may be housed in community cages with a maximum of five mice per cage and with rations and water available ad libitum for a period of 7 days. On the seventh day each mouse is weighed (to the nearest tenth of a gram), sacrificed in a humane manner, and the uterus removed, blotted, and weighed (to the nearest milligram).

   4. Evaluation of the Bioassay Results

a. *Negative assay*   When the ratio of the mean uterine weight to the mean terminal weight for a given sample is less than the ratio obtained with the positive control, the test shall be considered negative. That is, the total estrogenic activity is less than 5 ppb equivalents of DES and the diet is within the specifications and acceptable for use.

b. *Positive assay*   When the ratio of the mean uterine weight to the mean terminal body weight of a sample is more than the ratio for the positive control, the test shall be considered positive.

of DES and the diet is not within the specifications and should be
rejected for use in bioassays.

c. *Invalid assay*   When the ratio of the mean uterine weight to the
mean terminal body weight of the positive control is not at least
1.5 times the ratio obtained with the negative control, the entire
test shall be considered invalid.

    C. Minerals and Heavy Metals

    1. *Calcium and Zinc* [2,8]

a. *General description of method*   The sample is ashed at 550°C,
dissolved in HCl, filtered, diluted, and analyzed by atomic absorption spectrometry (air-acetylene flame) for calcium (422.7 nm) and
zinc (213.8 nm).

b. *Preparation of sample*   Place a well-glazed porcelain crucible
containing 2-10 g of the sample into a cold muffle furnace; slowly
increase the heat to 550°C and ash the sample for 4 hr. Allow the
crucible to cool, add 10 ml of 3 N HCl, cover the crucible with a
watch glass, and gently boil it for 10 min. After the crucible has
cooled, filter the contents into a 100-ml volumetric flask and
adjust the volume with water. Make any subsequent dilutions necessary to bring the concentration of calcium or zinc into the linear
range of the instrument by using 0.1 N HCl.

(1) Analysis of calcium. Set an atomic absorption spectrometer
equipped with a hollow-cathode calcium lamp and a 10-cm burner head
to previously established optimum conditions using a rich air-
acetylene flame and a wavelength of 422.7 nm. Read at least four
standard solutions within the linear range of the instrument (e.g.,
0, 5, 10, 15, and 20 µg of calcium per milliliter) before and after
each group of unknown samples (12 or less); flush the burner well
with water between samples. Prepare a calibration curve from the
mean of each standard determined before and after the group of
unknowns and calculate the calcium content of each sample by using
the following relationship:

$$Ca\ (ppm) = \frac{\mu g/ml\ in\ unknown\ (from\ curve)}{g/ml\ of\ sample\ analyzed}$$

(2) Analysis of zinc   Set an atomic absorption spectrometer equipped with a hollow-cathode zinc lamp and a 10-cm burner head to previously established optimum conditions using a lean air-acetylene flame and a wavelength of 213.8 nm. Prepare four standard solutions of zinc within the linear range of the instrument, construct a calibration curve (absorption versus concentration), analyze the samples of unknown zinc content, and perform calculations in a manner similar to that described for calcium.

   2. *Copper* [2,9]

a. *General description of method*   The sample is ashed, dissolved in HCL, reacted with tetraethylenepentamine, and the copper content determined spectrophotometrically at 620 nm.

b. *Preparation of sample*   Ash 8 g of sample at 600°C for 2 hr and transfer the residue to a 200-ml volumetric flask by using 20 ml of HCl and 50 ml of water. Boil the contents for 5 min, allow to cool, and adjust the volume to 200 ml with water. Transfer a 50-ml aliquot to a 100-ml volumetric flask for color development and subsequent analysis.

   Prepare standard solutions of copper in 100-ml volumetric flasks by using 1-10 ml of aqueous copper sulfate (1 mg of Cu per milliliter). Next, add 4 ml of HCl, dilute to 50 ml with water, then add 5 ml of tetraethylenepentamine. Finally, adjust the volume to 100 ml with water and mix thoroughly; also prepare a reagent blank using all of the reagents except the copper sulfate solution.

   Add 5 ml of tetraethylenepentamine to the 50-ml aliquots of samples of unknown copper content, adjust the volume to 100 ml with water, mix thoroughly, and filter the mixture prior to analysis.

c. *Analysis of copper*   Prepare a calibration curve (absorbance versus concentration) for copper by using a spectrophotometer set at 620 nm to measure the standard solutions. Correct all absorbance readings by subtracting the value obtained for the reagent blank.

Determine the absorbance of the samples for analysis and calculate
their copper content by using the following relationship:

$$\text{Cu (ppm)} = \frac{\mu g/ml \text{ in unknown (from curve)}}{g/ml \text{ of sample analyzed}}$$

3. *Arsenic*

a. *General description of method*   This modification of the method
of Hundley and Underwood [10] involves the very careful ashing of a
20-g sample, evolution of arsine, development of a colored complex
with silver diethyldithiocarbamate, and subsequent colorimetric
analysis at 540 nm.

b. *Preparation of sample*   Mix 20 g of the sample with 3 g of MgO
and 10 ml of cellulose powder in a porcelain dish then add 50 ml of
deionized water and stir to form a slurry. Rinse the stirring rod
with water and heat the dish at 110°C overnight or until the contents
are dry. Next, pre-char the sample in a muffle furnace at 300°C
until evolution of smoke ceases. Allow the dish to cool and overlay
the contents with 3 g of $Mg(NO_3)_2 \cdot 6H_2O$. Place the dish in a cool
furnace and slowly increase the heat to 550°C then ash the sample at
that temperature for 2 hr. Again, allow the dish to cool, moisten
the residue with deionized water and dissolve it with 50 ml of 6 N HCl.
Transfer the solution and any residue to a 250-ml flask used for evolution of arsine. Use two 20-ml portions of 6 N HCl and several small
portions of deionized water to rinse the contents of the dish into the
flask. The total volume added to the flask should be 90 ml of 6 N HCl
plus 85 ml of water.

c. *Apparatus for arsine evolution*   Use a 250-ml flask with a ground
glass neck (24/40 joint) for an evolution flask. Saturate glass wool
with a saturated aqueous solution of lead acetate and dry just to
touch in a 110°C oven. Use a delivery tube with a 24/40 joint to
connect to the flask and with an open end to dip into the trapping
solution contained in a 15-ml conical tube. Plug the 24/40 joint
with lead acetate-saturated glass wool and wrap the other end of the
delivery tube with unimpregnated glass wool to diffuse the bubbles
of gas.

d. *Evolution of arsine*   Pipet 5 ml of silver diethyldithiocarbamate
(Ag-DDC) solution (0.5% Ag-DDC in pyridine) into a 15-ml conical receiving tube. Add 2 ml of potassium iodide (KI) solution (15% KI in
deionized water) and 1 ml of stannous chloride ($SnCl_2$) solution
(40% $SnCl_2 \cdot 2H_2O$ in HCl) separately to the evolution flask and swirl
the contents after each addition. Finally, add 6 g of zinc to the
flask and quickly connect the delivery tube to the evolution flask
and place the receiving tube to allow the evolved arsine and hydrogen
to pass through the Ag-DDC solution. Analyze the Ag-DDC solution
colorimetrically for arsine content.

e. *Analysis of arsenic*   Prepare a series of standards for use in
constructing a calibration curve (absorbance versus concentration)
by spiking evolution flasks containing 90 ml of 6 N HCl and 85 ml of
water with various amounts of arsenic up to a total of 10 µg. Proceed with the generation of arsine and the trapping of the vapors
from each flask in Ag-DDC solution. Determine the absorbance of the
Ag-DDC solutions by using a spectrophotometer set at 540 nm employing
pyridine as a reference. Prepare a reagent blank in the same manner
and subtract its absorbance from that of each sample. Calculate the
arsenic content of the samples for analysis by relating their absorbance to the standard curve.

f. *Typical results*

(1) Five reagent blanks carried through the procedure gave
0.033 ± 0.009 ppm As.

(2) Five samples of laboratory chow 5010C (Ralston Purina Co.,
St. Louis, Mo.) unspiked and spiked with 0.1 ppm of arsenic gave
0.090 ± 0.004 and 0.167 ± 0.009 ppm As, respectively; therefore the
recovery of arsenic at the 0.100 ppm level was about 77%.

(3) Triplicate samples of laboratory chow 5010C assayed before
and after being autoclaved gave results of 0.114 ± 0.009 and 0.115
± 0.005 ppm as As corrected for 77% recovery.

4. *Cadmium and Lead* [11,12]

a. *General description of method*   The sample is ashed at 550°C,
dissolved in HNO_3, diluted, and analyzed for cadmium (228.8 nm) by

using an atomic absorption spectrometer equipped with a graphite
furnace. For the lead analysis, an aliquot of the solution is
reacted with ammonium pyrrolidine dithiocarbamate, extracted with
methyl isobutyl ketone, and analyzed in a similar manner at 283.3 nm.

b. *Analysis of cadmium*   Dry-ash 5 g of sample by slowly charring
it then heating at 550°C for 6 hr. Dissolve the residue by using
two 5-ml portions of 1 N HNO_3 and bringing each portion of acid to
a boil. Quantitatively transfer the solutions to a 50-ml volumetric
flask and adjust the contents to volume with deionized water. Analyze the solution for cadmium content by using an atomic absorption
spectrometer (228.8 nm) equipped with a graphite furnace. Calculate
the cadmium content by relating the absorbance to a standard curve
prepared from a series of cadmium solutions analyzed within the
linear range of the instrument.

c. *Analysis of lead*   Withdraw a 10-ml aliquot of the solution
analyzed for cadmium, add a drop of thymol blue, and dilute aqueous
ammonium hydroxide (1:9) dropwise until the color changes from yellow
to light blue. Add 2 ml of a 1% aqueous solution of ammonium pyrrolidine dithiocarbamate (APDC), mix, then add 4 ml of methyl isobutyl
ketone and thoroughly mix the preparation again. Extraction of the
sample solutions with APDC is necessary in the case of animal feed
to eliminate interferences. Set the instrument used for the cadmium
assay at 283.3 nm and analyze the organic phase for lead. Calculate
the lead content by relating the absorbance to a standard curve prepared from known concentrations of lead analyzed in the same manner.

d. *Typical results*

(1) Cadmium. (a) Reagent blanks for cadmium averaged about 11.1 ppb.
(b) Triplicate samples of unspiked laboratory chow 5010C analyzed
versus samples spiked with 100 ppb of cadmium yielded recoveries of
96.2 ± 1.9%. (c) Triplicate samples of laboratory chow 5010C (unspiked) contained 90.3 ± 1.1 ppb of cadmium, corrected for 96.2%
recovery.

(2) Lead. (a) Six reagent blanks yielded 24 ± 2 ppb. of lead.
(b) Triplicate samples of unspiked laboratory chow 5010C analyzed

versus samples spiked with 200 ppb of lead gave recoveries of 102
± 4%. (c) Triplicate samples of laboratory chow 5010C (unspiked)
contained 310 ± 20 ppb of lead. (d) Triplicate samples of rat and
mouse ration (unspiked) used by the National Institutes of Health
(NIH) contained 1240 ± 40 ppb of lead.

5. *Selenium* [13]

a. General description of method   The sample is prepared by wet
digestion with $HClO_4$-H_2SO_4-HNO_3 and treatment with H_2O_2. A complex
is then formed by using NH_4OH, 2,3-diaminonaphthalene (DAN), and
ethylenedinitrilotetraacetate (EDTA) reagents. The complex is extracted with hexane and selenium is determined by spectrophotofluorescence.

b. Special reagents

(1) The DAN reagent. Add 50 mg of DAN to a 125-ml separatory
funnel containing 50 ml of sulfuric acid solution (140 ml of concentrated H_2SO_4 added to water then diluted to 1 liter with water).
Shake the contents for 15 min, add 50 ml of hexane, and shake for an
additional 15 min. After the layers have separated, place a plug of
glass wool in the stem of the funnel and draw off the bottom layer
for immediate use.

(2) The EDTA reagent. Prepare a 0.02 M solution by dissolving
7.445 g of disodium-EDTA in water and diluting it to 1 liter.

c. Procedure   Accurately weigh 1 g or less of the sample, containing up to 0.5 μg of selenium, and place it into a 100-ml Kjeldahl
flask. Sequentially add 6 ml of concentrated NHO_3, 2 ml of 70%
$HClO_4$, and 5 ml of concentrated H_2SO_4. Use a micro Kjeldahl digestion unit to heat slowly in initial stages to avoid any loss and
slowly increase the heat to a vigorous boil. Add small amounts of
HNO_3 at first signs of charring. The solution will turn yellow and
then water white. Remove the flask and swirl the contents to contact
the bulb area and the lower neck; the yellow color may reappear.
(In some instances the solution may remain pale yellow; in those
cases a heating time of about 2.5 hr is considered sufficient.)

Remove the flask, add 1 ml of 30% H_2O_2 and swirl the contents; after
all action ceases return the flask to the heat until the contents
are boiling briskly and white fumes appear. Add H_2O_2 twice more and
continue final boiling for 5 min after the appearance of white fumes.
Cool the flask, carefully add 30 ml of water, and quantitatively
transfer the contents to a 250-ml Erlenmeyer flask by using two
10-ml portions and one 5-ml portion of water. Prepare DAN reagent.
as time permits. Add to the flask, with mixing, 10 ml of EDTA
reagent, 25 ml of aqueous NH_4OH (40 ml concentrated NH_4OH diluted
to 100 ml), and 5 ml of DAN reagent. Bring the mixture rapidly to
a vigorous boil by using a burner and place the flask on a preheated
hot plate to continue boiling. Boil the mixture for exactly 2 min
then set it aside for 1 hr. Add 6 ml of hexane, shake the contents
for 5 min, then transfer the mixture to a separatory funnel and
allow the phases to separate. Discard the aqueous phase (bottom),
collect the hexane layer in a tube, and centrifuge the contents at
about 1000 rpm for 5 min. Measure the relative fluorescent intensity
of the hexane extract by using a spectrophotofluorometer set with
excitation and emission wavelengths of 374 and 520 nm, respectively.
Calculate the selenium content of the sample by relating the relative intensity (corrected for the reagent blank) to a standard curve
prepared from known amounts of selenium analyzed in the same manner.

d. Typical results

(1) Quadruplicate reagent blanks yielded 180 ± 8 ppb of selenium.

(2) Quadruplicate samples of unspiked laboratory chow 5010C analyzed versus samples spiked with 200 ppb of selenium gave recoveries
of 104 ± 6%.

(3) Quadruplicate samples of laboratory chow 5010C (unspiked),
analyzed before and after being autoclaved, contained 420 ± 16 and
388 ± 2 ppb of selenium, respectively.

(4) Triplicate samples of NIH rat and mouse ration were found
to contain 383 ± 35 ppb of selenium.

6. Mercury

a. *General description of method*   This modified method of Hatch
and Ott [14] is based on wet digestion of the sample, acid oxidation
for dissolution, reduction of mercury to the elemental state, and
analysis of the vapors by flameless atomic absorption spectrometry.

b. *Procedure*   Accurately weigh 1 g of sample and transfer it to a
100-ml Kjeldahl flask containing three glass beads. Add, in sequence,
6 ml of concentrated HNO_3, 2 ml of $HClO_4$, 5 ml of concentrated H_2SO_4,
and 1 ml of 2% sodium molybdate. Using a micro Kjeldahl digestion
unit, slowly heat the flask in the initial stage to avoid any loss
and gradually increase the heat to a vigorous boil. If charring
occurs, add a few drops of concentrated HNO_3. The solution will turn
yellow and then water white. Remove the flask from the digestion
unit and swirl the contents; the yellow color may reappear. Continue
heating until the contents are water white and white fumes appear.
The total digestion time should be almost 2 hr. Remove the flask,
swirl the contents, cool, and add 1 ml of 30% hydrogen peroxide; the
contents will turn yellow. Heat the flask until white fumes again
appear then swirl and cool the contents. Repeat the hydrogen peroxide additions twice more and continue final boiling for 5 min
after the appearance of white fumes.

Quantitatively transfer the sample to a 100-ml volumetric flask
using several rinses of deionized water; adjust the solution to
100 ml. Use a Coleman Model MAS-50 Mercury Analyzer System (Coleman
Instruments Division, Perkin-Elmer Corp., Maywood, Ill.) to determine
the residue of mercury in the sample as described.

Pour the 100-ml sample solution into a BOD bottle and add
two drops of 5% potassium permanganate solution. Next, add 5 ml
of 5.6 N HNO_3 and swirl the contents, and after 15 sec add 5 ml
of 18 N H_2SO_4, swirl the contents, and wait for 45 sec. Add 5 ml
of 1.5% hydroxylamine hydrochloride and swirl the contents; the
sample should turn clear in about 15 sec. Finally, add 5 ml of
10% stannous chloride and immediately insert the bubbler of the

mercury analyzer into the BOD bottle and make sure that the stopper is tightly sealed. Record the highest meter reading and then place the bubbler into a BOD bottle containing 100 ml of 1 N HNO_3 and purge for several minutes to clean the system. (Note: The various reagents used in this procedure are available in a Mercury Analysis Reagent Kit; Coleman, No. 50-050.)

Although the instrument is designed to read total micrograms of mercury directly from the meter, it is suggested that a standard curve be prepared as follows. Prepare a series of BOD bottles containing 0.1-2.0 µg of mercury in a volume of 100 ml. Follow the procedure previously described beginning with the addition of two drops of potassium permanganate solution. Plot micrograms of mercury versus the meter reading. Calculate the mercury content in the samples for analysis by relating their meter readings to the standard curve.

c. Typical results

(1) Quadruplicate reagent blanks yielded 0.0435 ± 0.005 ppm of mercury.

(2) Triplicate samples of unautoclaved laboratory chow 5010C spiked with 0.2 and 0.5 ppm of mercury gave recoveries of 71.7 ± 2.6 and 87.3 ± 4.4%, respectively.

(3) Triplicate samples of unspiked laboratory chow 5010C analyzed before and after being autoclaved gave values essentially identical to the reagent blanks. Therefore, based on the criterion of twice background (reagent blank), all samples contained less than 0.1 ppm of mercury.

D. Vitamins

1. Vitamin A [15]

a. General description of method   The method is based on the saponification of vitamin A esters by reflux with alcoholic KOH, extraction of the retinol thus formed with hexane, cleanup on a column of alumina, development of a colored complex with antimony trichloride, and quantitation of the colored product at 620 nm by
        rophotometry.

b. Special reagents and apparatus

(1) Carr-Price reagent and dispenser. Add sufficient chloroform to 200 g of antimony trichloride to make 1 liter. Warm and shake to dissolve, cool, and add 30 ml of acetic anhydride (total volume = 1030 ml); store in a repipet-type dispenser to rapidly and accurately deliver 10.0 ml.

(2) Alumina. Dispense 5 ml of water in the inner surface of a glass-stoppered bottle and add 95 g of Woelm alumina (neutral). Mix the contents thoroughly by shaking and allow the mixture to stand with occasional shaking for 12 hr prior to use. Store in a tightly stoppered container.

(3) Preparation of vitamin A standard solution. Weigh 100 mg of vitamin A reference solution (obtained from USP Reference Standards, 12601 Twinbrook Parkway, Rockville, Md.) into a 125-ml Erlenmeyer flask and add 400 mg of fresh cottonseed oil. Carry this extraction through the saponification and extraction procedure and use aliquots of the resulting hexane solution to evaluate the performance of the alumina column.

(4) Spectrophotometer. For rapid absorbance determinations, use an instrument equivalent to a Turner Model 350 spectrophotometer (G. K. Turner Associates, Palo Alto, Calif.) equipped with 19-mm diameter cells; set the wavelength at 620 nm.

c. Preparation of standard vitamin A curve   Cut the tip from a capsule of USP reference solution and weigh 100-200 mg into a 50-ml beaker. Dissolve the solution in chloroform, quantitatively transfer it to a 50-ml volumetric flask, and dilute the contents to volume with chloroform. Prepare a series of dilutions in chloroform in such a manner that 2-ml aliquots treated with Carr-Price reagent give absorbances in the range of 0.1 to 0.8. Prepare a standard curve by plotting absorbances versus international units (IU) of vitamin A. (Note: 1 IU of vitamin A equals 0.3 μg.)

d. Preparation and evaluation of alumina cleanup column   Prepare a column [12 mm inside diameter (i.d.), No. 420,000, Kontes Glass Co.,

Vineland, N.J.] by successively adding a plug of glass wool, 5 g of
sodium sulfate, 1.2 g of Woelm alumina (5% water), and 5 g of sodium
sulfate; wash the column with 15 ml of hexane and discard the eluate.
Add 20 ml of the standard solution of saponified vitamin A obtained
as described. Immediately after the solution has percolated through
the column, add 25 ml of hexane-4% acetone. Check the column by
using a long-wave ultraviolet lamp; the vitamin A band should not
have moved more than about 2 mm below the surface of the alumina.
Elute and collect the vitamin A band by eluting the column with 60 ml
of hexane-15% acetone; check the column by using the ultraviolet lamp
to ensure that the vitamin A is completely eluted in this fraction.
Evaporate the eluate to dryness at 60°C under water pump vacuum;
dissolve the residue in 50 ml of chloroform and determine the vitamin A content by using a 2-ml aliquot. Determine the recovery of
vitamin A by relating the results from the saponified vitamin A after
column cleanup to the standard reference curve. Alternately, samples
of feed are spiked with known amounts of vitamin A acetate and the
results compared with those from unspiked samples.

e. *Procedure*

(1) Saponification and extraction procedure. Add 40 ml of 95% ethyl
alcohol and 8 ml of aqueous KOH [50%, weight/volume (w/v)] to an
Erlenmeyer flask containing 8 g of the sample for analysis. Reflux
the contents for 30 min on a steam bath or hot plate at a reflux
rate of about 2 drops per second; occasionally swirl the flask.
Remove the flask and rapidly cool it with tap water.

Transfer the extract to a 250-ml separatory funnel by using a
small funnel and a plug of glass wool to strain out the particles.
Extract the residue in the flask by using three 10-ml portions of
hexane and add each portion to the separatory funnel through the
plug of glass wool; discard the residue. Add 100 ml of water and
5 g of NaCl to the separatory funnel and gently shake the contents.
Separate the hexane layer and extract the aqueous layer with three
additional 20-ml portions of hexane. Combine the hexane extracts
in a 250-ml separatory funnel and wash with 100-ml portions of water

until the water phase is no longer basic to phenolphthalein; about
six washings are usually adequate. During the first several washings
mix the phases by gentle swirling and rotate the separatory funnel
to wash the inner surface. If in spite of gentle mixing an emulsion
forms, add 5 g of NaCl and gently shake the contents to dissolve the
salt; the emulsion should then break. After several washings the
phases may be mixed by vigorous shaking to ensure adequate washing.
After the final washing transfer the hexane layer to a 100-ml volumetric flask by percolating it through a plug of sodium sulfate
(ca. 25 mm diameter × 10 mm thick). Wash the flask and plug with
10 ml hexane.

(2) Cleanup and analysis. Add a 20-ml aliquot of the hexane solution to an alumina column prepared as previously described. Add
25 ml of hexane-4% acetone to elute yellow pigments; discard the
eluate. Finally elute and collect the vitamin A by using 60 ml of
hexane-15% acetone. Evaporate the eluate just to dryness at 60°C
under water pump vacuum and dissolve the residue in 4 ml of chloroform. Pipet 2 ml of this solution into a cuvette, quickly add 10 ml
of Carr-Price reagent, and immediately read the absorbance at 620 nm.
Since the color fades rapidly, use the maximum absorbance observed.
The absorbance reading should be within the range of 0.1 to 1.0; if
it is too high, a 1-ml aliquot of the chloroform solution may be
appropriately diluted. If the absorbance is too low, take a larger
aliquot of the hexane solution (e.g., 50 ml) and concentrate it to
about 20 ml by using water pump vacuum and a 60°C water bath; clean
up the concentrate on alumina and assay for vitamin A as described.
Calculate the vitamin A content (IU per gram of feed) by relating
the absorbance of the unknown sample to that of known amounts on
the standard curve.

All steps in the procedure should be carried out at low light
levels or in actinic glassware. Heating during solvent evaporation
should be minimal and all procedures should be completed within an
8-hr period for reliable results.

f. Typical results

(1) Six replicates of unspiked laboratory chow 5010C analyzed versus six spiked with 171 IU of retinol per 8 g yielded recoveries of 62.0 ± 5.3%.

(2) Quadruplicate samples of unspiked laboratory chow 5010C analyzed before and after being autoclaved were found to contain 41.7 ± 3.3 and 25.3 ± 1.7 IU/g, respectively (corrected for 62% recovery). The loss of vitamin A content in the chow from 40.3 to 25.3 IU/g upon autoclaving was expected. However, the amount of vitamin A remaining (25.3 IU/g) is sufficient for the nutritional need of mice since chow not intended for autoclaving contains only about 15 IU/g.

2. *Vitamin B$_1$* [16]

a. General description of method   Salient elements of the procedure include extraction of the sample with 0.1 N HCl, and oxidation of thiamine to thiochrome which is then extracted into isobutyl alcohol and analyzed by spectrophotofluorescence (excitation and emission wavelength maxima 374 nm and 426 nm, respectively). Three variations of the method are presented; they include (1) a short method, (2) an enzymatic hydrolysis method, and (3) an enzymatic hydrolysis method with a column cleanup of the thiochrome.

b. Special reagents and apparatus

(1) Enzyme solution. Prepare a 10% aqueous solution of Diastase (No. D-23, Fisher Scientific Co., Fair Lawn, N.J.) on the day it is to be used.

(2) Oxidizing reagent. Prepare a 1% aqueous solution of potassium ferricyanide; dilute 4 ml of the solution to 100 ml with 15% aqueous NaOH (freshly prepared prior to use).

(3) Thiamine hydrochloride standard solution. Dry thiamine hydrochloride under vacuum over silica gel, then weigh 50 mg and dissolve it in 500 ml of 20% ethyl alcohol in water previously adjusted to pH 3.5-4.3 with HCl. Store the solution in an actinic bottle.

(4) Potassium chloride-hydrochloric acid. Dissolve 250 g of KCl
in distilled water and dilute it to 1 liter; then add 8.5 ml of
concentrated HCl.

c. *Short method for thiamine analysis*   Transfer a 1-g sample of
the laboratory chow to a 20-ml culture tube equipped with a Teflon-
lined screw cap and add 15 ml of 0.1 N HCl. For each group of samples pipet 1 ml of thiamine stock solution (100 μg/ml) and 14 ml of
0.1 N HCl into a culture tube and carry the standard through the
procedure along with the samples.

Seal the tube, shake the contents well, and heat it in a boiling
water bath for 30 min with intermittent shaking. Centrifuge the tubes
for 10 min at 1000 rpm, pipet 5 ml of the supernatant liquid into a
50-ml volumetric flask, and dilute the contents to volume with 0.1
N HCl. Pipet two 5-ml aliquots into 20-ml culture tubes containing
0.5 g of NaCl. To one tube add 3 ml of the potassium ferricyanide
solution. (Note: This should be done rapidly and directly to the
aliquot of sample.) Immediately add 10 ml of isobutyl alcohol, seal
the tube, and shake it vigorously for 15 sec. To prepare a blank
add 3 ml of 15% aqueous NaOH to the other tube, then add 10 ml of
isobutyl alcohol and vigorously shake the contents for 15 sec. At
this point the samples can be stored up to 30 min in low light while
others are being made up. After all the samples have been prepared
(oxidized) shake them for an additional 2 min and centrifuge for
5 min at 1000 rpm.

Pipet about 2 ml of the top layer (isobutyl alcohol) from the
tube containing the oxidized standard into a fluorescence cell (1 cm,
square) and determine the relative intensity (RI) by using a spectrophotofluorometer set at 374 and 426 nm for excitation and emission,
respectively. Also determine the RI values of all samples and
blanks. Occasionally recheck the RI value of the standard and
adjust the instrument to the original intensity if necessary. Subtract the RI of the blank from those of the samples and calculate
the thiamine hydrochloride content as follows:

$$\text{Thiamine·HCl (ppm)} = \frac{\text{RI of sample}}{\text{RI of standard}} \times \frac{1.11}{0.84}$$

d. *Enzyme hydrolysis method*   Transfer a 0.5-g sample of the laboratory chow to a 20-ml culture tube and add 15 ml of 0.1 N HCl.
Prepare a standard in another tube by adding 0.5 ml of the thiamine
hydrochloride solution (100 μg/ml) and 14.5 ml of 0.1 N HCl. Seal
the tubes, shake the contents, and heat in a boiling water bath for
30 min with intermittent shaking.

Transfer the contents of the tube into a 100-ml round-bottom
flask by using 0.1 N HCl to rinse the tube. Dilute to about 65 ml
with 0.1 N HCl and add a sufficient amount of 2 N sodium acetate
solution (ca. 5 ml) to give a pH of 4.0-4.5. Add 5 ml of the enzyme
solution (10% aqueous diastase), seal the flask, and incubate the
contents for 3 hr at 45-50°C. Filter the digested mixture into a
100-ml volumetric flask by using 0.1 N HCl for rinsing and washing
the filter; after the filtrate has cooled, adjust the volume to
100 ml with 0.1 N HCl. Add two 5-ml aliquots of the solution to
culture tubes containing 0.5 g of NaCl and proceed with the oxidation employing potassium ferricyanide and subsequent steps as
described for the short method for thiamine analysis. Correct the
RI values of the samples by subtracting those of the blank and calculate the thiamine hydrochloride content as follows:

$$\text{Thiamine} \cdot \text{HCl (ppm)} = \frac{\text{RI of sample}}{\text{RI of standard}} \times \frac{1.00}{0.87}$$

e. *Enzyme hydrolysis method with thiochrome Decalso column cleanup*
Prepare the sample (0.5 g) and standard as described for the enzymatic hydrolysis method and carry them through the procedure to the
point where the digested mixture is adjusted to a volume of 100 ml.
Prepare a column by adding 1.5 g of Thiochrome Decalso (No. T-97,
Fisher) as an aqueous slurry to a column (12 mm i.d., No. 420,000,
Kontes) plugged with glass wool. (Note: Do not allow the liquid
in the column to fall below the Decalso.) Percolate a 50-ml portion
of the digested sample solution through the column and wash the
column with three 5-ml portions of hot water (near boiling).
Finally, elute the thiamine into a 50-ml volumetric flask by using
five 5-ml portions of hot KCl-HCl solution (near boiling). Allow

the eluate to cool and adjust the volume to 50 ml with 0.1 N HCl.
Add two 5-ml aliquots of the solution to culture tubes containing
0.5 g NaCl and proceed with the oxidation and subsequent steps as
described for the short method for thiamine analysis. Calculate
the thiamine hydrochloride content as described for the enzyme
hydrolysis method.

f. Typical results

(1) Blank samples for the short method and the enzyme method
using Decalso cleanup yielded 2.2 and 0.6 ppm of thiamine hydrochloride, respectively.

(2) Recoveries from laboratory chow 5010C spiked with 100 ppm
of thiamine hydrochloride and assayed by the short method and the
enzyme hydrolysis method were 84 and 87%, respectively.

(3) Typical assays of laboratory chow 5010C analyzed by the
short method, the enzyme hydrolysis method, and the enzyme method
using Decalso cleanup were 49.3, 58.4, and 47.2 ppm of thiamine
hydrochloride, respectively. After this chow was autoclaved, assays
were 29.9, 33.8, and 32.1 ppm, respectively.

g. Discussion Enzyme hydrolysis is necessary if part of the
thiamine is present as the pyrophosphate; however, for routine
analysis the short method is recommended. Results obtained with
the short method are consistent and readily corrected for recovery
and for the increase that would be obtained by enzyme hydrolysis.
In the case of laboratory chow 5010C, the results are multiplied
by 1.11 to give values equivalent to those of the enzyme method and
divided by 0.84 to correct for recovery of the thiamine hydrochloride.
The use of the Decalso cleanup column resulted in a lower recovery.
Although the cleanup column reduced the blank from about 2.2 to 0.6
ppm the benefit is considered marginal and the use of the column is
not recommended for routine analysis.

E. Total Protein, Fat, and Volatiles

1. *Total Protein* [2,17]

a. *General description of method*   The classical Kjeldahl procedure
is employed. The sample is digested with concentrated H_2SO_4, made
alkaline, and the nitrogen is distilled as ammonia and trapped in a
boric acid solution. The ammonia is titrated with standard H_2SO_4
and calculated as total crude protein.

b. *Special reagents*

(1) Sodium hydroxide-sodium thiosulfate solution. Dissolve 500 g
of NaOH and 25 g of $Na_2S_2O_3 \cdot 5H_2O$ in ammonia-free water and dilute
to 1 liter.

(2) Mixed indicator. Mix two volumes of 0.2% methyl red in 95%
ethyl alcohol with one volume of 0.2% methylene blue in 95% ethyl
alcohol. Prepare a fresh solution at least monthly.

(3) Standard sulfuric acid titrant. Prepare the titrant (ca. 0.2 N)
by diluting 6 ml of concentrated H_2SO_4 to 1 liter with water. Stan-
dardize the acid solution against 0.2 N Na_2CO_3 (1 ml of 0.2 N H_2SO_4 =
2.80 mg of nitrogen).

(4) Phenolphthalein indicator solution. Dissolve 5 g of phenolphthalein disodium salt in distilled water and dilute to 1 liter.
If necessary, add 0.02 N NaOH dropwise until a faint pink color
appears.

c. *Procedure*   Accurately weigh 1-1.2 g of the feed into an 800-ml
Kjeldahl flask; add 25 ml of concentrated H_2SO_4, 15 g of Na_2SO_4,
3 g of $HgSO_4$, and a few boiling chips and allow the mixture to boil
until white fumes appear. Let the mixture digest for an additional
30 min while frequently turning the flask to allow good contact of
the ingredients. Cool the flask and contents to room temperature
then carefully add 500 ml of ammonia-free water and 0.3 ml of phenolphthalein indicator solution; then add 75 ml of 50% NaOH-sodium thiosulfate solution taking care not to mix the contents. Quickly connect
the flask to a distillation apparatus and mix the contents. If the

mixture is not red, add more of the 50% NaOH-sodium thiosulfate
solution until a distinct red color persists. Distill 300 ml of
the contents and collect the distillate in a trap containing 50 ml
of a 2% solution of aqueous boric acid. Add about 10 drops of mixed
indicator and titrate the ammonia by using the standard H_2SO_4 solution. Carry a blank (feed absent) through the entire procedure for
use in correcting the results.

Calculate the nitrogen and crude protein content of the sample
as follows:

Nitrogen (%)

$$= \frac{[\text{sample - blank (ml acid)}] \times \text{normality (acid)} \quad 14.007}{\text{weight of sample (mg)}} \times 100$$

Crude protein (%) = % nitrogen × 6.25

2. *Total Fat* [2,18]

a. *General description of method* Crude fat is determined gravimetrically by extracting a vacuum-dried sample of the chow with
diethyl ether and weighing the residue.

b. *Special reagent: anhydrous ether* Wash ether with two or three
portions of distilled water then allow it to stand over NaOH or KOH
pellets until most of the water is abstracted from the ether. Decant
the ether into a dry bottle and carefully add small pieces of clean
metallic sodium, allowing the ether to stand until the evolution of
hydrogen ceases. Store the dehydrated ether over metallic sodium
in a loosely stoppered bottle.

c. *Procedure* Dry the sample of feed to a constant weight in a
vacuum oven (ca. 100 mmHg) for 5 hr at 95-100°C. Extract 2.00 g
of the dried feed in a Soxhlet apparatus for 4 hr with anhydrous
ether at a reflux rate of about 5-6 drops per second. Evaporate
the extract in a tared dish by using a boiling water bath. Cool
the dish in a desiccator and determine the weight of the residue.
Also determine the weight of residue obtained from a blank extraction (feed absent) for use in correcting the residue found in the
feed.

$$\text{Fat (\%)} = \frac{\text{residue from feed (g) - blank (g)}}{\text{dry weight of sample (g)}} \times 100$$

3. *Total Volatiles* [2,19]

a. General description of method   Total volatiles are determined gravimetrically as the percentage of sample weight lost in a 135°C oven for 2 hr.

b. Procedure   Accurately weigh approximately 5 g of the feed sample into a tared aluminum dish (with cover) and evenly distribute it on the bottom of the dish. With the cover removed, place the dish and cover in an oven set at 135 ± 2°C and allow the sample to dry for 2 hr. Place the cover on the dish and allow it to cool in a desiccator. Weigh the dish and calculate the loss in weight.

$$\text{Volatiles (\%)} = \frac{\text{loss in weight (g)}}{\text{initial weight of sample (g)}} \times 100$$

F.   Pesticides and Related Substances

1. *General Description of Method*

Elements of several procedures [2,20-23] were combined for the analysis of chlorinated and organophosphorus pesticides as well as polychlorinated biphenyl (PCB) compounds. The sample is extracted with 6% diethyl ether-hexane. The extract is cleaned up and the residues separated into five fractions on a column of Florisil. The separate fractions are then analyzed by electron-capture gas chromatography (EC-GC).

2. *Procedure*

Extract 10 g of the sample by mechanically shaking it overnight with 150 ml of 6% diethyl ether-hexane at a moderate speed. Filter the mixture by using Whatman No. 1 filter paper and a Buchner filter; rinse the filter with an additional 100-ml portion of the extraction solvent and concentrate the combined filtrate to about 10 ml by using water pump vacuum and a 50°C water bath. Reserve the concentrate for cleanup on Florisil.

Prepare a Shell-type column (400 mm × 22 mm i.d.) by successively adding a plug of glass wool, a 2-cm layer of sodium sulfate,
a 13-cm layer of Florisil (after lightly tapping the column), and
a 2-cm layer of sodium sulfate. [Note: The glass wool and sodium
sulfate are extracted with benzene and dried overnight in an oven
at 120°C prior to use. The Florisil (60-100 mesh) is activated
overnight in an oven at 130°C prior to use.] Prewet the column with
50 ml of hexane and allow the solvent level to drop about 1 cm from
the top of the sodium sulfate layer before adding the sample extract
and each subsequent elution fraction.

Transfer the concentrated sample extract (ca. 10 ml) to the
column, rinse the container and column with three 3-ml portions of
hexane, and elute the column with 150 ml of hexane and reserve the
eluate (fraction A). Sequentially elute the column with 200 ml of
6% diethyl ether-hexane (fraction B), 225 ml of 15% diethyl ether-
hexane (fraction C), 200 ml of 50% diethyl ether-hexane (fraction D),
and 150 ml of 10% acetone-hexane (fraction E). Evaporate the separate fractions to about 2 ml by using water pump vacuum and a 50°C
water bath and adjust the volumes to 10 ml with isooctane for subsequent analysis via EC-GC. (Note: Samples containing more than
8% fat may require a liquid partitioning cleanup prior to the Florisil column.) The Florisil column should be periodically evaluated
to ensure that the various compounds are eluted as follows:

Fraction A: PCBs   Fraction B: Lindane
            Heptachlor   Heptachlor epoxide
            Aldrin   p,p'-DDD (TDE)
            p,p'-DDE   p,p'-DDT
Fraction C: Dieldrin   Fraction D: Diazinon
            Endrin   Parathion
Fraction E: Malathion

Recoveries of 80% or better are expected for all of these compounds
in the fractions indicated.

Analyze each fraction from the Florisil column by injecting 5-μl amounts of the isooctane solution into a gas chromatograph equipped with an EC detector. For example, a typical system currently in use [2] is a Hewlett-Packard (Palo Alto, Calif.) Model 5840A instrument equipped with a linear ^{63}Ni EC detector. The 180-cm glass column (2 mm i.d.), packed with 10% SP 2100 on Supelcoport (100-120 mesh) is operated isothermally at 230°C with the carrier gas (argon-5% methane) flowing at 30 ml/min. The injection port and detector are operated at 250 and 350°C, respectively. Identification of the compounds is based on retention time, and residues are quantified by measuring either the peak height or the area under the peak.

Samples that indicate the presence of pesticides or PCBs are further analyzed and confirmed by using a similar EC-GC system except that a column of different polarity is employed [e.g., a 180-cm glass column packed with 5% QF-1 (or OV-210) on Supelcoport (or Gas Chrom Q)].

Partition values (p-values) also provide an excellent means for additional confirmation of the identity of peaks obtained via EC-GC [23-26].

In the procedure just described, emphasis is placed on the analysis of chlorinated compounds; only a few of the common organophosphorus insecticides that give a fairly good response with the EC detector have been evaluated. Therefore, a separate screening procedure for residues of the organophosphorus compounds is recommended. Procedures employing temperature-programmed GC with a flame photometric detector operated in the phosphorus (526 nm) and/or sulfur (394 nm) mode have been reported by the author [27-29].

III   ANALYSIS OF ANIMAL BEDDING, CARDBOARD FEEDER BOXES, AND WATER

A.   Animal Bedding and Cardboard Feeder Boxes

1.   *Pesticides and Related Substances*

Cut the cardboard into small pieces (ca. 5 mm × 5 mm) prior to weighing the sample. Weigh 10-g portions of the cardboard or bedding (hardwood chips) and extract them with 150 ml of 6% diethyl ether-hexane overnight by using a mechanical shaker operated at a moderate speed. Proceed with the analysis as previously described for animal feed.

2. Pentachlorophenol

a. *General description of method*   The sample is extracted with 10% methanol-benzene, subjected to liquid-liquid partitioning, acetylated by using pyridine-acetic anhydride, and analyzed by EC-GC [30].

b. *Procedure*   Extract 10 g of the animal bedding or cardboard (cut into pieces about 5 mm square) with 100 ml of 10% methanol-benzene for 4 hr on a mechanical shaker operated at a moderate speed. In order to ensure satisfactory recovery of the pentachlorophenol (PCP), e.g., 75% or better, allow the samples to soak overnight and shake them for an additional 30 min the next day. Filter the extract through a plug of sodium sulfate (ca. 5 g) and reserve the filtrate for subsequent analysis.

Transfer a 25-ml portion of the extract (2.5 g equivalents of sample) to a 100-ml round-bottom flask and concentrate the contents to about 3 ml by using water pump vacuum and a 40°C water bath. Transfer the contents to a 20-ml culture tube by using small portions of benzene; evaporate the contents of the tube just to dryness by using a stream of dry nitrogen and a 40°C water bath. (Note: All culture tubes are equipped with Teflon-lined screw caps.)

Add 5 ml of deionized water and 1 ml of 6 M H_2SO_4 to the tube and shake the contents vigorously for 1 min; then add 5 ml of hexane-isopropyl alcohol (5:3, v/v) and again shake the tube for 1 min. Centrifuge the mixture to separate the phases and quantitatively transfer the organic layer to an 8-ml culture tube; discard the aqueous layer. Extract the organic phase with two 2-ml portions of 0.1 M aqueous sodium tetraborate; centrifugation is usually required to separate the phases. Reserve the combined aqueous extracts in an 8-ml culture tube for subsequent derivatization and analysis.

Add 2.5 ml of hexane and 100 µl of fresh acetylating reagent (2 ml pyridine + 0.8 ml acetic anhydride) to the combined aqueous extracts, shake the contents for 1 min, and assay the hexane layer by EC-GC. Also, carry a reagent blank and a sample spiked with 1 ppm (µg/g) of PCP through the entire procedure. Prepare a standard equivalent to 1 ppm of PCP by adding 2.5 µg of the compound to 4 ml of sodium tetraborate solution and proceeding with the acetylation step as described; adjust the volume of the hexane layer to exactly 2.5 ml.

Analyze each sample by injecting 5-µl amounts into a gas chromatograph equipped with an EC detector. A typical system currently in use [30] is a Hewlett-Packard Model 5840A instrument equipped and operated exactly as described for pesticides except that the column is operated at 210°C. Under these conditions, the derivatized PCP has a retention time of 1.60 min. Calculations of residues of PCP are made by relating either the peak height or the area under the peak to those of standards; results are also corrected for the reagent blank and for recovery. Residues of PCP as low as 1 ppb (ng/g) can be detected by this procedure. The identity of peaks believed to be PCP may be confirmed by using the alternative EC-GC system equipped with a column of QF-1 as mentioned for pesticides.

B. Water

1. *Pesticides and Related Substances* [2,22]

Transfer a 1700-ml sample of the water for analysis to a 2-liter separatory funnel containing 200 ml of hexane. Shake the sample vigorously three times for 1 min each, allowing the layers to separate each time. Drain and discard the aqueous layer then percolate the hexane extract through a plug of sodium sulfate (ca. 7 g) and wash the plug twice with 20-ml portions of hexane. Evaporate the combined hexane filtrates just to dryness by using water pump vacuum and a 50°C water bath. Dissolve the residue in 10 ml of isooctane and perform the assays via EC-GC as described for animal feed.

2. *Chloroform* [2,22]

a. General description of method   Injections of the water sample
are made directly into a GC equipped with a linear [63]Ni EC detector.
The chloroform content of the sample is read from a standard curve
of peak area plotted versus ppb amounts of chloroform.

b. Procedure   Prepare a stock solution of chloroform in acetone
(1 mg/ml); then prepare a high-level aqueous solution of chloroform
(1 ng/μl) by injecting 100 μl of the stock solution into 100 ml of
organic-free water. (Note: A water system consisting of an ion-
exchange bed and an activated charcoal filter obtained from Conti-
nental Water Conditioning Corp., El Paso, Tex., was found to provide
organic-free water of acceptable quality.) Dilute the high-level
aqueous solution with organic-free water to provide standard aqueous
solutions of chloroform (1-100 pg/μl; 1-100 ppb) for direct analysis
by injecting 5-μl amounts into the GC. Prepare a standard curve
(peak area plotted versus ppb of chloroform).

   Inject 5 μl of the organic-free water for use as a blank correc-
tion then inject 5 μl of each sample of unknown chloroform content.
Subtract the peak area obtained with the blank from those of the
samples and determine chloroform content (ppb) by relating corrected
peak areas to the standard curve.

   A typical system currently in use [2] is a Hewlett-Packard
Model 5840A instrument equipped with a linear [63]Ni EC detector.
The 180-cm glass column (2 mm i.d.), packed with 5% SP 2100-5%
Benton 34 on Supelcoport (100-120 mesh), is operated isothermally
at 50°C with the carrier gas (argon-5% methane) flowing at 25 ml/min.
The injection port and detector are operated at 100 and 200°C,
respectively. Under these conditions the retention time of chloro-
form is 2.25 min and residues as low as 1 ppb can be detected.

3. *Metals* [2,31]

a. General description of method   The sample of water, stabilized
with nitric acid, is analyzed directly for 10 elements by atomic
absorption spectrometry. Quantitative results are obtained by relating absorbance values to standard curves prepared for each element.

Table 2.3. Analytical parameters and instrumental conditions
for the determination of 10 elements in water

Element	Flame	Wavelength (nm)	Linear Range (ppm)	Minimum detectable quantity (ppb)
Arsenic	$Ar-H_2$[a]	193.7	0.1 to 6	20
Beryllium	$N_2O-C_2H_2$	234.9	0.025 to 2	20
Cadmium	$Air-C_2H_2$	228.8	0.025 to 2	5
Chromium	$Air-C_2H_2$	357.9	0.1 to 5	20
Copper	$Air-C_2H_2$	324.7	0.1 to 5	20
Iron	$Air-C_2H_2$	248.3	0.1 to 5	20
Lead	$Air-C_2H_2$	283.3	0.5 to 20	20
Mercury	Flameless[b]	253.6	0.5 to 7	20
Nickel	$Air-C_2H_2$	232.0	0.1 to 5	20
Selenium	$Ar-H_2$[a]	196.0	0.1 to 6	50

[a]Gaseous hydride method.
[b]Cold vapor method.

b. Procedure   Prepare standard curves for all of the elements
sought by using an atomic absorption spectrometer and the analytical
parameters listed in Table 2.3. Aliquots of the water sample (stabilized by adding concentrated HNO_3 to produce a pH of 2 or below)
are then subjected to analysis for the 10 elements by using the
instrumental conditions given in the table.

REFERENCES

1. D. L. Greenman, N. A. Littlefield, and W. L. Oller, National
    Toxicological Research, Jefferson, Ark. Personal communication.

2. R. L. Lea and S. M. Billedeau, Gulf South Research Institute,
    Little Rock, Ark. Personal communication.

3. W. Horwitz (ed.). *Official Methods of Analysis of the Associa-
    tion of Official Analytical Chemists* 11th Ed. AOAC, Washington
    D.C., 1970, pp. 426-436.

4. L. M. Seitz and H. E. Mohr. Aflatoxin detection in corn: A rapid simple screening test convertible to a quantitative method. *Cereal chem. 51*, 487-491 (1974).

5. P. R. Beljaars, J. C. H. M. Schumans, and P. J. Koken. Quantitative fluorodensitometric determination and survey of aflatoxins in nutmeg. *J. Ass. Offic. Anal. Chem. 58*, 263-271 (1975).

6. W. Przybylski. Formation of aflatoxin derivatives on thin layer chromatographic plates. *J. Ass. Offic. Anal. Chem. 58*, 163-164 (1975).

7. National Center for Toxicological Research. *Animal Feed Estrogen Activity Bioassay and Report Standard* No. 2. NCTR, Jefferson, Ark., September 5, 1973.

8. W. Horwitz (ed.). *Official Method of Analysis of the Association of Official Analytical Chemists* 11th Ed. AOAC, Washington, D.C., 1970, p. 132.

9. W. Horwitz (ed.). *Official Method of Analysis of the Association of Official Analytical Chemists* 11th Ed. AOAC, Washington, D.C., 1970, p. 134.

10. H. K. Hundley and J. C. Underwood. Determination of total arsenic in total diet samples. *J. Ass. Offic. Anal. Chem. 53*, 1176-1178 (1970).

11. Anonymous. Atomic absorption spectrophotometric method. *J. Ass. Offic. Anal. Chem. 56*, 480-481 (1973).

12. Anonymous. Lead in evaporated milk: Atomic absorption spectrophotometric method. *J. Ass. Offic. Anal. Chem. 56*, 481-483 (1973).

13. I. Hoffman, R. J. Westerby, and M. Hidiroglou. Precise fluorometric microdetermination of selenium in agricultural materials. *J. Ass. Offic. Anal. Chem. 51*, 1039-1042 (1968).

14. W. R. Hatch and W. L. Ott. Determination of submicrogram quantities of mercury by atomic absorption spectrophotometry. *Anal. Chem. 40*, 2085-2087 (1968).

15. W. Horwitz (ed.). *Official Method of Analysis of the Association of Official Analytical Chemists* 11th Ed. AOAC, Washington, D.C., 1970, pp. 767-769.

16. W. Horwitz (ed.). *Official Method of Analysis of the Association of Official Analytical Chemists* 11th Ed. AOAC, Washington, D.C., 1970, pp. 771-774.

17. American Public Health Association. *Standard Methods for the Examination of Water and Wastewater* 13th Ed. Amer. Pub. Health Assc., Washington, D.C., 1974, pp. 255-257.

18. W. Horwitz (ed.). *Official Method of Analysis of the Association of Official Analytical Chemists* 11th Ed. AOAC, Washington, D.C., 1970, p. 128.

19. W. Horwitz (ed.). *Official Method of Analysis of the Association of Official Analytical Chemists* 11th Ed. AOAC, Washington, D.C., 1970, p. 130.

20. Food and Drug Administration. *Pesticide Analytical Manual* Vol. 1. FDA, Washington, D.C., 1971.

21. J. F. Thompson (ed.). *Manual of Analytical Methods*. U.S. Environmental Protection Agency, Research Triangle Park, N.C., 1974.

22. Gulf South Research Institute. *Standard Operating Procedure Manual*. Gulf South Res. Inst., New Iberia, La., 1974.

23. M. Beroza and M. C. Bowman. Identification of pesticides at nanogram level by extraction p-values. *Anal. Chem. 37*, 291-292 (1965).

24. M. C. Bowman and M. Beroza. Extraction p-values of pesticides and related materials in six binary solvent systems. *J. Ass. Offic. Anal. Chem. 48*, 943-952 (1965).

25. M. C. Bowman and M. Beroza. Identification of compounds by extraction p-values using gas chromatography. *Anal. Chem. 38*, 1544-1549 (1966).

26. M. Beroza, M. N. Inscoe, and M. C. Bowman. Distribution of pesticides in immiscible binary solvent systems for cleanup and identification and the extraction of pesticides from milk. *Res. Rev. 30*, 1-61 (1969).

27. M. C. Bowman and M. Beroza. GLC retention times of pesticides and metabolites containing phosphorus and sulfur on four thermally stable columns. *J. Ass. Offic. Anal. Chem. 53*, 499-508 (1970).

28. M. C. Bowman, M. Beroza, and K. R. Hill. Chromatograms of foods for multicomponent residue analyses determination of pesticides containing phosphorus and/or sulfur by GLC flame photometric detection. *J. Ass. Offic. Anal. Chem. 54*, 346-358 (1971).

29. M. C. Bowman and M. Beroza. Use of Dexsil 300 on specially washed chromosorb W for multicomponent residue determinations of phosphorus- and sulfur-containing pesticides by flame photometric GLC. *J. Ass. Offic. Anal. Chem. 54*, 1086-1092 (1971).

30. F. R. Fullerton, National Center for Toxicological Research, Jeferson, Ark. Personal communication.

31. Environmental Protection Agency. *Manual of Methods for Chemical Analysis of Water and Wastewater*. EPA, Nat. Environ. Res. Center, Cincinnati, Ohio, 1974.

3

ANALYSIS OF THE TEST SUBSTANCES

I INTRODUCTION

The chemical analysis of the test compound and assays for
traces of the substance in a variety of substrates are required for
all toxicological tests with hazardous substances if such tests are
to be valid and safe. In Chapter 1 the necessity for providing
assurance of the identity, purity, and stability of the substance;
its homogeneity, stability, and proper concentration in the dosage
form; safe usage in the workplace; and safe disposal were previously
discussed. In order to meet these requirements adequate analytical
chemical methods must be available for the particular test substance.
Moreover, these methods must be employed to evaluate the various
chemical aspects of an experiment prior to the initiation of animal
tests.

This chapter describes analytical procedures for several of the
test substances studied at the National Center for Toxicological
Research (NCTR) during the past 5 years. Although emphasis is
placed on the analysis of the dosage form, procedures for other
substrates and data concerning analytical chemical properties of
the compounds are also included.

In toxicological experiments the test substance is usually
administered to an animal either by gavage, injection, inhalation
(as particles, aerosols, or vapors), application to the skin, or
orally as a solid or liquid. Oral administration of the substance
via the diet or drinking water is most convenient for long-term
experiments with large numbers of animals receiving multiple doses.

Although oral doses may be given in the form of a liquid, pellet,
granule, emulsion, agar block, microencapsulation, etc., thus far
only granular animal feed and drinking water have been used as
vehicles for dosing animals in large-scale tests at the NCTR.
Details concerning the analysis of some aromatic amines, estrogens,
pesticides, and other compounds in one of these dosage forms and
other substrates are given later (Sections II-V). In addition, the
Salmonella typhimurium test for mutagenicity (Ames test), although
bacteriological in nature, is also described (Section VI) since it
is rapidly becoming a standard screening procedure in toxicological
research.

II   AROMATIC AMINES

A.   2-Acetylaminofluorene [1]

1. General Description of Method
Procedures are described for determining residues of 2-acetylamino-
fluorene (2-AAF) in laboratory chow and six different microbiological
media by spectrophotofluorescence (SPF) and gas chromatography (GC).
The salient elements of the SPF method are extraction, a rapid cleanup on alumina, acid hydrolysis of 2-AAF to 2-aminofluorene (2-AF),
further cleanup by organic solvent, extraction of interferences from
the aqueous amine hydrochloride, conversion of the hydrochloride to
the free base (2-AF), and its extraction and finally quantification
of 2-AAF as 2-AF by SPF. In the GC method, the extract is cleaned
up by solvent partitioning followed by silica gel chromatography
with residues being determined directly as 2-AAF. Additional data
are presented concerning partition values (p-values), GC and SPF
characteristics and adsorption liquid chromatographic properties of
2-AAF, 2-AF, and fluorene, and solubility values for 2-AAF in various solvents.

2. Introduction
2-Acetylaminofluorene (N-2-fluorenylacetamide) is a carcinogen that
has been widely studied and is known to produce tumors in specific

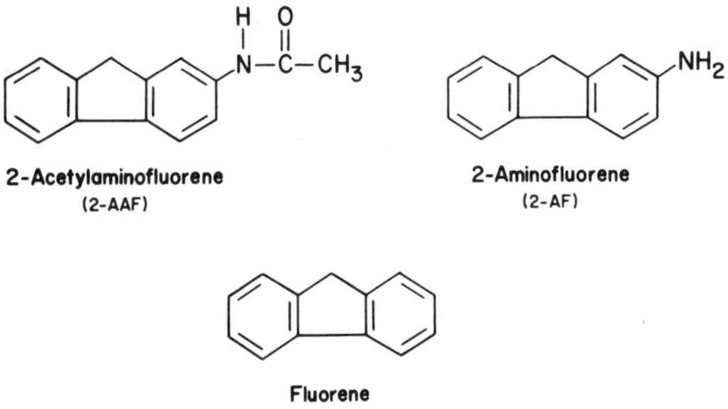

2-Acetylaminofluorene
(2-AAF)

2-Aminofluorene
(2-AF)

Fluorene

Figure 3.1. Formulas of 2-AAF, 2-AF, and
fluorene. (From Bowman and King [1].)

organs [2,3]. As part of a long-term, low-dose study of 2-AAF in
mice, an analytical method was required for monitoring residues of
the compound added to the animal's diet in order to ensure the requisite dosage as well as the homogeneity and stability of 2-AAF in the
diet. In addition, microbiological systems that will degrade 2-AAF
and thus destroy its carcinogenic activity were being sought, and a
method for analyzing traces of the compound in the growth media was
required. Formulas of 2-AAF and two of its degradation products,
2-AF and fluorene, are shown in Figure 3.1.

Several methods for determining residues of 2-AAF have been
reported. Westfall [4] devised a colorimetric method for estimating
2-AF in biological material by diazotizing the amino group and coupling with sodium 2-naphthol-3,6-disulfonate. Later, Westfall and
Morris [5] used the method to analyze for 2-AAF after hydrolyzing
it to 2-AF; their reagent blanks for tissue extracts were equivalent
to 1-5 µg of 2-AF. Sandin et al. [6] determined the molar extinction
coefficient and absorption maximum of 2-AAF to be 4.46 and 288 nm,
respectively. Irving [7] determined 2-AAF and 2-AF in urine extracts
by ultraviolet absorption after separating them by solvent partitioning. The analysis of 2-AAF and its degradation products (particularly the hydroxylated metabolites) has depended mostly on the use
of ^{14}C-labeled material [8,9]. None of these procedures, however,

were sufficiently specific and sensitive for our substrates; therefore, the following procedures were developed.

3. Experimental

a. *Materials*   Fluorene (melting point, mp, 114-115°C) and 2-AF
(mp 126-127°C) were purchased from Eastman Organic Chemicals,
Rochester, N.Y.   The 2-AAF (mp 193-195°C) was purchased from Aldrich
Chemical Co., Milwaukee, Wis.   The fluorene and 2-AAF were used as
received since they contained no extraneous GC peaks and recrystallization failed to change their GC or SPF response.   The 2-AF (light
brown) was recrystallized from methanol-water prior to use; although
a white crystalline product was obtained, the melting point remained
essentially unchanged.   Purification of the 2-AF removed extraneous
GC peaks and enhanced the GC and SPF responses by about 5%.

Adsorbents were silica gel (No. 3405) from J. T. Baker Chemical
Co., Phillipsburg, N.J.; basic alumina, Brockman Activity I (No.
A-941), and Hyflo Super Cel (No. H-333) from Fisher Scientific Co.,
Fair Lawn, N.J.; and charcoal (Darco KB) from Atlas Chemical Indus-
tries, Wilmington, Del.   The silica gel was dried overnight at 130°C,
adjusted to 7% moisture with buffer pH 7 (Fisher Scientific Co.,
No. SO-B-108), mixed well and allowed to stand overnight prior to
use.   The other adsorbents were used as received.   The sodium sulfate
was anhydrous.   All reagents were CP (chemically pure) grade and
solvents were pesticide grade.   The laboratory chow (type 5010C,
Ralston Purina Co., St. Louis, Mo.) contained about 6% fat and had
a pH of 5.5; 93.3% was not volatile at 110°C overnight.   All ingredients for the microbiological culture media were purchased from
Difco Laboratories, Detroit, Mich.   The media were prepared in
accordance with the directions supplied by the manufacturer except
that the proteose peptone was a 2% aqueous solution of Bacto-Proteose
Peptone No. 3.

b. *Preparation of samples for GC*

(1)   Laboratory Chow.   A 20-g portion of the sample was deactivated
by the addition of 20 ml of distilled water, then extracted with

100 ml of chloroform-methanol [9:1, volume/volume (v/v)] in a 150-ml
bottle sealed with a Teflon-lined cap by shaking for 2 hr at 200
excursions per minute on an Eberbach shaker (No. 205-575, Curtin
Scientific Co.). The supernatant was then percolated through a plug
of anhydrous sodium sulfate (25 mm diameter × 30 mm thick), and 50 ml
of the extract (equivalent to 10 g of sample) was evaporated to dryness on a 60°C water bath under water pump vacuum. The residue was
dissolved in 10 ml of acetonitrile and extracted twice with 20-ml
portions of hexane, then the acetonitrile phase was evaporated to
dryness as described. The residue was dissolved in 20 ml of benzene
by using the 60°C water bath and a Teflon policeman, and the solution was reserved for subsequent silica gel cleanup.

A silica gel column was prepared by adding successively to a
12-mm inside diameter (i.d.) glass tube (No. 420,000, Kontes Glass
Co., Vineland, N.J.) a plug of glass wool, 5 g of sodium sulfate,
5 g of silica gel (7% buffer, pH 7), and 5 g of sodium sulfate. The
column was washed with 20 ml of benzene and the eluate discarded.
The benzene solution of the chow extract was added to the column
and, after it had percolated into the adsorbent, the container and
the column were washed with five 10-ml rinses of 2% acetone in benzene (the combined eluates contain residues of fluorene and 2-AF if
any were present in the extractive). Finally, the column was eluted
with 60 ml of 5% acetone in benzene (this eluate contains 2-AAF).
The fractions were then evaporated to dryness as described and the
residues dissolved in an appropriate volume of chloroform (e.g.,
2-5 ml) for injection into the GC.

(2) Microbiological media. Twenty millileters of the medium was
mixed with 1 g of sodium chloride in a 125-ml separatory funnel,
extracted three times with 10-ml portions of chloroform, and each
portion successively percolated through a plug of sodium sulfate
(25 mm diameter × 10 mm thick). The combined extracts were evaporated to dryness as described; the residue was dissolved in 20 ml
of benzene and reserved for silica gel cleanup.

A silica gel column was prepared as described for analysis of
the laboratory chow except that 2 g of silica gel was used and the

column was washed with 10 ml of benzene prior to use. The benzene
solution of the extract was added to the column, allowed to percolate
into the adsorbent, then the container and the column were washed
twice with 10-ml portions of 2% acetone in benzene (the combined
eluates contain fluorene and 2-AF). The column was then eluted with
20 ml of 8% acetone in benzene (contains residues of 2-AAF). The
fractions were evaporated to dryness as described and the residue
dissolved in chloroform (ca. 1-2 ml) for injection into the GC.

c. Preparation of samples for analysis by SPF

(1) Laboratory chow. A 3-g portion of the sample was deactivated
by the addition of 3 ml of distilled water, then extracted on the
shaker as previously described except with 15 ml of chloroform-
methanol (9:1, v/v) in a culture tube (20 x 150 mm) sealed with a
Teflon-lined cap. The supernatant was decanted through a plug of
sodium sulfate (15 mm diameter x 10 mm thick) and the percolate centrifuged at 1000 revolutions per minute (rpm) for 10 min. Five milliliters of the extract (1 g equivalent of chow) was then added to a
column (Kontes, No. 420,000) consisting of 2 g of basic alumina supported by a plug of glass wool. The column was washed twice with 2-ml
portions of chloroform and the total effluent collected in a culture
tube, evaporated to near dryness with a jet of dry air, and finally
to dryness with water pump vacuum and a 60°C water bath. Hydrolysis
of 2-AAF to 2-AF was then accomplished by adding 4 ml of methanol and
2 ml of concentrated HCl to the dry residue and heating it in the
sealed tube at 85°C for 2 hr by using a tube heater (Kontes, No.
720,000). After the tube had cooled, 3 ml of distilled water was
added and the contents extracted three times with 7-ml portions of
benzene; each portion of benzene was carefully withdrawn and discarded by using a 10-ml syringe and cannula. Next, 4 ml of 10 N
sodium hydroxide was added and the contents extracted three times
with 7-ml portions of benzene. Each portion was successively percolated through a plug of sodium sulfate (15 mm diameter x 10 mm thick)
and collected in a 50-ml glass-stoppered flask containing a boiling
bead and one drop of diethylene glycol to serve as a "keeper." The

contents were evaporated just to dryness under water pump vacuum at 60°C and the residue dissolved in an appropriate volume of methanol (5 ml or more) for SPF analysis.

(2) Microbiological media. Ten milliliters of the medium in a culture tube containing 1 g of sodium chloride was extracted with two 10-ml portions of benzene, which were successively percolated through a plug of sodium sulfate (15 mm diameter x 10 mm thick). The total extractive was then percolated through a 2-g alumina column and the benzene effluent discarded. The column was then washed with 5 ml of chloroform-methanol (9:1, v/v) and two 2-ml portions of chloroform; the combined washings were evaporated, hydrolyzed, extracted, and prepared for SPF analysis as described for laboratory chow except that only two extractions of the acid phase were required.

d. *Solubility and p-value determinations* The solubility of 2-AAF in several solvents was determined by preparing supersaturated solutions (5 ml) in 10-ml flasks by alternately heating them in a water bath at 50°C and shaking them with a vortex mixer during a period of 4 hr. The solutions were then mechanically shaken at ambient temperature (25 ± 2°C) for 6 days. The supernatant was decanted into glass-stoppered tubes and centrifuged at 2000 rpm for about 4 hr. Portions of the supernatant were appropriately diluted and anlyzed by GC.

Extraction p-values for the three compounds in several immiscible binary solvent systems were determined by GC as described by Beroza and Bowman [11,12].

e. *Gas chromatographic analysis* A Hewlett-Packard (Palo Alto, Calif.) Model 5750 gas chromatograph with a flame ionization detector (FID) was fitted with a 100-cm glass column (4 mm i.d., 6 mm o.d.) containing 10% OV-101 [weight/weight (w/w)] on 80-100 mesh Gas Chrom Q (Applied Science Lab, State College, Pa.) and operated under the following conditions after preconditioning the column overnight at 275°C: helium carrier gas, 75 ml/min; column, 250°C; injection port, 275°C; detector, 290°C. Under these conditions, retention times (t_R) for fluorene, 2-AF, and 2-AAF were 0.55, 1.45, and 3.60 min, respectively.

Five microliters of the cleaned-up extract dissolved in chloroform were injected for analysis. Quantification of the unknown was
based on the peak height of known amounts of standard; peak height to
about 1×10^{-8} amp full scale was proportional to concentration of
sample. Initial conditioning of the GC column by repeatedly injecting
2-AAF and the extracts was required for reproducible, linear, and
sensitive responses.

f. *Spectrophotofluorimetric analysis*   An Aminco-Bowman instrument
(American Instrument Co., Silver Spring, Md.) equipped with a xenon
lamp and a 1P28 detector was used with 1-cm cells and a 2-2-2-mm slit
program to measure fluorescence. Excitation (λ_{Ex}) and emission (λ_{Em})
maxima for the three compounds were as follows.

2-AAF: λ_{Ex} = 296 nm, λ_{Em} = 328 nm
2-AF: λ_{Ex} = 297 nm, λ_{Em} = 366 nm
fluorene: λ_{Ex} = 266 nm, λ_{Em} = 307 nm

All dilutions were made with methanol. During operation, the instrument was calibrated frequently to produce a relative intensity (RI)
of 5.0 with a solution of 0.3 μg quinine sulfate per milliliter of
0.1 N sulfuric acid (λ_{Ex} = 350 nm, λ_{Em} = 450 nm). Readings were
corrected for the solvent blank and RI was plotted versus concentration of the three compounds on log-log paper to produce standard
curves.

All samples were diluted to contain extract equivalent to 0.2 g
of chow per milliliter or to 2 g of medium per milliliter or diluted
further as required. To be certain that the RI was within the linear
range of the standard curve and thus unaffected by concentration
quenching, samples were diluted with an equal volume of solvent; the
RI of the diluted samples should have been about half that of the
undiluted solution. If it was not, dilution was continued until RI
was halved by dilution. After the untreated control sample (diluted
in the same manner as the unknown) was subtracted, concentration in
micorgrams per milliliter was determined from the standard curve.
Since residues of 2-AAF are analyzed as 2-AF, the analytical results
are multiplied by a factor of 1.23 to express them as 2-AAF.

4. *Results and Discussion*

In studies concerning the efficiency of extracting residues of 2-AAF
from aged samples of spiked chow, higher recoveries were obtained
from portions shaken at room temperature than from those extracted
in a Soxhlet apparatus. The addition of water to deactivate the
sample greatly enhanced recovery (up to 30% enhancement), particularly from autoclaved samples. The reason for lower recoveries from
the Soxhlet extractions is not known; however, the prolonged exposure
of the sample at the reflux temperature of the solvent may have caused
partial degradation and/or conjugation of the residue.

Recoveries from chow spiked with 5, 50, and 250 parts per million
(ppm) of 2-AAF and analyzed by the GC procedure (partitioning and
silica gel cleanup) averaged 63, 87, and 97%, respectively. Samples
from the GC analysis were not sufficiently clean for SPF. However,
a satisfactory additional cleanup was achieved by adding a benzene
solution (5 ml) of the GC sample to a column (12 mm i.d.) containing
1.25 g of Darco KB-Hyflo Super Cel (1:4, w/w) and eluting the 2-AAF
with 25 ml of benzene-acetone (1:1, v/v); the eluate was evaporated
to dryness and analyzed by SPF as 2-AAF per se as described. This
cleanup further reduced recoveries to about 52, 67, and 69% for the
5-, 50-, and 250-ppm samples, respectively. Sensitivities (based on
twice the interference from untreated samples) of both the GC and SPF
procedures for chow and the GC procedure for biological media were
about 1 and 0.1 ppm, respectively. Figure 3.2 shows typical gas
chromatograms of the analytical standards and extracts of chow and
a biological growth medium (Rogosa). A comparison of Figure 3.2B
(solvent partitioning only) and 3.2C illustrates the reduction in
interference accomplished by the silica gel chromatography; the 2-AAF
residues in chow (Figure 3.2D) could not be analyzed without the
silica gel cleanup.

Adsorption liquid chromatography of the three compounds on
silica gel was investigated as a cleanup procedure for GC. A 1-ml
solution containing 500 µg of each of the three compounds was placed
on the column and washed into the adsorbent with 5 ml of benzene.
The eluate was then analyzed by GC of 5-ml aliquots as the column

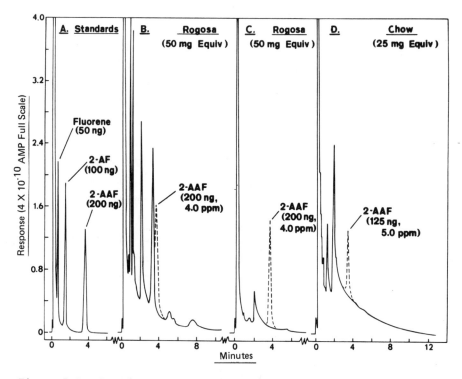

Figure 3.2. Gas chromatograms of 2-AAF and two of its analogs. Solid lines in chromatograms B, C, and D are unspiked extracts carried through the method (exception: B was not cleaned up with silica gel); broken lines are the same solutions spiked with 2-AAF. (From Bowman and King [1].)

was sequentially eluted with a total of 60 ml of benzene, 50 ml of 2% acetone in benzene, and finally 65 ml of 5% acetone in benzene. As shown in Figure 3.3, fluorene and 2-AF were completely separated and eluted with the benzene, nothing emerged in the 2% acetone effluent, and the 2-AAF was completely eluted by the 5% acetone mixture. These results may be useful for metabolic studies or for the adaptation of our method or of others to other substrates. In studies with spiked extracts, it was found that the 2% acetone mixture eluted much of the interfering materials but no 2-AAF; accordingly, this solvent mixture was used in our GC cleanup. When the silica gel was partially deactivated by adding 7% water, some decomposition of 2-AAF

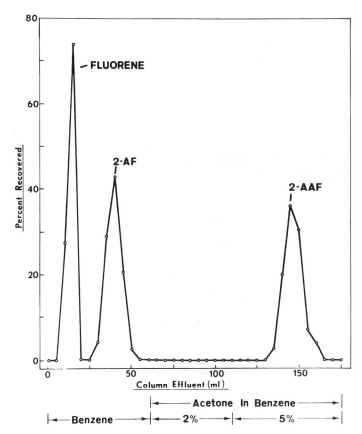

Figure 3.3. Separation of 2-AAF, 2-AF, and
fluorene on a column of silica gel. (From
Bowman and King [1].)

was observed; the use of pH 7 buffer, rather than water alone,
corrected the difficulty.

Later, a more rapid and sensitive method was required for the
analysis of 2-AAF residues in smaller-size samples. The strong
fluorescence of 2-AF and its properties as an organic base formed
the basis of the SPF method. Figure 3.4 shows the excitation and
emission spectra of the three compounds and Figure 3.5 is a plot of
RI versus concentration of the compounds.

Acid hydrolysis of 2-AAF to 2-AF increased the fluorescence of
the residue about 50-fold and provided a sensitivity that could not

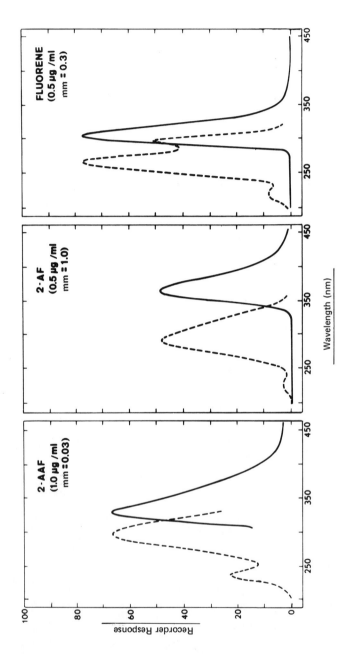

Figure 3.4. Excitation (dotted line) and emission (solid line) spectra of 2-AAF, 2-AF, and fluorene in methanol. In this and other figures, mm denotes instrument meter multiplier setting. (From Bowman and King [1].)

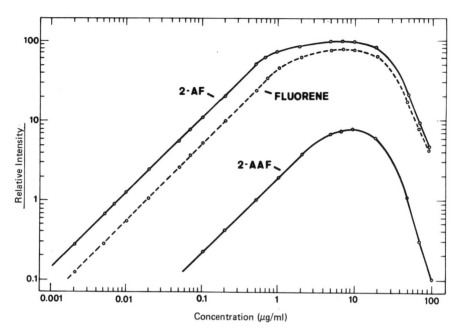

Figure 3.5. Standard curves for 2-AAF, 2-AF, and
fluorene in methanol. (From Bowman and King [1].)

be obtained by a direct SPF assay of 2-AAF. In addition, the acid
hydrolysis of the acetyl group followed by the organic-solvent extraction of the aqueous phase containing 2-AF as the amine hydrochloride
provided a cleanup far superior to that obtained in the GC method.
Therefore, the SPF procedure is preferred to GC for analyzing low
levels of residues.

Quadruplicate samples of laboratory chow untreated and spiked
with 2-AAF at 2.0, 20, and 200 ppm were analyzed by the SPF procedure;
the results are presented in Table 3.1. Based on twice the SPF reading
obtained from the untreated chow, the limit of sensitivity would be set
at about 0.5 ppm, but because its fluorescence was highly reproducible
and the excitation and emission maxima from the chow did not correspond
to those of 2-AF, identification and estimation of residues as low as
0.1 ppm level may be possible.

Four replicates of the six microbiological media untreated and
spiked with 2-AAF at 0.10 and 1.0 ppm were also analyzed by the SPF

Table 3.1. Spectrophotofluorimetric and GC analyses of extracts of laboratory chow spiked with 2-AAF

Added		Recovered ($\bar{x} \pm$ SE)[a]		
ppm	μg[b]	μg[b]		%
SPF Analysis				
0	0	0.243 $\pm$ 0.022		--
2.0	2.0	1.53	$\pm$ 0.03	76.5 $\pm$ 1.5
20	20	17.3	$\pm$ 0.1	86.5 $\pm$ 0.5
200	200	170.0	$\pm$ 1.3	85.0 $\pm$ 0.7
GC Analysis[c]				
20	20	16.8	$\pm$ 0.3	84.2 $\pm$ 1.5
200	200	165.0	$\pm$ 2.6	82.3 $\pm$ 1.3

Source: Bowman and King [1].

[a]Mean ($\bar{x}$) and standard error (SE) of four samples.

[b]Per gram of sample.

[c]Methanol solutions from the SPF analysis were evaporated to dryness, dissolved in chloroform, and the 2-AF analyzed by GC

method and the results are presented in Table 3.2. Limits of sensitivity (based on twice the SPF reading of the untreated medium) varied from about 14 parts per billion (ppb) for Rogosa to 52 ppb for the thioglycolate medium. Again, the fluorescence of the untreated samples was highly reproducible and did not correspond to that of 2-AF.

The SPF procedure for both chow and media detects residues of 2-AAF and 2-AF. Recoveries of 2-AF are generally about 10% lower than those of 2-AAF, probably because of its greater volatility. Studies with chow and media spiked with 2-AAF and autoclaved have indicated that the compound is stable; however, if residues of 2-AF are sought, the analysis may be performed by omitting the 2-hr hydrolysis at 85°C and immediately extracting the acidified extract at ambient temperature to remove any residues of 2-AAF before hydrolysis occurs. The behavior of the hydroxylated metabolites of 2-AAF in the analytical procedure is not known since analytical standards are not

Table 3.2. Spectrophotofluorimetric analysis of six different biological growth media spiked with 2-AAF at 0.0, 0.1, and 1.0 ppm

Biological medium	Added ppm	Added μg^{b}	Recovered ($\bar{x} \pm$ SE)[a] μg^{b}	%
Rogosa	0	0	0.057 ± 0.003	--
	0.10	1.0	0.805 ± 0.024	80.5 ± 2.4
	1.00	10.0	8.76 ± 0.155	87.6 ± 1.6
Lactobacillus MRS	0	0	0.067 ± 0.005	--
	0.10	1.00	0.846 ± 0.012	84.6 ± 1.2
	1.00	10.0	8.79 ± 0.113	87.9 ± 1.1
Brain heart infusion	0	0	0.200 ± 0.005	--
	0.10	1.0	0.901 ± 0.013	90.1 ± 1.3
	1.00	10.0	9.07 ± 0.229	90.7 ± 2.3
Proteose peptone	0	0	0.114 ± 0.008	--
	0.10	1.00	0.702 ± 0.020	70.2 ± 2.0
	1.00	10.0	8.25 ± 0.286	82.5 ± 3.9
Trypticase soy dextrose	0	0	0.127 ± 0.003	--
	0.10	1.00	0.864 ± 0.153	86.4 ± 1.5
	1.00	10.0	8.73 ± 0.090	87.3 ± 0.9
Thioglycolate	0	0	0.234 ± 0.012	--
	0.10	1.00	0.897 ± 0.031	89.7 ± 3.2
	1.00	10.0	8.89 ± 0.106	88.9 ± 1.1

Source: Bowman and King [1].

[a]Mean and standard error of four samples.

[b]Per 10 ml of medium.

Table 3.3. Solubility data for 2-AAF in some common organic
solvents and in vegetable oils

Solvent	Solubility of 2-AAF (mg/ml) at 25 ± 2°C
Acetone	42.0
Acetonitrile	16.3
Benzene	27.4
Chloroform	36.0
Corn oil	2.26
Dimethyl sulfoxide	>200
Ethyl acetate	56.6
Ethyl alcohol	22.2
Hexane	0.02
Methyl alcohol	24.2
Peanut oil	2.46
Propylene glycol	11.1
Soybean oil	2.00
Water	0.007

available. However, any residues of these compounds extracted by the
procedure might be lost during the adsorption column cleanup. For
example, N-OH-2-AAF is apparently irreversibly sorbed by alumina and
silica gel on thin-layer plates [10].

The SPF method for media, with minor modifications, has been
applied to the analysis of 2-AF and 2-AAF at the low ppb level in
wastewater, human urine, fixatives, and other aqueous substrates.

The possibility of analyzing for traces of the compounds by
preparing electron-capturing derivatives was investigated. When the
three compounds were dissolved in 1 ml of chloroform and reacted with
50 μl of liquid bromine for 5 min at ambient temperature, derivatives
with high electron-capturing properties were obtained. Presumably,
two bromine atoms were added to the fluorene ring of each compound.
Unfortunately, this technique had to be rejected because cleaned-up

extracts of the brominated samples contained electron-capturing
interferences.

Solubility data for 2-AAF in the common organic solvents and in
vegetable oils were required before analytical method development and
the formulation of animal diets could be undertaken; such values could
not be found in the literature. Results of our determinations are
presented in Table 3.3.

Partition values (the fraction of solute partitioning into the
nonpolar phase of an equivolume immiscible binary solvent system) are
useful in developing extraction and cleanup procedures and in confirming the identities of GC peaks [11-14]. The following values were
obtained for the compounds listed: (1) in chloroform-aqueous NaOH,
HCl, or H_2SO_4 (0.001, 0.1, or 10 N), p-values for fluorene and 2-AAF
are 1.0; (2) in chloroform-aqueous NaOH (0.001, 0.1, or 10 N), aqueous
HCl, or H_2SO_4 (0.001 N), the p-value for 2-AF is 1.0; (3) in chloroform-aqueous HCl or H_2SO_4 (10 N), for 2-AF it is 0.01 or less; and
(4) in chloroform-aqueous HCl or H_2SO_4 (0.1 N), for 2-AF it is about
0.17. Values for 2-AAF were determined in several other solvent
systems as follows: hexane-acetonitrile, 0.008; chloroform-water,
1.0; chloroform-60% methanol (40% water), 0.94; hexane-dimethylform-
amide, 0.004; benzene-water, 1.0; and hexane-80% acetone (20% water),
0.24.

The analysis of 2-AAF in wastewater via SPF is discussed in
Chapter 5 and a procedure for determining 2-AF and 2-AAF in human
urine and wastewater via electron-capture (EC) GC of pentafluoropropionyl derivatives is presented in Chapter 4.

B. Benzidine, Diorthotoluidine, and Dianisidine [15]

1. *General Description of Method*
Spectrophotofluorimetric methods are described for the trace analysis
of benzidine, 3,3'-dimethylbenzidine (diorthotoluidine), 3'3-dimethoxy-
benzidine (dianisidine), and their dihydrochloride salts in microbiological growth media, wastewater, potable water, human urine, and rat
blood. The salient elements of the methods for these known or suspected carcinogens are extraction of the residues as the free amine

with benzene, rapid cleanup on an alumina column, and quantification
of the free amine in methanol via SPF. Potable water solutions of
the salts are diluted with buffer (pH 4) and quantified directly by
SPF. Ancillary analytical information concerning the solubility and
stability of these compounds, p-values, GC analysis of the free amines,
and thin-layer chromatographic (TLC) data in 10 solvent systems are
also presented.

2. *Introduction*

Urinary bladder tumors in human subjects exposed to chemicals utilized
in the synthesis of dyes were first reported by Rehn [16] in 1895.
Rehn called the lesions "aniline tumors"; however, subsequent research
proved that aniline was not the causative agent and other aromatic
amines, such as benzidine and its congeners, were then indicated. The
toxicological effects of compounds in the benzidine family have been
widely studied for several years, and in 1974, the U. S. Department
of Labor called for the regulation of benzidine, 3,3'-dichlorobenzi-
dine, and 4-aminobiphenyl by placing them on the list of chemical compounds known to, or suspected to, cause human cancer from occupational
exposure [17]. A comprehensive overview of the literature and problems
associated with the use of benzidine and its congeners was recently
reported by Haley [18].

Before proposed long-term feeding studies with benzidine, diorthotoluidine, and dianisidine could be initiated at the NCTR, analytical
methods were sought to satisfy all of the experimental requirements
previously discussed. In addition, a procedure was also needed for
evaluating the microbiological systems which were then being tested
in an attempt to discover a means of destroying the carcinogenic
effects of the chemicals. The formulas of the three compounds are
shown in Figure 3.6. In order to improve their water solubility and
chemical stability and reduce volatility, the chemicals are administered to the animals as aqueous solutions of dihydrochlorides; therefore, analytical methods for these salts were also required.

Several colorimetric methods for benzidine, based on diazotization and coupling reactions, have been reported [19-21]; also

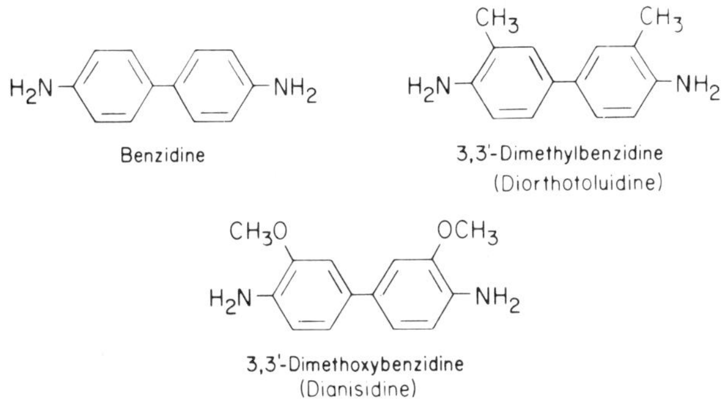

Figure 3.6. Formulas of benzidine, 3,3'-dimethyl-benzidine, and 3,3'-dimethoxybenzidine. (From Bowman et al. [15].)

Chloramine-T reagent was employed to determine benzidine and its congeners [22,23]. Clayson et al. [24] reported a qualitative method for benzidine and its metabolites based on reversed phase paper chromatography. Rinde [25] used 2,4,6-trinitrobenzenesulfonic acid and fluorescamine to detect benzidine on TLC plates; spectrophoto-metric and fluorimetric methods employing these reagents were also used to quantitate benzidine excretion following feeding of benzidine dyes. None of these methods, however, provide the sensitivity, speci-ficity, accuracy, and precision required for our use. The following procedures were therefore developed for use in conjunction with the toxicological tests with the three compounds.

3. *Experimental*

a. *Materials*   Benzidine (mp 127-129°C) was purchased from Fisher Scientific Co., Fair Lawn, N.J., and the benzidine dihydrochloride was Matheson, Coleman, Bell chemical No. B-260. The 3,3'-dimethyl-benzidine (mp 129-131°C) and 3,3'-dimethoxybenzidine dihydrochloride were purchased from Pfaltz and Bauer Co., Flushing, N.Y. The 3,3'-dimethylbenzidine dihydrochloride was prepared from the corresponding amine (2 g in 50 ml of benzene) by bubbling an excess of anhydrous HCl through the solution to precipitate the salt; the 3,3'-dimethoxy-benzidine (mp 137-139°C) was prepared from an aqueous solution of the

corresponding salt by making it strongly alkaline with NaOH and extracting the free amine with benzene. All six chemicals were vacuum
dried overnight at 60°C prior to use. The high purity of the amines
was demonstrated by the absence of extraneous GC peaks; the salts,
after conversion to the free amines, were also free of extraneous
peaks and yielded the correct amount of product.

    The adsorbent (basic alumina, Brockman Activity I) from Fisher
Scientific Co. (No. A-941) was used as received. Sodium sulfate was
anhydrous; all reagents were CP grade and all solvents were pesticide
grade. Ingredients for the microbiological culture media were purchased from Difco Laboratories, Detroit, Mich., and the media were
prepared in accordance with the instructions supplied by the manufacturer. The TLC plates (20 x 20 cm, Fisher, No. 6-601A), precoated
with Silica Gel GF (250 μm thick), were activated in an oven at 130°C
for 1 hr and allowed to cool in a desiccator prior to use. All culture tubes were of borosilicate glass and equipped with Teflon-lined
screw caps. The buffer (pH 4, potassium biphthalate, 0.05 M) was
Fisher Chemical No. SO-B-98.

b. Preparation of sample for SPF analysis

(1) Microbiological growth media. Ten milliliters of the trypticase
soy dextrose (TSD) or brain heart infusion (BHI) medium was added to
a 30-ml culture tube and 1 g of NaCl, 0.2 ml of 10 N NaOH, and 10 ml
of benzene were added. The tube was sealed, shaken vigorously for 2
min, and centrifuged for 10 min at 2000 rpm. The benzene layer was
carefully withdrawn by using a syringe and cannula and percolated
through a plug of sodium sulfate (25 mm diameter x 10 mm thick) in
tandem with a glass column (12 mm i.d., Kontes, No. 420,000) prepared
by adding successively, a plug of glass wool, 5 g of sodium sulfate,
1 g of basic alumina, and 5 g of sodium sulfate. The medium was extracted with two additional 10-ml portions of benzene, which were
successively percolated through the plug and column. Finally, the
column was washed with 10 ml of dichloromethane-10% methanol to ensure complete elution of the free amine residue from the column. The
combined eluates, after the addition of one drop of diethylene glycol

to serve as a keeper, were evaporated just to dryness by using water pump vacuum and a 60°C water bath. The dry residue was dissolved in an appropriate amount of methanol for SPF analysis as the free amine.

(2) Wastewater. One hundred milliliters of the sample, 2 g of NaCl, and 0.5 ml of 10 N NaOH were added to a 160-ml culture tube. The sample was then shaken, centrifuged, cleaned up, and prepared for analysis as described for media. (Exception: Three 15-ml portions of benzene were used for the extraction.)

(3) Urine. Procedures utilizing alkaline hydrolysis or acid hydrolysis prior to extraction, as well as no hydrolysis, were tested: (a) No hydrolysis--analyses were performed exactly as described for wastewater; (b) Alkaline hydrolysis--analyses were performed exactly as described for wastewater except the alkaline solution in the tube was sealed, heated in a water bath at 80°C for 2 hr, then cooled prior to the extraction with benzene; (c) Acid hydrolysis--these analyses were also performed as described for wastewater, except that 0.5 ml of concentrated HCl was substituted for the 10 N NaOH, then the mixture was heated at 80°C for 2 hr, cooled, and made alkaline with 1 ml of 10 N NaOH prior to extraction with benzene.

(4) Blood. Procedures employing no hydrolysis of the sample prior to extraction, as well as alkaline or acid hydrolysis, were tested: (a) No hydrolysis--6 ml of distilled water, 1 ml of 10 N NaOH, and 1 g of NaCl were added to a 20-ml culture tube containing 1 ml of whole rat blood. The contents were mixed, and then extracted with three 10-ml portions of benzene, cleaned up, and prepared for SPF analysis as described for media; (b) Alkaline hydrolysis--samples were analyzed as for no hydrolysis except that the mixture in the sealed tube was held in an 80°C heating block for 2 hr with frequent shaking, then cooled prior to extraction with benzene; (c) Acid hydrolysis--analyses were performed as for no hydrolysis except that 1 ml of concentrated HCl was substituted for the NaOH and the sealed tube was then heated at 80°C for 2 hr, cooled, and made alkaline by adding 2 ml of 10 N NaOH. The mixture was then extracted, cleaned up, and prepared for SPF analysis as described.

(5) Potable water. Aqueous solutions of the dihydrochloride salts
slated for use as the animals' drinking water to administer the proper
dosage of test chemical are assayed for proper concentrations after
sequential dilutions with water containing 2% (v/v) of buffer (pH 4).
The fluorescence of the diluted sample (e.g., 1 ppm) is compared
directly with that of a standard solution prepared in the same manner.

(6) Recovery experiments. Triplicate samples of both biological
media were separately spiked with 100 µl of methanol (or water) containing the appropriate amount of the free amine (or its salt) to
produce residues of 0, 0.1, and 1.0 ppm. The samples were allowed
to stand in the refrigerator (5°C) overnight prior to extractions.
Samples (1 ml) of whole rat blood were spiked in the same manner at
0 and 10 ppm, held at 5°C overnight, and analyzed as described.
Wastewater and urine samples (100 ml) were spiked at 0 and 20 ppb by
adding 1 ml of methanol (or water) containing the appropriate amount
of the test compound, held at 5°C overnight, and analyzed as described.

c. *Stability of aqueous solutions of the test compounds* Aqueous
solutions of the three amines (ca. 50 ppm) and of their dihydrochloride
salts (ca. 50 and 500 ppm) were prepared for use in tests to determine
the chemical stability of the test compounds under simulated animal
test conditions. The animal drinking water dispenser for each cage
(four mice per cage) consisted of a glass bottle (500 ml, 62 mm
square x 180 mm high) fitted with a No. 8 rubber stopper and a stainless steel "sipper tube" (8 mm o.d. x 90 mm long) containing a steel
ball to serve as a valve. Triplicate dispensers, each containing
375 ml of the various test solutions, were placed in cages and exposed
to ambient conditions (25 ± 2°C and continuous fluorescent lighting)
in the animal room. Samples (10 ml) were taken from each dispenser
immediately and 1, 2, 4, 8, and 16 days later. The pH of each sample
was determined and solutions of the salts were diluted and anlyzed as
described for potable water. Solutions of the free amines were diluted with methanol to an appropriate concentration (e.g., 0.5 µg/ml)
and the fluorescence related to standards of the free amines diluted
in the same manner.

d. Gas chromatographic analysis   A Hewlett-Packard Model 5750 gas chromatograph equipped with a flame ionization detector was fitted with a 100-cm glass column (4 mm i.d., 6 mm o.d.) containing 10% OV-101 (w/w) on Gas Chrom Q (80-100 mesh) and operated with a helium carrier flow of 100 ml/min. The injection port and detector temperatures were 275 and 290°C, respectively. The column oven was operated isothermally for the quantitative analysis of the individual free amines (e.g., p-value determinations) as follows: benzidine, 215°C; 3,3'-dimethylbenzidine, 235°C; and 3,3'-dimethoxybenzidine, 240°C; under these conditions, their retention times (t_R) were 2.35, 2.25, and 2.70 min, respectively. In assays concerning the GC purity of the free amines, the oven was temperature-programmed from 200 to 280°C at the rate of 10°C/min. A typical temperature-programmed chromatogram of the three compounds is shown in Figure 3.7.

e. Spectrophotofluorometric analysis   An Aminco-Bowman instrument (American Instrument Co., Silver Spring, Md.), equipped with a xenon lamp and a 1P28 detector, was used with 1-cm square cells and a 2-2-2-mm slit program to measure fluorescence. All dilutions of the free amines were freshly prepared in methanol and those of the salts were in water-2% buffer (pH 4). Excitation (λ_{Ex}) and emission (λ_{Em}) wavelengths and relative intensities are presented in Table 3.4.

The instrument was frequently calibrated to produce a RI of 5.0 with a dilution of 0.3 μg quinine sulfate per milliliter of 0.1 N sulfuric acid (λ_{Ex} = 350 nm, λ_{Em} = 450 nm). Readings were corrected for solvent blanks and RI was plotted versus concentration of the six compounds on log-log paper to produce a standard curve.

To ensure that the RI was within the linear range of the standard curve and thus unaffected by concentration quenching, samples were diluted with an equal volume of solvent to ascertain whether the RI was about half of the undiluted solution. If it was not, dilution was continued until the RI was halved by dilution. Extracts of wastewater and urine, medium, and blood for SPF analysis were first diluted to contain 10, 1, and 0.2 g equivalents of sample per milliliter, respectively; further dilutions were made as required to be certain

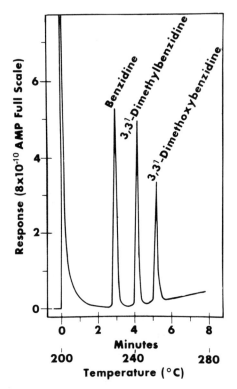

Figure 3.7. A typical temperature-programmed chromatogram of 500-ng amounts of benzidine, 3,3'-dimethylbenzidine, and 3,3'-dimethoxybenzidine injected in 5 μl of chloroform as determined by a flame ionization detector. (From Bowman et al. [15].)

the RI was within the linear range of the standard curve. The RI of the untreated control samples was then subtracted from that of the unknown and the concentration in micrograms per milliliter was determined from the standard curve. In the instances where salts are assayed as the free amines, the analytical results for benzidine, 3,3'-dimethylbenzidine, and 3,3'-dimethoxybenzidine are multiplied by the factors 1.40, 1.34, and 1.30, respectively to express them on the proper basis.

Table 3.4. Spectrophotofluorimetric data for benzidine and some
of its derivatives

Compound	λ_{Ex} (nm)	λ_{Em} (nm)	RI (1 µg/ml)
Benzidine	295	396	33.5
Benzidine·2HCl	302	410	7.45
3,3'-Dimethylbenzidine	300	384	51.8
3,3'-Dimethylbenzidine·2HCl	310	410	12.2
3,3'-Dimethoxybenzidine	312	380	64.3
3,3'-Dimethoxybenzidine·2HCl	318	422	8.25

f. *Solubility, p-value, and TLC determinations*   The solubilities
of benzidine, 3,3'-dimethylbenzidine, 3,3'-dimethoxybenzidine, and
their salts in water at 25 ± 2°C were determined by SPF as described
by Bowman and King [1].

Extraction p-values for the three amines were determined in
several solvent systems by GC in the manner described by Bowman and
Beroza [13].

The TLC determinations were made by using a Gelman Model 51325-1
apparatus and activated glass plates precoated with silica gel GF.
The plates were spotted with 5 µl (5 µg) of methanol solutions of the
free amines or anthracene (reference compound). After the developing
solvent had ascended 13 cm above the spotting line (ca. 25 min), the
plates were removed and the solvent allowed to evaporate. The spots
were made visible by viewing them under ultraviolet light (254 nm)
and the R_f (retention factor) values calculated.

4. *Results and Discussion*

In preliminary studies of the analytical chemical properties of these
compounds, the free amines were found to gas chromatograph well with
minimal column conditioning; the three compounds were also readily
separated (Figure 3.7) and quantified. Gas chromatographic analysis
was therefore employed for p-value determinations and purity assays;

however, the FID lacked the sensitivity and specificity required
for trace analysis of residues in a variety of substrates. The
possibility of oxidizing the free amines to their corresponding
dinitro analogs was investigated, since these derivatives might then
be assayed by EC-GC with higher sensitivity and specificity. The use
of m-chloroperbenzoic acid, hydrogen peroxide, and potassium permanganate under various conditions, however, produced no more than a
20% yield of the derivative. The portion of the free amines not
derivatized remained unchanged or was converted to products that did
not emerge from the gas chromatograph, depending on the severity of
the oxidation reaction.

Tests pertaining to the SPF properties of the compounds revealed
that all six fluoresce strongly. The RI values of the free amines in
methanol were about five times greater than those of the salts in
aqueous buffer. Limits of detection and linearity of the amines and
salts were about 2 and 10 ng/ml, respectively. As expected, the SPF
response of aqueous solutions of the salts varied with pH, and assays
of these compounds diluted with water alone were not reproducible.
This problem was overcome by using an aqueous solution containing 2%
buffer (v/v, pH 4) for dilutions and SPF measurements. Excitation
and emission spectra and standard curves for the six compounds are
presented in Figures 3.8-3.10. The SPF method was selected for subsequent assays because of its high sensitivity and the specificity
afforded of the characteristic excitation and emission maxima of each
compound. Determination of the three amines or the three salts in   .
admixture was attempted by measuring the RI at the excitation and
emission maxima for each compound and calculating the amount of each
constituent by using simultaneous equations. However, this was not
successful because of the large differences in specific RI and extensive overlap of the spectra.

Results from the assays of microbiological growth media are presented in Table 3.5. Recoveries averaged 68 and 80% for samples
spiked with 0.10 and 1.0 ppm, respectively. The SPF background for
unspiked BHI and TSD media was about 0.04 and 0.02 ppm, respectively.

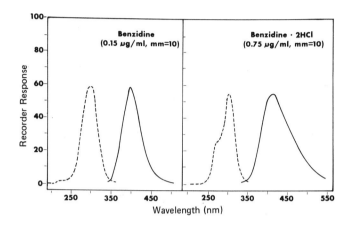

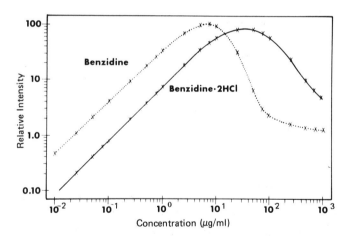

Figure 3.8. Top: Excitation (dotted line) and emission (solid line) spectra of benzidine and its dihydrochloride salt. Bottom: Standard curves for the two compounds. (From Bowman et al. [15].)

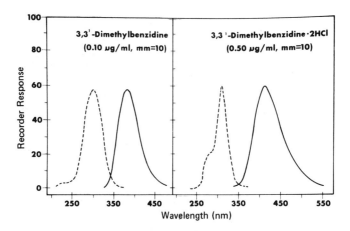

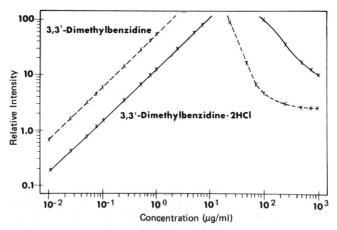

Figure 3.9. Top. Excitation (dotted line) and emission (solid line) spectra of 3,3'-dimethylbenzidine and its dihydrochloride salt. Bottom: Standard curves for the two compounds. (From Bowman et al. [15].)

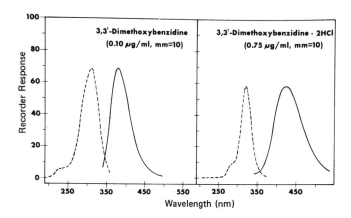

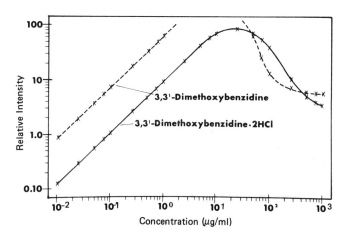

Figure 3.10. Top: Excitation (dotted line) and emission (solid line) spectra of 3,3'-dimethoxybenzidine and its dihydrochloride salt. Bottom: Standard curves for the two compounds. (From Bowman et al. [15].)

Table 3.5. Analysis of two biological growth media spiked with benzidine, two congeners, and their salts at 0, 0.10, and 1.0 ppm

Compound	Medium	Added[a]		Recovered ($\bar{x}$ ± SE)[b]	
		ppm	µg	ppm	%
Benzidine	BHI	0.0	0.0	0.040 ± 0.000	--
		0.10	1.0	0.070 ± 0.000	70.0 ± 0.0
		1.00	10.0	0.780 ± 0.004	78.0 ± 0.4
	TSD	0.0	0.0	0.019 ± 0.000	--
		0.10	1.0	0.075 ± 0.000	75.0 ± 0.0
		1.00	10.0	0.787 ± 0.012	78.7 ± 1.2
Benzidine·2HCl	BHI	0.0	0.0	0.040 ± 0.000	--
		0.10	1.0	0.073 ± 0.002	73.0 ± 2.0
		1.00	10.0	0.795 ± 0.000	79.5 ± 0.0
	TSD	0.0	0.0	0.019 ± 0.002	--
		0.10	1.0	0.073 ± 0.001	73.0 ± 1.0
		1.00	10.0	0.778 ± 0.004	77.8 ± 0.4
3,3'-Dimethylbenzidine	BHI	0.0	0.0	0.037 ± 0.001	--
		0.10	1.0	0.074 ± 0.005	74.0 ± 5.0
		1.00	10.0	0.839 ± 0.010	83.9 ± 1.0
	TSD	0.0	0.0	0.029 ± 0.004	--
		0.10	1.0	0.073 ± 0.002	73.0 ± 2.0
		1.00	10.0	0.902 ± 0.009	90.2 ± 0.9

Compound	Medium				
3,3'-Dimethylbenzidine·2HCl	BHI	0.0	0.0	0.045 ± 0.004	--
		0.10	1.0	0.070 ± 0.002	70.0 ± 2.0
		1.00	10.0	0.777 ± 0.006	77.7 ± 0.6
	TSD	0.0	0.0	0.036 ± 0.003	--
		0.10	1.0	0.064 ± 0.001	64.0 ± 1.0
		1.00	10.0	0.710 ± 0.003	61.0 ± 0.3
3,3'-Dimethoxybenzidine	BHI	0.0	0.0	0.031 ± 0.003	--
		0.10	1.0	0.078 ± 0.001	78.0 ± 1.0
		1.00	10.0	0.923 ± 0.007	92.3 ± 0.7
	TSD	0.0	0.0	0.019 ± 0.001	--
		0.10	1.0	0.055 ± 0.000	55.0 ± 0.0
		1.00	10.0	0.829 ± 0.008	82.9 ± 0.8
3,3'-Dimethoxybenzidine·2HCl	BHI	0.0	0.0	0.030 ± 0.003	--
		0.10	1.0	0.057 ± 0.005	57.0 ± 5.0
		1.00	10.0	0.715 ± 0.002	71.5 ± 0.2
	TSD	0.0	0.0	0.027 ± 0.003	--
		0.10	1.0	0.052 ± 0.001	52.0 ± 1.0
		1.00	10.0	0.770 ± 0.006	77.0 ± 0.6

Source: Bowman et al. [15].

[a]Per 10 ml of sample.

[b]Mean and standard error from triplicate assays; spiked samples are corrected for controls. Controls and 0.10 ppm samples contained 1 g equivalent of medium per milliliter for the SPF reading; the 1.0 ppm samples contained 0.2 g equivalent/ml.

Table 3.6. Analysis of wastewater spiked with benzidine, two
congeners, and their salts at 0 and 20 ppb

| Compound | Added[a] | | Recovered $(\overline{x} \pm SE)$[b] | |
	ppb	µg	ppb	%
Benzidine	0	0.0	4 ± 1	--
	20	2.0	17 ± 0	85
Benzidine·2HCl	0	0.0	4 ± 1	--
	20	2.0	15 ± 1	75
3,3'-Dimethylbenzidine	0	0.0	4 ± 1	--
	20	2.0	15 ± 0	75
3,3'-Dimethylbenzidine·2HCl	0	0.0	3 ± 1	--
	20	2.0	13 ± 1	65
3,3'-Dimethoxybenzidine	0	0.0	3 ± 0	--
	20	2.0	16 ± 0	80
3,3'-Dimethoxybenzidine·2HCl	0	0.0	3 ± 0	--
	20	2.0	14 ± 1	70

Source: Bowman et al. [15].

[a]Per 100 ml of sample.

[b]Mean and standard error from triplicate assays; spiked samples are
corrected for controls. Samples contained 10 g equivalents of water
per milliliter for the SPF reading.

Lowest recoveries were obtained with 3,3'-dimethoxybenzidine and its
salt. Assays of samples of wastewater (collected from the decontamination of control animal cages) separately spiked with 20 ppb of each
compound gave recoveries averaging 75% (Table 3.6). The precision
was excellent and the background was about 4 ppb.

Table 3.7 lists the results of SPF assays of whole rat blood
spiked with 10 ppm of the six compounds. Recoveries without hydrolysis of the sample and after alkaline or acid hydrolysis averaged about
14, 19, and 63%, respectively. Acid hydrolysis is therefore required
to recover a substantial portion of the residue; control background
was about 0.15 ppm. Recovery of the compounds from blood varied
inversely with their polarity.

Data from human urine spiked with 20 ppb of the compounds are
presented in Table 3.8. Recoveries of the free amines from urine
without hydrolysis and after alkaline hydrolysis were 90 and 68%,
respectively; those for the salts were 38 and 57%. It is apparent
that the procedure employing no hydrolysis should be used when residues of the free amines are sought, since alkaline hydrolysis diminished the recovery by about 20%. On the other hand, alkaline hydrolysis enhanced the recovery of the salts by about 20%; the reason for
this behavior is not fully understood. Acid hydrolyses of urine were
also performed, but, formation of a purple-colored product in both
control and spiked samples prevented the assay by SPF.

Results of 16-day stability studies with aqueous solutions of
benzidine (50 ppm) and its salt (50 and 500 ppm) under simulated
animal test conditions are presented in Table 3.9. The solutions
of the salt were essentially stable with a decrease in concentration
of less than 2% during the test period, whereas the free amine declined about 11%. In similar tests, 3,3'-dimethylbenzidine and its
salt declined about 9%, and 3,3'-dimethoxybenzidine and its salt
declined about 64 and 9%, respectively. The results in Table 3.9
illustrate the excellent precision of the SPF procedure for the
analysis of these compounds in potable water. The p-values (Table
3.10), which are useful in developing extraction and cleanup methods

Table 3.7. Analysis of whole rat blood spiked with benzidine, two congeners, and their salts at 0 and 10 ppm

Compound	Hydrolysis	Added[a]		Recovered ($\bar{x}$ ± SE)[b]	
		ppm	μg	ppm	%
Benzidine	None	0.0	0.0	0.051 ± 0.013	--
		10.0	10.0	0.668 ± 0.216	6.7 ± 2.2
	Alkaline	0.0	0.0	0.063 ± 0.013	--
		10.0	10.0	2.52 ± 0.34	25.2 ± 3.4
	Acid	0.0	0.0	0.048 ± 0.005	--
		10.0	10.0	7.39 ± 0.09	73.9 ± 0.9
Benzidine·2HCl	None	0.0	0.0	0.045 ± 0.007	--
		10.0	10.0	0.563 ± 0.108	5.6 ± 1.1
	Alkaline	0.0	0.0	0.086 ± 0.028	--
		10.0	10.0	2.49 ± 0.31	24.9 ± 3.1
	Acid	0.0	0.0	0.052 ± 0.008	--
		10.0	10.0	7.57 ± 0.125	75.7 ± 1.2
3,3'-Dimethylbenzidine	None	0.0	0.0	0.152 ± 0.052	--
		10.0	10.0	1.58 ± 0.13	15.8 ± 1.3
	Alkaline	0.0	0.0	0.276 ± 0.044	--
		10.0	10.0	2.16 ± 0.10	21.6 ± 1.0
	Acid	0.0	0.0	0.223 ± 0.006	--
		10.0	10.0	6.55 ± 0.09	65.5 ± 0.9

3,3'-Dimethylbenzidine·HCl	None	0.0	0.0	0.152 ± 0.052	--
		10.0	10.0	2.85 ± 0.19	28.5 ± 1.9
	Alkaline	0.0	0.0	0.276 ± 0.044	--
		10.0	10.0	2.11 ± 0.006	21.1 ± 0.6
	Acid	0.0	0.0	0.223 ± 0.006	--
		10.0	10.0	6.04 ± 0.37	60.4 ± 3.7
3,3'-Dimethoxybenzidine	None	0.0	0.0	0.128 ± 0.049	--
		10.0	10.0	0.464 ± 0.098	4.6 ± 1.0
	Alkaline	0.0	0.0	0.236 ± 0.034	--
		10.0	10.0	1.19 ± 0.47	11.9 ± 4.7
	Acid	0.0	0.0	0.192 ± 0.006	--
		10.0	10.0	5.35 ± 0.06	53.5 ± 0.6
3,3'-Dimethoxybenzidine·2HCl	None	0.0	0.0	0.128 ± 0.049	--
		10.0	10.0	2.10 ± 0.020	21.0 ± 2.0
	Alkaline	0.0	0.0	0.236 ± 0.034	--
		10.0	10.0	1.01 ± 0.18	10.1 ± 1.8
	Acid	0.0	0.0	0.192 ± 0.006	--
		10.0	10.0	4.64 ± 0.14	46.4 ± 1.4

Source: Bowman et al. [15]

[a] Per milliliter of sample.

[b] Mean and standard error from triplicate assays; spiked samples are corrected for controls. Control and spiked samples contained 200 and 20 mg equivalents of blood per milliliter, respectively, for the SPF readings.

Table 3.8. Analysis of human urine spiked with benzidine, two
congeners, and their salts at 0 and 20 ppb

Compound	Hydrolysis[a]	Added[b] ppb	Added[b] µg	Recovered ($\bar{x} \pm$ SE)[c] ppb	Recovered ($\bar{x} \pm$ SE)[c] %
Benzidine	None	0	0.0	5 ± 0	--
		20	2.0	18 ± 1	90
	Alkaline	0	0.0	6 ± 1	--
		20	2.0	13 ± 1	65
Benzidine·2HCl	None	0	0.0	5 ± 0	--
		20	2.0	7 ± 1	35
	Alkaline	0	0.0	6 ± 1	--
		20	2.0	11 ± 1	55
3,3'-Dimethylbenzidine	None	0	0.0	5 ± 0	--
		20	2.0	18 ± 1	90
	Alkaline	0	0.0	6 ± 1	--
		20	2.0	14 ± 1	70
3,3'-Dimethylbenzidine·2HCl	None	0	0.0	5 ± 0	--
		20	2.0	8 ± 1	40
	Alkaline	0	0.0	6 ± 1	--
		20	2.0	11 ± 2	55
3,3'-Dimethoxybenzidine	None	0	0.0	4 ± 1	--
		20	2.0	18 ± 2	90
	Alkaline	0	0.0	5 ± 1	--
		20	2.0	14 ± 1	70
3,3'-Dimethoxybenzidine·2HCl	None	0	0.0	4 ± 0	--
		20	2.0	8 ± 1	40
	Alkaline	0	0.0	5 ± 1	--
		20	2.0	12 ± 1	60

Source: Bowman et al. [15].

[a]Development of purple-colored product upon acid hydrolysis of
unspiked urine prevented the assay via SPF.

[b]Per 100 ml of sample

[c]Mean and standard error of triplicate assays; spiked samples are
corrected for controls. Control and spiked samples contained 10 g
equivalents of urine per milliliter for the SPF readings.

Table 3.9. Stability of aqueous solutions of benzidine and its dihydrochloride after exposure to simulated animal test conditions for 16 days

	Concentration and pH of solution indicated[a]					
	Benzidine		Benzidine·2HCl			
	50 ppm solution		50 ppm solution		500 ppm solution	
Sampling interval (days)	ppm	pH	ppm	pH	ppm	pH
0	54.0 ± 0.0	6.70 ± 0.10	49.7 ± 0.2	3.95 ± 0.01	507 ± 3	3.30 ± 0.02
1	52.0 ± 0.2	6.35 ± 0.15	49.6 ± 0.2	3.95 ± 0.01	496 ± 2	3.26 ± 0.01
2	53.8 ± 2.9	6.65 ± 0.12	49.7 ± 0.3	4.00 ± 0.21	493 ± 3	3.25 ± 0.02
4	52.8 ± 0.5	6.45 ± 0.10	49.4 ± 0.5	4.07 ± 0.02	498 ± 4	3.34 ± 0.02
8	50.2 ± 0.7	6.35 ± 0.30	49.9 ± 0.1	4.10 ± 0.02	504 ± 4	3.35 ± 0.05
16	47.8 ± 0.7	6.25 ± 0.18	48.9 ± 0.2	3.98 ± 0.07	497 ± 4	3.35 ± 0.03

Source: Bowman et al. [15].

[a]Mean and standard error from triplicate assays.

Table 3.10. Partition values of benzidine, 3,3'-dimethylbenzidine, and 3,3'-dimethoxybenzidine in various solvent systems

Solvent system	Partition value		
	Benzidine	3,3'-Dimethyl-benzidine	3,3'-Dimethoxy-benzidine
Hexane-acetonitrile	0.02	0.01	0.03
Hexane-80% acetone (20% water)	0.08	0.16	0.15
Chloroform-water	1.0	1.0	1.0
Chloroform-60% methanol (40% water)	0.85	0.96	0.97
Chloroform-aqueous NaOH (5.0, 0.5, or 0.05 N)	1.0	1.0	1.0
Chloroform-aqueous HCl (5.0, 0.5, or 0.05 N)	0.00	0.00	0.00
Hexane-dimethylformamide	0.00	0.00	0.00

for confirmatory tests [11-14], were obtained from the three free amines by GC.

Solubility data for the three amines and their dihydrochloride salts were required before analytical method development or formulation of the spiked animal drinking water could be undertaken; precise values could not be found in the literature. Results of our determinations via SPF are given in Table 3.11.

Thin-layer chromatographic R_f values for the three free amines and anthracene (included as a reference compound) in 10 solvent systems are reported in Table 3.12. These data are useful in the development of cleanup procedures and for the separation and identification of the compounds in admixture. The three compounds were separated by using 10% acetone or methanol in chloroform or benzene. Aqueous solutions of the salts, spotted and developed as described, gave R_f values identical to those of the free amines in all of the solvent systems tested.

Table 3.11. Solubility data for benzidine, 3,3'-dimethylbenzidine, 3,3'-dimethoxybenzidine, and their dihydrochloride salts

Compound	Solubility in water (mg/ml) at 25 ± 2°C
Benzidine	0.52
Benzidine·2HCl	61.7
3,3'-Dimethylbenzidine	1.3
3,3'-dimethylbenzidine·2HCL	76.7
3,3'-Dimethoxybenzidine	0.06
3,3'-Dimethoxybenzidine·2HCL	41.4

At the onset of animal tests with benzidine·2HCl-treated drinking water, routine monitoring of the air and work areas was also initiated to signal any accidental exposure of our personnel to traces of the compound. Air samples were collected by using a Model No. EMWL-2000H High Volume Air Sampler (General Metal Works, Inc., Cleves, Ohio) equipped with a No. 3000 (20 x 25 cm) fiberglass filter (retains 99.9% of particles larger than 0.3 µm in diameter) and operated continuously during the work day with an air flow of 1.42 m^3/min; the filter was removed weekly for chemical analysis and a new one was installed. For analysis, the filter was cut into small pieces, mechanically shaken with 250 ml of 0.1 HCl for 1 hr, filtered, made alkaline with 5 ml of 10 N NaOH, and extracted three times with 25-ml portions of chloro- form. The combined chloroform extracts successively percolated through a plug of sodium sulfate were evaporated to dryness in the presence of one drop of keeper; the dry residue was dissolved in benzene for cleanup and analysis as described for wastewater. The SPF background of a new filter is equivalent to about 0.4 µg of benzidine, whereas after a week in the sampling device, it averages about 10 µg. This background fluorescence has not exhibited the characteristic excitation and emission maxima of the compound sought and, thus far, all filters except those spiked in the laboratory have contained no detectable residues of the test chemical.

Table 3.12. Thin-layer chromatographic R_f values of benzidine, 3,3'-dimethylbenzidine, 3,3'-dimethoxybenzidine, and anthracene in 10 solvent systems

Solvent system (v/v)	R_f values (x 100) of compound indicated			
	Benzidine	3,3'-Dimethyl-benzidine	3,3'-Dimethoxy-benzidine	Anthracene
Chloroform	10	14	11	100
Chloroform–ethyl acetate (9:1)	20	29	29	92
Chloroform–diethyl ether (9:1)	21	32	32	100
Chloroform–acetone (9:1)	24	33	38	83
Chloroform–methanol (9:1)	70	80	85	97
Benzene	2	2	2	69
Benzene–ethyl acetate (9:1)	9	11	13	73
Benzene–diethyl ether (9:1)	6	10	11	75
Benzene–acetone (9:1)	16	21	26	76
Benzene–methanol (9:1)	33	45	50	81

Source: Bowman et al. [15].

The monitoring of work areas (cages, floors, benches, apparatus, etc.) suspected of being contaminated with benzidine·2HCl (or benzidine) is accomplished by using kits consisting of a cotton applicator and a 5-ml culture tube containing exactly 2 ml of the aqueous buffer. The applicator is moistened with the aqueous buffer and used to swab a specific area then the applicator is vigorously stirred in the buffer after each of several subsequent swabbings of the same area. The tube and contents are then centrifuged at 2000 rpm for 10 min to remove any suspended material. Then 1 ml of the supernatant is either analyzed directly or appropriately diluted as described for the analysis of potable water. Background fluorescence is generally equivalent to 0.10 µg of benzidine; areas contaminated with as little as 0.30 µg of the salt are readily detected and the identity of the chemical is confirmed by its characteristic excitation and emission maxima.

Subsequent procedures, which are based on EC-GC of pentafluoropropionyl derivatives of the three compounds in wastewater and human urine, are described in Chapter 4.

C. 3,3'-Dichlorobenzidine [26]

1. *General Description of Method*

Gas chromatographic procedures are described for the trace analysis of 3,3'-dichlorobenzidine and its dihydrochloride salt in animal feed, wastewater, and human urine. Salient elements of the method for these known carcinogens in feed are extraction of the residues as the free amine and a cleanup via acid-base liquid-liquid partitioning with benzene followed by a silica gel column. With wastewater and human urine, residues are adsorbed by percolating the sample through a column of XAD-2, eluted with acetone, and cleaned up with acid-base partitioning and a silica gel column. Residues are assayed by GC either as the free amine or after conversion to the pentafluoropropionyl (PFP) derivative by using an EC or a rubidium-sensitized thermionic-type (N/P) detector. Minimum detectable residues in feed, wastewater, and human urine are about 3 ppb, 18 ppt, and 60 ppt, respectively, as determined by EC-GC of the PFP derivative.

2. *Introduction*

Benzidine and certain related 3,3'-disubstituted analogs such as
3,3'-dichlorobenzidine (3,3'-dichloro-4,4'-diaminobiphenyl), hereafter referred to as DiClBzd, have been used for more than 60 years
as intermediates in the manufacture of organic pigments [22,23,27]
and the toxicological effects of compounds in the benzidine family
were widely studied for many years. In 1974 the U. S. Department
of Labor called for the regulation of benzidine and DiClBzd by placing them on a list of 14 chemical compounds known to cause, or suspected of causing, cancer from occupational exposure [17]. An excellent review of the literature and problems associated with the
use of benzidine and its congeners was given by Haley [18].

Since long-term feeding studies with DiClBzd using large numbers
of mice were proposed at the NCTR, analytical methods for the compound
were sought. Colorimetric methods for benzidine and other aromatic
amines based on diazotization and coupling reactions have been reported [20,21]; however, DiClBzd was not included. Other researchers
[22,23] used Chloramine-T reagent to determine benzidine, DiClBzd,
and congeners. Clayson et al. [24] quantitated benzidine and its
metabolites via reversed phase paper chromatography but DiClBzd was
not studied. Sawicki et al. [28] studied the fluorimetric behavior
of 45 polynuclear aromatic amines and heterocyclic imines; later,
Bowman et al. [15] and Holder et al. [29] reported sensitive SPF
procedures for benzidine, its congeners, and other aromatic amines
in a variety of substrates. 3,3'-Dichlorobenzidine was not included
in any of these studies, probably because of its low fluorescence.
None of these methods are suitable for the trace analysis of DiClBzd
in our substrates. The following procedures were therefore developed
for analyzing trace amounts of DiClBzd or its dihydrochloride salt
(hereafter, DiClBzd·2HCl) in animal feed, wastewater, and human urine.
The formulas of DiClBzd, its dihydrochloride salt, and its PFP derivative are presented in Figure 3.11.

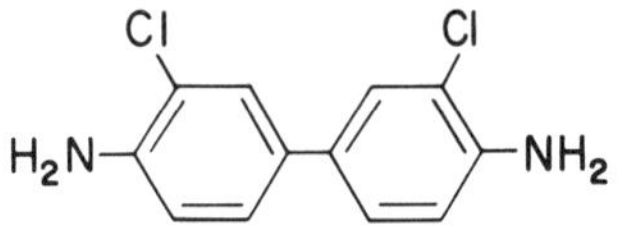

Figure. 3.11. Formulas of 3,3'-dichlorobenzidine
(I), its dihydrochloride salt (II), and its PFP
derivative (III). (From Bowman and Rushing [26].)

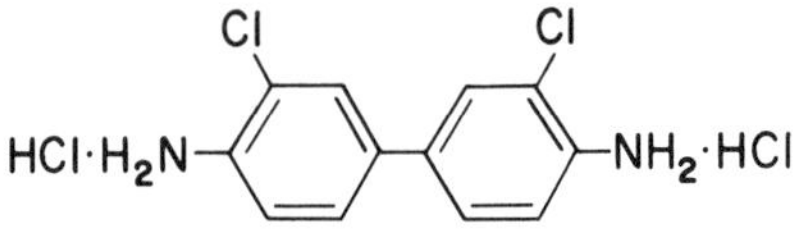

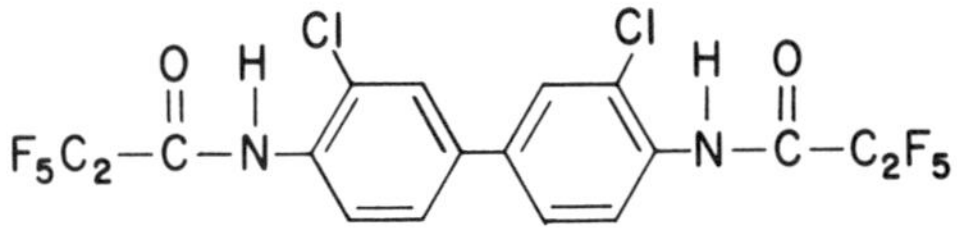

3. *Experimental*

a. *Materials*   The DiClBzd·2HCl (Lot No. 12414, Pfaltz and Bauer Co.,
Flushing, N.Y.) was washed several times with aqueous 1 N HCl, fil-
tered, and dried in a vacuum oven at ambient temperature for 3 days.
The DiClBzd was prepared by dissolving DiClBzd·2HCl in aqueous 1 N
NaOH and extracting the free amine with benzene; the solvent was then
evaporated and the product dried overnight in a vacuum oven at 60°C.
The DiClBzd contained no extraneous GC peaks (via EC, N/P, and FID).
The DiClBzd·2HCl, after conversion to the free amine, was also free
of extraneous GC peaks and yielded the correct amount of product.

Silica gel (No. 3405, J. T. Baker Chemical Co., Phillipsburg,
N.J.) was heated overnight in an oven at 130°C and stored in a desiccator prior to use. The silica gel was then partially deactivated
with 4% water for use in the analytical procedure by adding 24 g of
the dry material to a glass-stoppered bottle containing 1.0 ml of
water dispersed on its inner surface; the contents were mixed well
and allowed to stand for 24 hr with occasional shaking prior to use.

The XAD-2 resin, ca 450 g (No. 3409, Mallinckrodt Chemical Co.,
St. Louis, Mo.) was transferred to a 2000-ml flask and washed by
swirling it with 500 ml of distilled water for about 1 min; the
supernatant was then decanted and discarded. The process was

repeated by using three additional 500-ml portions of water followed by five 200-ml portions of acetone. The resin was transferred to a Buchner funnel to remove most of the acetone, then dried overnight in an oven at 70°C.

Trifluoracetic (TFA) anhydride (No. 67364) and PFP anhydride (No. 65193) were obtained from Pierce Chemical Co., Rockford, Ill.; the heptafluorobutyric (HFB) anyhydride (No. 270085) was obtained from Regis Chemical Co., Morton Grove, Ill. The 1-g ampules were opened immediately prior to use and a 50-µl Hamilton syringe was used to withdraw the derivatizing agent from the vial and deliver it into the reaction vessel.

Trimethylamine (TMA) reagent was prepared by dissolving 2.0 g of the hydrochloride salt in 5 ml of 5 N NaOH and extracting the free amine with four 5-ml portions of benzene which were successively per-colated through a plug of sodium sulfate (ca. 25 mm diameter x 20 mm thick); the volume of the combined extracts was adjusted to 20 ml with benzene. This stock solution (ca. 1 M) was stored at 5°C; por-tions were diluted 20-fold with benzene immediately prior to use.

The buffer solution (pH 6.0) was prepared by dissolving 136 g of KH_2PO_4 in 900 ml of distilled water and adjusting the pH to exactly 6.0 with 10 N NaOH. The volume was then adjusted to exactly 1 liter.

The keeper solution was paraffin oil (No. 01762, Applied Science Lab., State College, Pa.), 20 mg/ml of benzene.

The animal chow (Laboratory Chow, Type 5010C, Ralston Purina Co., St. Louis, Mo.) contained 6% fat, had a pH of 5.5, and 6.7% of it was volatile at 100°C overnight.

All solvents were pesticide grade and all reagents were CP grade.

b. *Preparation of cleanup columns*

(1) Silica gel. Columns (12 mm i.d., No. 420,000, Kontes Glass Co, Vineland, N.J.) equipped with a 50-ml reservoir were prepared by suc-cessively adding a plug of glass wool, 2 g of Na_2SO_4, 2 g of silica gel (4% water), and 2 g of Na_2SO_4. A separate drying tube containing a plug of Na_2SO_4 (ca. 25 mm diameter x 15 mm thick) was placed at the

top of each column. The columns and drying tubes were prepared immediately prior to use and washed with five 5-ml portions of benzene
which were discarded. (Note: The silica gel must be evaluated prior
to use to provide assurance that DiClBzd elutes as indicated in the
procedure. The container is kept tightly sealed to avoid changes in
moisture content.)

(2) XAD-2. Columns (12 mm i.d.), as previously described, were prepared by inserting a ball of glass wool (ca. 3 mm diameter) into the
stem to support the resin and to restrict the solvent flow; 2 g of
the dry XAD-2 resin was then added to the column by using 5 ml of
acetone. After a plug of glass wool was placed on top of the resin
to hold it in place, the column was washed with five additional 5-ml
portions of acetone followed by 5-ml portions of distilled water
prior to use.

c. *Extraction and cleanup of animal chow*   A 2-g portion of animal
chow weighed into a 100-ml glass-stoppered flask was made alkaline
by adding 5 ml of aqueous 0.2 N NaOH; 50 ml of benzene was added and
the sample was mechanically extracted for 2 hr on a reciprocating
shaker (No. 6000, Eberbach Corp., Ann Arbor, Mich.) at a rate of 200
excursions per minute. The supernatant extract was decanted into a
50-ml culture tube and centrifuged at 1200 rpm for 15 min to remove
any suspended particles of chow. (Note: All culture tubes were borosilicate glass equipped with Teflon-lined screw caps.) A 25-ml portion of the extract (1 g equivalent of sample) was transferred to a
50-ml round-bottom flask and evaporated to dryness using a 60°C water
bath and water pump vacuum. The residue was dissolved in 5 ml of
benzene, transferred to an 18-ml culture tube containing 5 ml of 4 N
HCl, vigorously shaken by hand for 5 min, and the benzene layer was
discarded. Two additional 5-ml portions of benzene were used to
sequentially wash the flask and to extract the acid phase in the
tube; the benzene layers were discarded. (Note: At this point the
sample may be stored in a refrigerator overnight.)

Benzene (8 ml) and 3 ml of 10 N NaOH were then added to the tube;
the contents were vigorously shaken by hand for 5 min and then centri-

fuged at 1000 rpm for 2-5 min to separate the layers. The benzene
layer (containing DiClBzd) was withdrawn and transferred to a silica
gel column, and two additional extractions with 8-ml portions of
benzene were performed in the same manner. Finally, the column was
washed with three 5-ml portions of benzene. All effluent from the
column except the first 5 ml was collected in a 50-ml round-bottom
flask containing 0.5 ml of keeper solution, evaporated to dryness
under water pump vacuum at 60°C as described, and the residue was
dissolved in an appropriate volume of benzene (e.g., 1 ml) for direct
analysis via EC-GC or N/P-GC, or for derivatization to PFP-DiClBzd
prior to GC analysis.

d. Extraction and cleanup of wastewater The sample of wastewater
(100 ml) was allowed to percolate through an XAD-2 column prepared
as described and two 10-ml portions of distilled water were used to
successively wash the sample container and the column; the column
was then washed with an additional 80 ml of distilled water and a
rubber bulb was used to force most of the water from the resin. The
DiClBzd and/or DiClBzd·2HCl residues were eluted from the column by
using four 4-ml portions of acetone and the effluent was collected
in an 18-ml culture tube; a rubber bulb was used to force most of the
acetone from the resin.

One milliliter of 12 N HCl was added and the tube was vigorously
shaken by hand for 5 min. The contents of the tube were then concentrated to about 4 ml using a tube heater (Kontes, No. 720,000) set at
60°C and a gentle stream of nitrogen. Benzene (4 ml) and 0.5 ml of
12 N HCl were added, the contents were shaken for 2 min, and the
benzene layer was discarded. The extraction was repeated with two
additional 4-ml portions of benzene which were also discarded. Next,
2 ml of 10 N NaOH and 5 ml of benzene were added, the contents were
shaken for 5 min, and the benzene layer was transferred to a silica
gel column. The contents of the tube were extracted with two additional 5-ml portions of benzene which were successively added to the
column. The column was eluted with five additional 5-ml portions of
benzene and all of the effluent except the first 5 ml was collected

in a 50-ml round-bottom flask containing "keeper" and evaporated to
dryness as described for chow and the residue was dissolved in an
appropriate volume of benzene (e.g., 2 ml) for direct analysis or
for derivatization to PFP-DiClBzd prior to GC analysis.

e. *Extraction and cleanup of human urine*   A sample of 100 ml of
human urine was percolated through XAD-2, the column was washed with
water, the residues were eluted with acetone, and the acetone eluate
was concentrated using a tube heater and a stream of nitrogen exactly
as described for wastewater except that the volume of the acetone
eluate was concentrated to about 2 ml. Benzene (2 ml) was added, the
contents were shaken for 2 min and the benzene layer was discarded;
the extraction was repeated with two additional 2-ml portions of
benzene which were also discarded. Benzene (4 ml) and 1.5 ml of 10 N
NaOH were added to the acid phase, the contents were shaken for 5 min,
centrifuged to separate the layers, and the benzene layer was transferred to a silica gel column. The extraction was repeated twice
with 3-ml portions of benzene which were also added to the column.
Finally, the column was eluted with five 6-ml portions of benzene and
all of the effluent except the first 5 ml was collected, evaporated
to dryness, and the residues were dissolved in benzene for analysis
as described for wastewater.

f. *Gas chromatographic assays*

(1) Electron-capture detection. A Hewlett-Packard (Palo Alto, Calif.)
Model 5750B instrument equipped with a ^{63}Ni EC detector (Tracor Inc.,
Austin, Tex.) and a 100-cm glass column (4 mm i.d.) containing 5%
OV-101 on 80-100 mesh Gas Chrom Q, conditioned at 275°C overnight
prior to use, was operated at 215°C in the DC mode with a nitrogen
carrier flow of 160 ml/min. The detector temperature was 270°C and
the injection port was 235°C. Under these conditions the retention
time (t_R) of DiClBzd was 2.35 min and those of its TFA, PFP, and HFB
derivatives were 2.10, 2.00, and 2.45 min, respectively. The t_R of
a reference standard of p,p'-DDT used to monitor the performance of
the EC-GC system was 1.85 min.

(2) N/P detection. A Perkin-Elmer (Norwalk, Conn.) Model 3920B instrument equipped with a rubidium-sensitized N/P detector and a 90-cm glass column (2 mm i.d.) containing 5% OV-101 on 80-100 mesh Gas Chrom Q, conditioned at 275°C overnight prior to use, was operated at 245°C with a nigrogen carrier gas flow of 15 ml/min. The injection port and interface (transfer line and detector) temperatures were 250 and 260°C, respectively. Gas flows for hydrogen and air were 1.1 and 64 ml/min, respectively. The temperature controller for the rubidium bead was set at 525. Under these conditions the t_R values for DiClBzd, its PFP derivative, and p,p'-DDT were 2.80, 2.30, and 2.20 min, respectively.

All injections were in 5 µl of benzene. Samples of unknown residue content were quantitated by relating peak heights to those of a known amount of the compound. The DiClBzd was expressed in terms of DiClBzd·2HCl and vice versa, through the following relationship: DiClBzd x 1.29 = DiClBzd·2HCl.

g. Derivatization of DiClBzd

(1) Preparation of various derivatives for EC-GC evaluation. The TFA, PFP, and HFB derivatives of DiClBzd were prepared by our modifications of the procedure described by Walle and Ehrsson [30] and Ehrsson et al. [31]. Trimethylamine solution (0.5 ml, 0.05 M) was added to an 8-ml culture tube containing the DiClBzd (1 µg or less) dissolved in exactly 1.5 ml of benzene (total benzene = 2.0 ml) and followed by 50 µl of the appropriate fluorinated anhydride reagent. The tube was sealed, shaken, heated in a 50°C water bath for 15 min, cooled, and the reaction was terminated by the addition of 1 ml of phosphate buffer (pH 6.0). The tube was shaken for 1 min, centfifuged for 1 min at 1000 rpm, and the lower aqueous layer was discarded; the extraction was repeated with an additional 1-ml portion of buffer. The upper benzene layer was transferred to a dry 8-ml culture tube containing 0.5 g of Na_2SO_4, shaken, and injected into the GC either directly or after appropriate dilution with benzene.

(2) Derivatization of cleaned-up extracts for analysis. Appropriate portions of the cleaned-up extracts of chow, wastewater, or human

urine were adjusted to exactly 1.5 ml of benzene in a 8-ml culture tube and subjected to derivatization by using TMA solution and PFP reagent. For example, with extracts of wastewater or human urine, 50 g equivalents were derivatized and with chow containing 1 ppm of residue or less, a 0.5 g equivalent was used. Correspondingly smaller amounts of chow extract were derivatized for samples containing higher levels of DiClBzd or its salt; however, such samples may also be analyzed without being derivatized.

h. *Recovery experiments*

(1) Animal chow. Triplicate 2-g samples of chow were spiked with 0, 0.01, 0.10, 1.0, 10, 100, and 1000 ppm of DiClBzd·2HCl by adding an appropriate amount of the chemical in 1 ml of methanol. The solvent was then removed by using a 60°C water bath and water pump vacuum to simulate the conditions under which bulk amounts of the diet will be prepared for use in animal tests. The samples were then allowed to cool, extracted, cleaned up, and assayed to determine the accuracy and precision of the procedure.

(2) Wastewater and human urine. Triplicate 100-ml samples of wastewater or human urine in 180-ml culture tubes were spiked with 0, 0.10, 1.0, 10, or 20 ppb of DiClBzd or DiClBzd·2HCl by adding an appropriate amount of the chemical in 0.5 ml of methanol. The tubes were sealed, mixed, and allowed to stand overnight at 5°C prior to analysis.

4. *Results and Discussion*

In feeding studies with carcinogens administered to large numbers of mice at our laboratory, animals are dosed either via their drinking water or their diet, and the use of drinking water is generally the method of choice if the chemical is sufficiently soluble and stable. Unfortunately, the solubilities of DiClBzd and DiClBzd·2HCl in water at 25 ± 2°C, which were approximated at 3.0 and 30 ppm, respectively, precluded the use of this medium. However, the solubility of DiClBzd· 2HCL (preferred to DiClBzd because of its lower volatility) in 95% ethanol at 25 ± 2°C, which was approximated at 12.6 mg/ml, was sufficient to permit the use of the solvent in the preparation of dosed diet.

3,3'-Dichlorobenzidine gives good response to EC-GC, and samples
of chow and wastewater containing residues as low as 1.0 ppm and 20
ppb, respectively, may be accurately assayed by the procedures described. The sensitivity of DiClBzd via N/P-GC was about the same as
EC-GC; however, the specificity of N/P-GC permitted injections of
larger amounts of sample extractives, and assays of lower levels of
residues could be achieved. Nevertheless, the limited sensitivities
of DiClBzd with both detectors and the somewhat temperamental characteristics of the N/P system led us to investigate the possibility of
derivatizing DiClBzd to enhance its electron-capturing properties.
Typical EC gas chromatograms of PFP and HFB derivatives of DiClBzd
are presented in Figure 3.12 along with DiClBzd per se and a p,p'-DDT
reference standard. The PFP and HFB derivatives gave about equal
responses and TFA-DiClBzd was about half as sensitive. The PFP
derivative was therefore selected for use in the analytical procedure
since it enhanced detector responses about 300-fold.

The spectrum of the PFP derivative of DiClBzd from a GC-mass
spectrometer indicated the presence of two PFP groups, probably one
on each of the amino groups (see formula III, Figure 3.11); this was
consistent with the molecular weight of 544.

Tests with benzene solutions of DiClBzd and its PFP derivative
stored at 5°C and assayed periodically by EC-GC indicated that both
compounds were stable for at least 22 days. The derivatization procedure as described yields excellent results and essentially no PFP-
DiClBzd is lost by washing the benzene reaction mixture with phosphate
buffer (pH 6). The use of aqueous ammonia as a washing agent was discussed by Walle and Ehrsson [30] and it should be avoided. In tests
where 3.0 and 0.75 N ammonium hydroxide were substituted for the
phosphate buffer, recoveries of the PFP-DiClBzd were only 8 and 38%,
respectively.

Results from triplicate samples of chow spiked with DiClBzd·2HCl
at 0, 0.010, 0.10, 1.00, 10.0, 100, and 1000 ppm as determined by the
three procedures are presented in Table 3.13. At levels of 1.0 ppm
or more, recoveries and precision were good and the three procedures

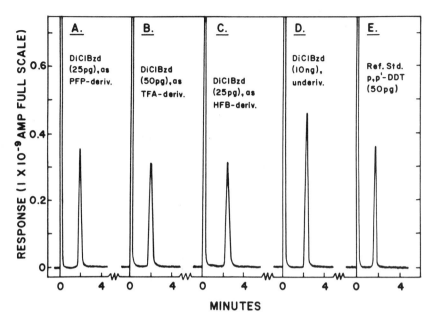

Figure 3.12. Electron-capture gas chromatograms.
A, B, and C are the PFP, TFA, and HFB derivatives
of DiClBzd; D is DiClBzd per se; and E is a p,p'-
DDT reference standard. All injections are in
5 μl of benzene. (From Bowman and Rushing [26].)

yielded comparable results. Therefore, for samples containing residues of this magnitude, analyses of underivatized extracts via EC-GC
or N/P-GC are the procedures of choice. For levels below 1.0 ppm,
analysis of the PFP derivatized sample via EC-GC is recommended.
Minimum levels of DiClBzd·2HCl detectable in chow (based on twice
background) via EC-GC of DiClBzd and PFP-DiClBzd were 120 and 3 ppb,
respectively; values from N/P-GC of either the free amine or the PFP-
derivative were about 40 ppb.

Data from samples of wastewater spiked with either the free
amine or the salt at levels of 0, 0.1, 1.0, and 10.0 ppb and human
urine spiked at 0, 1.0, and 20.0 ppb are presented in Table 3.14.
Recoveries from wastewater spiked with 1.0 ppb or more were 75% or
better and those spiked at 0.10 ppb gave recoveries of 55 ± 5%.
Wastewater containing as much as 10 ppb of residue may be analyzed

Table 3.13. Gas chromatographic analysis of 3,3'-dichlorobenzidine dihydrochloride in animal chow spiked at various levels as determined by three procedures

Added[a]		Procedure[b]	Equivalents of chow used per analysis	Recovered ($\bar{x}$ ± SE)[c]		
μg	ppm			μg	ppm	%
2000	1000	EC-underiv.	10 μg	1830 ± 12	914 ± 6	91.4 ± 0.6
		EC-PFP-deriv.	33.3 ng	1780 ± 26	891 ± 13	89.1 ± 1.3
		N/P-underiv.	1.0 mg	1880 ± 20	940 ± 10	94 ± 1
200	100	EC-underiv.	100 μg	185 ± 0.6	92.7 ± 0.3	92.7 ± 0.3
		EC-PFP-deriv.	500 ng	181 ± 1.4	90.4 ± 0.7	90.4 ± 0.7
		N/P-underiv.	1.0 mg	184 ± 4	92 ± 2	92 ± 2
20.0	10.0	EC-underiv.	1.0 mg	18.1 ± 0.38	9.07 ± 0.19	90.7 ± 1.9
		EC-PFP-deriv.	5.0 μg	17.9 ± 0.34	8.95 ± 0.17	89.5 ± 1.7
		N/P-underiv.	1.0 mg	18.2 ± 0.2	9.1 ± 0.1	91 ± 1
2.0	1.00	EC-underiv.	5.0 mg	1.38 ± 0.06	0.69 ± 0.03	69 ± 3
		EC-PFP-deriv.	25.0 μg	1.57 ± 0.014	0.785 ± 0.007	78.5 ± 0.7
		N/P-underiv.	5.0 mg	1.56 ± 0.06	0.78 ± 0.03	78 ± 3
0.200	0.100	EC-PFP-deriv.	250 μg	0.158 ± 0.003	0.0792 ± 0.0015	79.2 ± 1.5
0.020	0.010	EC-PFP-deriv.	1.25 mg	0.0126 ± 0.0004	0.0063 ± 0.0002	63 ± 2
0.000	0.000	EC-underiv.	5.0 mg	0.124 ± 0.038	0.06 ± 0.02	--
		EC-PFP-deriv.	1.25 mg	0.0026 ± 0.0018	0.0013 ± 0.0010	--
		N/P-underiv.	5.0 mg	0.04 ± 0.02	0.02 ± 0.01	--

Source: Bowman and Rushing [26].

[a]Per 2 g of chow.

[b]Abbreviations: EC-underiv., EC-GC of the free amine; EC-PFP-deriv., EC-GC of the pentafluoropropionyl derivative; N/P-underiv., GC of the underivatized sample using a rubidium-sensitized thermionic-type (N/P) detector.

[c]Mean and standard error from triplicate assays; spiked samples are corrected for background of control chow.

Table 3.14. Gas chromatographic analysis of 3,3'-dichlorobenzidine or its dihydrochloride salt in wastewater and human urine

Added[a]		Procedure[b]	Equivalents of sample used per analysis	Recovered ($\bar{x}$ ± SE)[c]		
μg	ppb			μg	ppb	%
Wastewater						
1.0	10.0	EC-underiv.	250 mg	0.78 ± 0.02	7.8 ± 0.2	78 ± 2
		N/P-underiv.	250 mg	0.82 ± 0.02	8.2 ± 0.2	82 ± 2
0.10	1.0	EC-PFP-deriv.	25 mg	0.0749 ± 0.0054	0.749 ± 0.054	74.9 ± 5.4
0.10[d]	1.0	EC-PFP-deriv.	25 mg	0.0785 ± 0.0016	0.785 ± 0.016	78.5 ± 1.6
0.01	0.1	EC-PFP-deriv.	125 mg	0.0055 ± 0.0005	0.055 ± 0.005	55 ± 5
0	0	EC-underiv.	250 mg	0.04 ± 0.00	0.4 ± 0.0	--
		N/P-underiv.	250 mg	0.03 ± 0.01	0.3 ± 0.1	--
		EC-PFP-deriv.	125 mg	0.0009 ± 0.0001	0.009 ± 0.001	--
Human Urine						
2.0[d]	20.0	EC-PFP-deriv.	2.5 mg	0.776 ± 0.139	7.76 ± 1.39	38.8 ± 7
		N/P-underiv.	250 mg	0.74 ± 0.16	7.4 ± 1.6	37 ± 8
0.10	1.0	EC-PFP-deriv.	25 mg	0.047 ± 0.008	0.47 ± 0.08	47 ± 8
0	0	EC-PFP-deriv.	25 mg	0.003 ± 0.000	0.03 ± 0.00	--
		N/P-underiv.	250 mg	0.09 ± 0.03	0.9 ± 0.3	--

Source: Bowman and Rushing [26].

[a] Per 100 g of sample

[b] Abbreviations as for Table 3.13.

[c] Mean and standard error from triplicate assays; spiked samples are corrected for background of control samples.

[d] Spiked as DiClBzd·2HCl

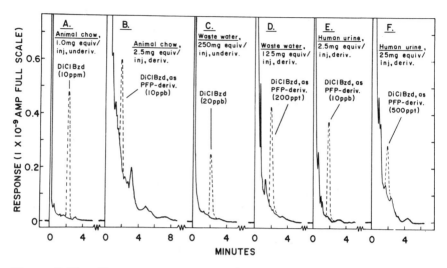

Figure 3.13. Electron-capture gas chromatograms. Solid lines are untreated sample extracts; broken lines (superimposed) illustrate responses of residues spiked into the extracts. In A and C neither the extract nor the DiClBzd were derivatized, all others were derivatized. All injections are in 5 μl of benzene. (From Bowman and Rushing [26].)

by EC-GC or N/P-GC without derivatization. At levels below 10 ppb, EC-GC assays of the PFP derivative are recommended. Minimum levels of the free amine detectable in wastewater (based on twice background) by EC-GC of DiClBzd or PFP-DiClBzd were 0.80 and 0.018 ppb, respectively; the level from N/P-GC was 0.60 ppb.

Recoveries from human urine spiked with 0, 1.0, and 20 ppb of the free amine or salt averaged 41 ± 8%. These losses occurred mostly during evaporation of the acidified acetone eluate from the XAD-2 column to a volume of 2 ml. The step is necessary to allow sufficient vaporization of volatile interferences from the sample to permit analysis at the 1.0-ppb level; unfortunately, some of the residue is also lost in the process. Nevertheless, recoveries and sensitivity are sufficient to signal any accidental exposure of an employee to the chemical. Minimum amounts of DiClBzd detectable in human urine (based on twice background) were about 0.060 ppb via EC-GC of the PFP derivative and 1.8 ppb by N/P-GC.

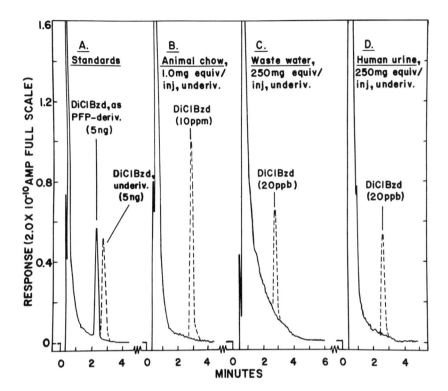

Figure 3.14. Gas chromatograms via nitrogen-phosphorus thermionic detection. A shows standards of DiClBzd and its PFP derivative; in B, C, and D, solid lines are underivatized extracts of untreated samples; broken lines (superimposed) illustrate responses of underivatized DiClBzd spiked into the extracts. All injections are in 5 μl of benzene. (From Bowman and Rushing [26].)

Typical EC gas chromatograms of various untreated control extracts (derivatized or underivatized) before and after being spiked with DiClBzd or its PFP derivative are presented in Figure 3.13. Chromatograms of extracts (underivatized) spiked in a similar manner as determined by N/P-GC are presented in Figure 3.14 with standards of DiClBzd and PFP-DiClBzd. Sensitivities of equal amounts of Cl-and/or N-containing compounds were compared by using the N/P detector and adjusting all responses (peak heights) in terms of the t_R of DiClBzd; the results are given in Table 3.15.

Table 3.15. Relative GC responses of equal amounts of chlorine-
and/or nitrogen-containing compounds

Compound	Response (peak height relative to DiClBzd = 1.0)
3,3'-Dichlorobenzidine	1.0
3,3'-Dichlorobenzidine, PFP derivative	0.83
4,4'-Dichlorobiphenyl	0.028
Benzidine	0.59
p,p'-DDT	0.080

Table 3.16. Partition values for 3,3'-dichlorobenzidine

Solvent system	Partition value
Hexane-acetonitrile	0.015
Hexane-80% acetone (20% water)	0.478
Chloroform-60% methanol (40% water)	0.974
Benzene-aqueous HCl (1 N)	0.093
Benzene-aqueous HCl (2 N)	0.0092
Benzene-aqueous HCl (4 N)	<0.0003
Benzene-aqueous NaOH (0.1 N)	0.98
Benzene-aqueous NaOH (1 N)	1.00
Chloroform-water	1.00
Chloroform-aqueous NaOH (0.1, 1, and 10 N)	1.00

It is interesting to note that the response of DiClBzd is greater than would be expected from the chlorine response of 4,4'-dichlorobiphenyl plus the nitrogen response from benzidine; also the response from PFP-DiClBzd was not as great as that from DiClBzd. Appreciable responses were also obtained from the compounds that contained chlorine and no nitrogen.

Partition values for DiClBzd, which were determined during the course of developing the procedure, are useful in selecting extraction and cleanup methods and for confirmation of identity. Since the values may also be useful to other investigators they are given in Table 3.16.

D. 4-Aminobiphenyl, 2-Naphthylamine, and Analogs [29]

1. *General Description of Method*
Spectrophotofluorimetric methods for monitoring trace levels of 4-aminobiphenyl, 2-naphthylamine, and their hydrochloride salts in wastewater, microbiological growth media, potable water, human urine, and mouse blood are described. The salient elements of the methods are extraction of the residues as the free amine with benzene, rapid cleanup on an alumina column, and quantification of the free amine in methanol via SPF. Potable water solutions of the salts are diluted with 0.01 N aqueous HCl and quantified directly by SPF. Ancillary analytical information concerning GC of the free amines, partitioning properties of the compounds between solvent pairs, their solubility and stability in water, and TLC data is presented. The compositions of various admixtures of 1- and 2-naphthylamine or their salts were determined by using SPF with calculations based on simultaneous equations.

2. *Introduction*
Long term feeding studies of two known carcinogens, 4-aminobiphenyl and 2-naphthylamine, against large numbers of mice were proposed at the NCTR and analytical methodology capable of satisfying the requirements of the experiment were sought. The formulas of these two carcinogens and four analogs are shown in Figure 3.15.

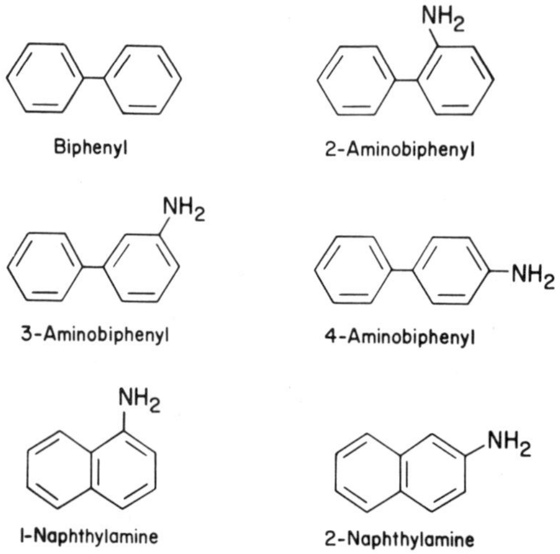

Biphenyl   2-Aminobiphenyl

3-Aminobiphenyl   4-Aminobiphenyl

l-Naphthylamine   2-Naphthylamine

Figure 3.15. Formulas of the carcinogens
4-aminobiphenyl and 2-naphthylamine, and
four analogs. (From Holder et al. [29].)

Several analytical methods for aromatic amines have been
reported in the literature. Lugg [32] described optimum reaction
conditions for the colorimetric determination of 24 phenols and
aromatic amines by using commercially available stabilized diazonium
salts. Bridges et al. [33] investigated the variation with pH of the
excitation and fluorescence wavelengths and fluorescence intensity of
several hydroxy- and aminobiphenyls with a view to using the data for
determining hydroxybiphenyls in biological material; however, no
actual substrates were assayed. Sawicki et al. [28] investigated
column, TLC, and fluorometric behavior of 45 polynuclear aromatic
amines and heterocyclic imines; Shimomura and Walton [34] studied the
effects of zinc, cadmium, and nickel nitrates on the TLC separation
of aromatic amines with silica gel and aluminum oxide. Masuda and
Hoffmann [35] described a method for determining 1- and 2-naphthyl-
amine in cigarette smoke. The compounds were derivatized by using
PFP anhydride and the neutral fraction was cleaned up on Florisil;
the N-pentafluoropropionamide was then assayed by EC-GC. Knight [36]
assayed aminoaromatic compounds by GC with FID. Gupta and Srivastava

[37] reacted acetic acid solutions of 48 substituted anilines and
other aromatic amines with an aqueous peroxydisulfate solution to
form colored products with differing absorption maxima in the visible
range, and El-Dib [21] reported a colorimetric procedure based on
diazotization of primary aromatic amines and coupling with resorcinol
or 1-naphthol. More recently, Jakovljevic et al. [38] described a
method for assaying traces of 4-aminobiphenyl in 2-aminobiphenyl
based on the separation of the free amines using TLC, extractions of
the isolated materials from the plates, and fluorometric determination. However, none of these methods possess all of the qualities
(specificity, sensitivity, accuracy, precision, versatility, and
speed) required for our substrates. The following procedures were
therefore developed for use with the toxicological experiments.

3. Experimental

a. *Materials*   4-Aminobiphenyl (mp 52-54°C; Aldrich Chemical Co.,
Milwaukee, Wis.), 1-naphthylamine (mp 49.1-50.3°C; Fisher Scientific
Co., Pittsburgh, Pa.), and 2-naphthylamine (mp 111-113°C; Sigma
Chemical Co., St. Louis, Mo.) were used as received since they contained no extraneous GC peaks. The salts of the amines were prepared
by bubbling an excess of anhydrous HCl through benzene solutions of
each amine to precipitate its corresponding salt; these were then
vacuum dried overnight at ambient temperature prior to use. Portions
of the salts, after conversion back to the free amine, yielded the
correct amount of product and were also void of extraneous GC peaks.
The adsorbent (basic alumina, Brockman Activity I; Fisher, No. A-941)
was used as received. Sodium sulfate was anhydrous; all reagents
were CP grade and all solvents were pesticide grade. Ingredients
for the microbiological culture media were purchased from Difco
Laboratories, Detroit, Mich. and the media were prepared in accordance with the instructions supplied by the manufacturer. All culture
tubes were of borosilicate glass and equipped with Teflon-lined screw
caps. The TLC plates (20 x 20 cm, Fisher, No. 6-601A), precoated
with silica gel GF (250 μm thick), were activated in an oven at 140°C
for 1 hr and allowed to cool in a desiccator prior to use.

Table 3.17. Spectrophotofluorimetric data for biphenyl and related
compounds

Compound	λ_{Ex} (nm)	λ_{Em} (nm)	RI (0.5 µg/ml)
Biphenyl	260	312	3.90
2-Aminobiphenyl	312	392	6.25
3-Aminobiphenyl	255	398	5.50
3-Aminobiphenyl·HCl	260	410	7.0
4-Aminobiphenyl	290	368	55.0
4-Aminobiphenyl·HCl	260	382	7.80
1-Naphthylamine	332	425	14.6
1-Naphthylamine·HCl	285	444	2.1
2-Naphthylamine	242	400	18.5
2-Naphthylamine·HCl	286	406	10.4

b. Spectrophotofluorimetric analysis   An Aminco-Bowman instrument
equipped with a xenon lamp and a 1P28 detector was used with 1-cm^2
cells and a 2-2-2-mm slit program to measure fluorescence. All dilutions of free amine were freshly prepared in methanol and those of
the salts were in 0.01 N HCl solution. Excitation and emission wavelengths for maximum fluorescence and the corresponding RI values are
presented in Table 3.17.

The instrument was frequently calibrated to produce an RI of
5.0 with a solution of 0.3 µg quinine sulfate per milliliter of 0.1 N
sulfuric acid (λ_{Ex} = 350 nm, λ_{Em} = 450 nm). Readings were corrected
for solvent blanks and RI was plotted versus concentration of the six
compounds on log-log paper to produce a standard curve. To ensure
that the RI was within the linear range of the standard curve and
thus unaffected by concentration quenching, samples were diluted
with an equal volume of solvent to ascertain whether the RI was about
half that of the undiluted solution. If it was not, dilution was
continued until the RI was halved. Preparation of samples for SPF
analysis is fully described later in this section. Extracts of
wastewater, urine, medium, and blood for SPF analyses were first

diluted to contain the equivalents of 10, 1, and 0.2 g of sample per
milliliter, respectively; further dilutions were made as required to
be certain that the RI was within the linear range of the standard
curve. The RI of the untreated control sample was then subtracted
from that of the unknown and the concentration (in micrograms per
milliliter) was determined from the standard curve. In the instances
where the salts were assayed as the free amines, the analytical results were multiplied by the factors 1.22 for 4-aminobiphenyl and
1.25 for 2-naphthylamine to express them in terms of the salts.

Determinations of 1- and 2-naphthylamine or their salts in
admixtures were performed by measuring the RI at the λ_{Ex} and λ_{Em}
maxima for each compound and calculating the amount of each constituent by using the simultaneous equations

$$I_a = F_{1a}C_a + F_{1b}C_b \tag{1}$$
$$I_b = F_{2a}C_a + F_{2b}C_b \tag{2}$$

where I_a and I_b are the observed RI values at the λ_{Em} maxima of compounds a and b, respectively; C_a and C_b are the respective concentrations; and the F factors (1a, 2a, 1b, 2b) are proportionality constants
for each constituent at each wavelength combination. The proportionality constants for each compound (0.1 μg/ml) were determined by
measuring the RI at the wavelength maxima for both compounds.

c. *Gas chromatographic analysis*   A Hewlett-Packard (Palo Alto,
Calif.) Model 5750 instrument equipped with a FID and a 100-cm glass
column (4 mm i.d., 6 mm o.d.) containing 10% OV-101 (w/w) on Gas
Chrom Q (80-100 mesh) was operated either isothermally or temperature-
programmed from 100 to 250°C at the rate of 10°C/min. The helium
carrier flow was 100 ml/min and the injection port and detector temperatures were set at 275 and 295°C, respectively. Temperature-
programmed analyses, which were used to determine whether our standards contained extraneous GC peaks, yielded t_R values in minutes
as follows: biphenyl, 5.30; 2-aminobiphenyl, 7.20; 3-aminobiphenyl,
8.50; 4-aminobiphenyl, 8.75; 1-naphthylamine, 6.50; and 2-naphthyl-
amine, 6.65. Typical chromatograms are presented in Figure 3.16.

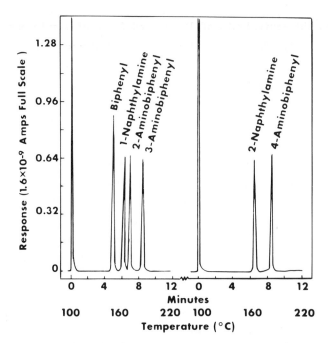

Figure 3.16. Typical temperature-programmed gas chromatograms (FID) of 500-ng amounts each of the six aromatic compounds shown in Figure 3.15 injected in 5 μl of chloroform. (From Holder et al. [29].)

For quantitative analysis of the individual free amines (e.g., for p-value determinations, the fraction of solute partitioning into the nonpolar phase of an equivolume immiscible binary solvent system), the column oven was operated isothermally at a temperature that resulted in a t_R of about 2 min. These temperatures (°C) were as follows: biphenyl, 140; 2-aminobiphenyl, 165; 3-aminobiphenyl, 180; 4-aminobiphenyl, 185; and 1- and 2-naphthylamine, 160.

d. *Solubility, p-value, and TLC determinations*   The solubilities of 4-aminobiphenyl, 2-naphthylamine, and their hydrochloride salts in water at 25 ± 2°C were determined by SPF in a manner similar to that described by Bowman and King [1] for 2-acetylaminofluorene.

Extraction p-values for the aromatic amines were determined in several solvent systems by GC in the manner described by Bowman and

Beroza [13]. The TLC determinations were made by using a Gelman
Model 51325-1 apparatus (Ann Arbor, Mich.) and glass plates precoated
with silica gel GF. The plates were spotted with 5 µl of methanol
solutions 1 µg/µl) of the test compounds (biphenyl was used as a
reference compound). After the developing solvent had ascended 13 cm
above the spotting line (ca. 25 min), the plates were removed and the
solvent allowed to evaporate. The spots were made visible by viewing
them under ultraviolet light (254 nm) and the R_f values were calculated.

e. *Preparation of samples for SPF analysis*

(1) Microbiological growth media. Ten milliliters of the trypticase
soy dextrose (TSD) or brain heart infusion (BHI) medium was added to
a 30-ml culture tube containing 1 g of NaCl and 10 ml of benzene.
After the addition of 0.2 ml of 10 N NaOH, the tube was sealed,
shaken vigorously for 2 min, and centrifuged for 10 min at about
625 x G. The benzene layer was carefully withdrawn by using a syringe
and cannula and percolated through a plug of sodium sulfate (25 mm
diameter x 10 mm thick) in tandem with a glass column (12 mm i.d.,
Kontes, No. 420,000) prepared by adding successively a plug of glass
wool, 5 g of sodium sulfate, 1 g of basic alumina, and 5 g of sodium
sulfate. The medium was extracted with two additional 10-ml portions
of benzene that were also percolated through the plug and column.
Finally, the column was washed with 10 ml dichloromethane-10% methanol
to ensure complete elution of the free amine residue from the column.
After the addition of one drop of diethylene glycol to serve as a
keeper, the combined eluates were evaporated just to dryness by using
water pump vacuum and a 60°C water bath. The dry residue was dissolved in an appropriate amount of methanol for SPF analysis as the
free amine.

(2) Wastewater. One hundred milliliters of sample was added to a
160-ml culture tube containing 2 g of NaCl then made alkaline with
0.5 ml of 10 N NaOH. The sample was then shaken for 2 min, centrifuged at about 50 x G for 10 min, cleaned up, and prepared for

analysis as described for media except that three 15-ml portions of benzene were used for extraction.

(3) Blood. Procedures employing no hydrolysis, as well as those involving alkaline or acid hydrolysis, of the sample prior to extraction were conducted as follows: (a) No hydrolysis--1 ml heparinized whole mouse blood was added to a 20-ml culture tube containing 6 ml distilled water and 1 ml of 10 N NaOH. The contents were mixed, extracted three times with 10-ml portions of benzene, and prepared for SPF analysis as described for media; (b) Alkaline hydrolysis-- samples were analyzed as described under no hydrolysis except that the mixture in the sealed tube was held in an 80°C heating block for 2 hr with gentle shaking at about 10-min intervals then cooled to ambient temperature prior to extraction with benzene; (c) Acid hydrolysis--analyses were performed as mentioned under no hydrolysis except that 1 ml of 12 N HCl was substituted for the NaOH and the sealed tube was then heated at 80°C for 2 hr, cooled, and then made alkaline by adding 2 ml of 10 N NaOH. The mixture was then extracted and prepared for SPF analysis as described for media.

(4) Potable water. Aqueous solutions of the hydrochloride salts, slated for use as the animals' drinking water, were assayed for proper concentration after sequential dilutions with 0.01 N HCl solution. The fluorescence of diluted sample (e.g., 0.1 ppm) was compared directly with that of a standard solution prepared in the same manner.

(5) Human urine. Procedures utilizing alkaline, acid, or no hydrolysis prior to extraction were employed for urine as follows: (a) No hydrolysis--analyses were performed exactly as described for wastewater; (b) Alkaline hydrolysis--analyses were performed exactly as described for wastewater except that the alkaline solution in the sealed tube was heated in a water bath at 80°C for 2 hr with gentle shaking at about 10-min intervals, then cooled to ambient temperature prior to extraction with benzene; (c) Acid hydrolysis--these analyses were also performed as described for wastewater except that 0.5 ml of

12 N HCl was substituted for the 10 N NaOH. This mixture was then
heated at 80°C for 2 hr, cooled, and made alkaline with 1 ml of
10 N NaOH prior to extraction with benzene.

f. Recovery experiments   Triplicate samples of both biological
media were separately spiked with 100 μl of methanol (or water) containing the appropriate amount of the free amine (or its salt) to
produce concentrations at 0, 0.1, and 1.0 ppm. The samples were
allowed to stand in the refrigerator (5°C) overnight prior to extraction. Samples (1 ml) of heparinized mouse blood were spiked
in the same manner at 0 and 2.0 ppm, held at 5°C overnight, and
analyzed as described. Wastewater and urine samples (100 ml) were
spiked at 0 and 20 ppb by adding 1 ml of methanol (or water) containing the appropriate amount of compound, held at 5°C overnight,
and analyzed as described.

g. Stability experiments   Aqueous 4-aminobiphenyl (ca. 1.0 and
100 ppm) dissolved in either deionized water or 0.01 N HCl (pH 2)
was tested to determine the chemical stability of the compound and
its acceptability to the animals under simulated test conditions.
The drinking water dispenser for each cage (four mice per cage) consisted of a rubber stopper and a stainless steel sipper tube (8 mm
o.d. x 90 mm long) containing a steel ball to serve as a valve.
Triplicate dispensers, each containing 325 ml of the various levels
of test solution, were placed in cages and exposed to ambient conditions (25 ± 2°C) and continuous fluorescent lighting in the animal
room. Samples (10 ml) were taken from each dispenser immediately
and 1, 2, 4, 8, and 16 days later. The pH of each sample was determined and solutions of the salt were diluted and analyzed as described
for potable water.

   4. Results and Discussion
The use of SPF as a means of assaying these compounds is indicated
by their strong fluorescence intensities, which result in high sensitivity, and by the inherent specificity of the method. The RI values
of the free amines in methanol are as much as seven times greater

than those of the corresponding hydrochloride salts in 0.01 N HCl
solutions. In these solvents the limit of detection, expressed as
twice background, were about 1-2 and 2-5 ng/ml for the free amines
and salts, respectively. As expected, the SPF response of the salts
was highly dependent on pH, and assays of these compounds diluted
with water alone were not reproducible. Excitation and emission
spectra and standard curves for 4-aminobiphenyl, 1-naphthylamine,
2-naphthylamine, and their hydrochloride salts are presented in
Figures 3.17-3.19.

The choice of 0.01 N HCl as the solvent for administering
4-aminobiphenyl·HCl to the animals via their drinking water was based
on results from stability studies presented in Table 3.18. Aqueous
solutions containing 1.0 and 100 ppm of the salt diminished in concentration by about 72 and 43%, respectively, during the 16-day
simulated test, whereas similar solutions in 0.01 N HCl diminished
only 5% at the 1.0 ppm level and were essentially unchanged at 100
ppm. The high accuracy and precision of the results obtained with
0.01 N HCl solutions of 4-aminobiphenyl·HCl illustrate the utility
of the method for obtaining rapid and reliable assays of the potable
water formulations for use in animal experiments. Tests with other
aqueous solutions [0.3% NaCl-HCl (0.5 N NaCl, 0.01 N HCl, pH 2) and
0.9% NaCl-HCl (0.15 N NaCl, 0.01 N HCl, pH 2)] of 4-aminobiphenyl
salt yielded about the same stabilizing effects as 0.01 N HCl; however, they were not as palatable to the animals.

Results from assays of the two microbiological growth media are
presented in Table 3.19. Recoveries from samples spiked with 0.10
and 1.0 ppm of 4-aminobiphenyl and its salt were 81-95%. However,
low recoveries (44-85%) were obtained for 2-naphthylamine and its
salt. The background fluorescence of unspiked media was 20-30 ppb.
Data from wastewater collected from the decontamination of control
animal cages (total solids content and pH were 217 ppm and 7.33,
respectively), unspiked and spiked with 20 ppb of the two amines and
their salts, are presented in Table 3.20. Recoveries averaged 89%,
precision was excellent, and the background of unspiked samples was
0.2-0.3 ppb.

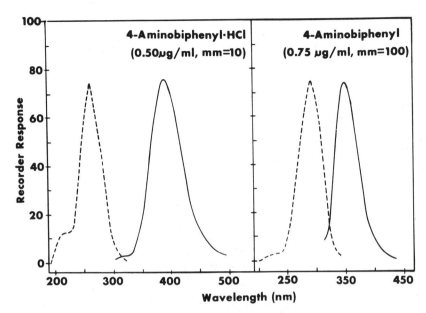

Figure 3.17a. Excitation (broken line) and
emission (solid line) spectra of 4-aminobiphenyl
and its hydrochloride salt. (From Holder et al.
[29].)

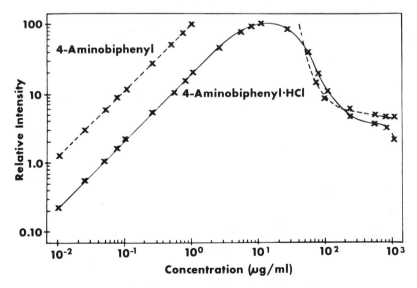

Figure 3.17b. Standard curves of 4-aminobiphenyl
and its hydrochloride salt in methanol and 0.01 N
aqueous HCl, respectively. (From Holder et al.
[29].)

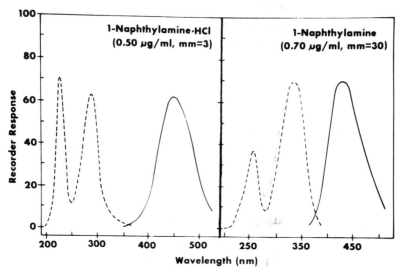

Figure 3.18a. Excitation (broken line) and
emission (solid line) spectra of 1-naphthylamine
and its hydrochloride salt. (From Holder et al.
[29].)

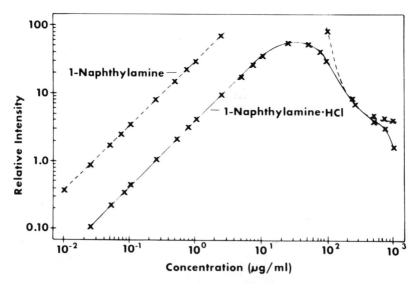

Figure 3.18b. Standard curves of 1-naphthylamine
and its hydrochloride salt in methanol and 0.01 N
aqueous HCl, respectively. (From Holder et al.
[29].)

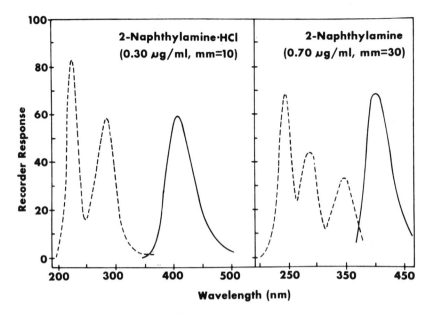

Figure 3.19a. Excitation (broken line) and
emission (solid line) spectra of 2-naphthylamine
and its hydrochloride salt. (From Holder et al.
[29].)

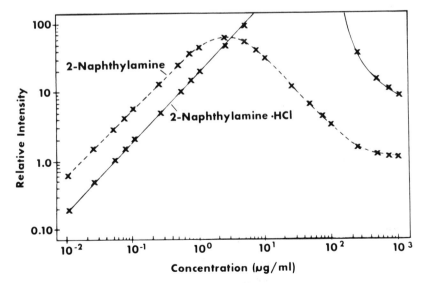

Figure 3.19b. Standard curves of 2-naphthylamine
and its hydrochloride salt in methanol and 0.01 N
aqueous HCl, respectively. (From Holder et al.
[29].)

Table 3.18. Stability of aqueous solutions of 4-aminobiphenyl hydrochloride after exposure to simulated test conditions for 16 days

Sampling interval (days)	1.0 ppm solution[b]		100 ppm solution[b]		1.0 ppm solution[c]		100 ppm solution[c]	
	ppm	pH	ppm	pH	ppm	pH	ppm	pH
0	0.989 ± 0.003	2.03 ± 0.01	98.9 ± 0.35	2.02 ± 0.01	1.01 ± 0.001	7.47 ± 0.01	93.8 ± 0.001	4.17 ± 0.01
1	0.973 ± 0.012	2.07 ± 0.01	99.2 ± 0.42	2.03 ± 0.01	0.781 ± 0.001	7.03 ± 0.02	79.7 ± 0.06	4.08 ± 0.06
2	0.968 ± 0.005	2.04 ± 0.02	97.9 ± 0.90	2.06 ± 0.01	0.649 ± 0.019	6.70 ± 0.02	73.5 ± 0.17	3.95 ± 0.06
4	0.976 ± 0.021	2.05 ± 0.02	98.6 ± 1.00	2.02 ± 0.03	0.459 ± 0.020	6.63 ± 0.04	60.4 ± 2.30	4.01 ± 0.01
8	0.950 ± 0.001	2.04 ± 0.03	98.3 ± 0.31	2.00 ± 0.01	0.365 ± 0.023	6.81 ± 0.02	62.4 ± 0.66	3.94 ± 0.08
16	0.936 ± 0.002	2.06 ± 0.01	98.9 ± 0.50	2.05 ± 0.02	0.282 ± 0.011	6.45 ± 0.04	57.4 ± 1.10	3.91 ± 0.06

Concentration and pH of solutions indicated ($\bar{x} \pm SE$)[a]

Source: Holder et al. [29].

[a]Mean and standard error from triplicate assays.

[b]Aqueous HCl solution (0.01 N, pH 2); samples adjusted for control.

[c]Deionized water solution; samples adjusted for control.

Table 3.19. Analysis of two biological growth media spiked with 4-aminobiphenyl, 2-naphthylamine, and their hydrochloride salts at 0, 0.10, and 1.0 ppm

Compound	Medium[a]	Added[b] ppm	Added[b] μg	Recovered ($\bar{x}$ ± SE)[c] ppm	Recovered ($\bar{x}$ ± SE)[c] %
4-Aminobiphenyl	BHI	0	0	0.031 ± 0.001	--
		0.10	1.0	0.086 ± 0.001	86 ± 1.0
		1.00	10.0	0.948 ± 0.033	94.8 ± 3.3
	TSD	0	0	0.024 ± 0.001	--
		0.10	1.0	0.081 ± 0.002	81 ± 2.0
		1.00	10.0	0.810 ± 0.006	81 ± 0.6
4-Aminobiphenyl·HCl	BHI	0	0	0.031 ± 0.001	--
		0.10	1.0	0.087 ± 0.001	87 ± 1.0
		1.00	10.0	0.855 ± 0.014	85.5 ± 1,4
	TSD	0	0	0.024 ± 0.001	--
		0.10	1.0	0.090 ± 0.003	90 ± 3.0
		1.00	10.0	0.908 ± 0.010	90.8 ± 1.0
2-Naphthylamine	BHI	0	0	0.015 ± 0.001	--
		0.10	1.0	0.070 ± 0.005	70 ± 5.0
		1.00	10.0	0.853 ± 0.030	85.3 ± 3.0
	TSD	0	0	0.018 ± 0.00	--
		0.10	1.0	0.051 ± 0.006	51 ± 6.0
		1.00	10.0	0.712 ± 0.035	71.2 ± 3.5
2-Naphthylamine·HCl	BHI	0	0	0.015 ± 0.001	--
		0.10	1.0	0.053 ± 0.001	53 ± 1.0
		1.00	10.0	0.701 ± 0.002	70.1 ± 0.2
	TSD	0	0	0.018 ± 0.00	--
		0.10	1.0	0.044 ± 0.007	44 ± 7.0
		1.00	10.0	0.646 ± 0.003	64.6 ± 0.3

Source: Holder et al. [29].

[a]BHI, brain heart infusion; TSD, trypticase soy desxtrose.

[b]Per 10 ml of sample.

[c]Mean and standard error from triplicate assays; spiked samples are corrected for controls. Methanol solutions from controls and 0.10-ppm samples for SPF readings contained an equivalent of 1.0 g of medium per milliliter; the 1.0-ppm samples contained 0.2 g/ml.

Table 3.20. Analysis of wastewater spiked with 4-aminobiphenyl,
2-naphthylamine, and their hydrochloride salts at 0 and 20 ppb

Compound	Added[a] ppb	Added[a] µg	Recovered ($\bar{x}$ ± SE)[b] ppb	Recovered ($\bar{x}$ ± SE)[b] %
4-Aminobiphenyl	0	0	0.3 ± 0.00	--
	20	2.0	19 ± 0.00	95
4-Aminobiphenyl·HCl	0	0	0.3 ± 0.00	--
	20	2.0	18 ± 0.00	90
2-Naphthylamine	0	0	0.2 ± 0.00	--
	20	2.0	18 ± 0.00	90
2-Naphthylamine·HCl	0	0	0.2 ± 0.00	--
	20	2.0	16 ± 0.00	80

Source: Holder et al. [29].

[a] Per 100 ml of sample.

[b] Mean and standard error from triplicate assays; spiked samples are
corrected for controls. Methanol solutions for SPF readings contained an equivalent of 10 g of water sample per milliliter.

Whole mouse blood unspiked or spiked with 2.0 ppm of the two
amines and their salts were assayed without hydrolysis or after
alkaline or acid hydrolysis; results of these tests are presented
in Table 3.21. Acid hydrolysis yielded the best recoveries (namely,
62-76%) and is therefore considered the method of choice; under those
conditions the background fluorescence of unspiked samples was about
0.03 ppm.

Data from human urine unspiked and spiked with 20 ppb of the
amines and salts are presented in Table 3.22. Better recoveries of
the free amines were obtained without hydrolysis than by utilizing
an alkaline hydrolysis step. On the other hand, alkaline hydrolysis
enhanced recoveries of the salts; the reason for this behavior is
not known. Acid hydrolysis of the urine was also performed; however,
formation of a purple-colored product in both control and spiked
samples prevented the assay by SPF.

Table 3.21. Analysis of whole mouse blood (heparinized) spiked with
4-aminobiphenyl, 2-naphthylamine, and their hydrochloride salts at
0 and 2.0 ppm

Compound	Hydrolysis	Added[a] ppm	μg	Recovered ($\bar{x}$ ± SE)[b] ppm	%
4-Aminobiphenyl	None	0	0	0.022 ± 0.007	--
		2.0	2.0	0.206 ± 0.063	10 ± 3
	Alkaline	0	0	0.048 ± 0.001	--
		2.0	2.0	0.727 ± 0.081	36 ± 4
	Acid	0	0	0.034 ± 0.008	--
		2.0	2.0	1.51 ± 0.01	76 ± 0.5
4-Aminobiphenyl·HCl	None	0	0	0.022 ± 0.007	--
		2.0	2.0	0.115 ± 0.007	6 ± 0.4
	Alkaline	0	0	0.048 ± 0.001	--
		2.0	2.0	0.542 ± 0.020	27 ± 1
	Acid	0	0	0.034 ± 0.008	--
		2.0	2.0	1.23 ± 0.11	62 ± 6
2-Naphthylamine	None	0	0	0.021 ± 0.001	--
		2.0	2.0	0.088 ± 0.010	4.4 ± 0.5
	Alkaline	0	0	0.039 ± 0.004	--
		2.0	2.0	0.482 ± 0.046	24.1 ± 2.3
	Acid	0	0	0.027 ± 0.002	--
		2.0	2.0	1.37 ± 0.08	68.5 ± 4.2
2-Naphthylamine·HCl	None	0	0	0.021 ± 0.001	--
		2.0	2.0	0.160 ± 0.012	8 ± 0.6
	Alkaline	0	0	0.039 ± 0.004	--
		2.0	2.0	0.332 ± 0.034	16.6 ± 1.7
	Acid	0	0	0.027 ± 0.002	--
		2.0	2.0	1.51 ± 0.03	75.3 ± 1.3

Source: Holder et al. [29].

[a]Per milliliter of sample.

[b]Mean and standard error from triplicate assays; methanol solutions
of control and spiked samples for SPF readings contained an equivalent of 200 and 20 mg of blood per milliliter, respectively. Spiked
samples are corrected for controls.

Table 3.22. Analysis of human urine spiked with 4-aminobiphenyl,
2-naphthylamine, and their hydrochloride salts at 0 and 20 ppb

Compound	Hydrolysis	Added[a] ppm	Added[a] µg	Recovered ($\bar{x} \pm$ SE)[b] ppm	Recovered ($\bar{x} \pm$ SE)[b] %
4-Aminobiphenyl	None	0	0	0.008 ± 0.001	--
		20	2.0	0.019 ± 0.001	95 ± 1
	Alkaline	0	0	0.002 ± 0.000	--
		20	2.0	0.012 ± 0.000	60 ± 0
4-Aminobiphenyl·HCl	None	0	0	0.008 ± 0.001	--
		20	2.0	0.009 ± 0.001	45 ± 1
	Alkaline	0	0	0.002 ± 0.000	--
		20	2.0	0.011 ± 0.000	55 ± 0
2-Naphthylamine	None	0	0	0.003 ± 0.000	--
		20	2.0	0.016 ± 0.001	80 ± 1
	Alkaline	0	0	0.001 ± 0.000	--
		20	2.0	0.013 ± 0.001	65 ± 1
2-Naphthylamine·HCl	None	0	0	0.003 ± 0.000	--
		20	2.0	0.010 ± 0.001	50 ± 1
	Alkaline	0	0	0.001 ± 0.000	--
		20	2.0	0.015 ± 0.001	75 ± 1

Source: Holder et al. [29].

[a]Per 100 ml of sample.

[b]Mean and standard error of triplicate assays; spiked samples are
corrected for controls. Methanol solutions of control and spiked
samples for SPF readings contained an equivalent of 10 g of urine
per milliliter. Development of interferences upon acid hydrolysis
of unspiked urine prevented the assay via SPF.

Table 3.23. Solubilities of 4-aminobiphenyl, 2-naphthylamine, and their hydrochloride salts.

Compound	Solubility in water (mg/ml) at 25 ± 2°C
4-Aminobiphenyl	0.18
4-Aminobiphenyl·HCl	4.14
2-Naphthylamine	0.22
2-Naphthylamine·HCl	26.1

Source: Holder et al. [29].

Water solubilities of the two aromatic amines and their salts were required before analytical method development or formulation of spiked animal drinking water could be undertaken; however, these values could not be found in the literature. Results of our solubility tests, determined as described by Bowman and King [1], analyzed via SPF are given in Table 3.23.

Thin-layer chromatographic R_f values for the aromatic amines (biphenyl was used as a reference compound) in 10 solvent systems are reported in Table 3.24. Anthracene may be substituted for biphenyl as the reference compound since their R_f values were identical in all of the systems tested. These data are useful in the development of cleanup procedures and for the separation and identification of the compounds in mixtures. Any two of the compounds tested may be separated from each other by choosing the appropriate solvent system. Aqueous solutions of the salts spotted and developed, as described, gave R_f values identical to those of the free amines.

Partition values are useful in developing extraction and cleanup methods and for confirmatory tests; the p-values for the compounds of interest were therefore determined via FID-GC, and the results are presented in Table 3.25. It is interesting to note that in the chloroform-aqueous NaOH systems, all normalities of NaOH tested (0.05-5.0 N) yielded p-values of 1.0. On the other hand, with chloroform-aqueous HCl, 0.5 N HCl was not sufficient to completely

Table 3.24. Thin-layer chromatographic R_f values of the carcinogens 4-aminobiphenyl and 2-naphthylamine, and four analogs, in 10 solvent systems

Solvent system (v/v)	R_f values (x 100) of compound indicated					
	4-Amino-biphenyl	3-Amino-biphenyl	2-Amino-biphenyl	Biphenyl	1-Naphthyl-amine	2-Naphthyl-amine
Chloroform	31	38	57	83	34	31
Chloroform-ethyl acetate (9:1)	58	61	79	94	61	57
Chloroform-diethyl ether (9:1)	58	62	83	97	62	57
Chloroform-acetone (9:1)	68	70	88	100	71	65
Chloroform-methanol (9:1)	90	90	96	100	90	85
Benzene	13	12	24	73	16	13
Benzene-ethyl acetate (9:1)	29	33	52	72	36	29
Benzene-diethyl ether (9:1)	30	33	56	77	36	29
Benzene-acetone (9:1)	43	46	65	75	47	41
Benzene-methanol (9:1)	62	63	73	78	63	58

Source: Holder et al. [29].

Table 3.25. Partition values for the carcinogens 4-aminobiphenyl and 2-naphthylamine, and four analogs, in seven solvent systems

Solvent system	Partition value[a]					
	Biphenyl	2-Amino-biphenyl	3-Amino-biphenyl	4-Amino-biphenyl	1-Naphthyl-amine	2-Naphthyl-amine
Hexane-acetonitrile	0.38	0.11	0.03	0.24	0.08	0.03
Hexane-80% acetone (20% water)	0.90	0.73	0.53	0.51	0.48	0.44
Chloroform-water	0.98	1.00	1.00	1.00	1.00	1.00
Chloroform-60% methanol	1.00	1.00	0.98	0.99	0.95	0.94
Chloroform-aqueous NaOH						
(5.0 N)	--	1.0	1.0	1.0	1.0	1.0
(0.5 N)	--	1.0	1.0	1.0	1.0	1.0
(0.05 N)	--	1.0	1.0	1.0	1.0	1.0
Chloroform-aqueous HCl						
(5.0 N)	--	0.03	0.01	0.01	0.00	0.00
(0.5 N)	--	0.47	0.10	0.10	0.03	0.02
(0.05 N)	--	0.96	0.82	0.81	0.57	0.42
Hexane-dimethylformamide	0.21	0.04	--	0.01	--	--

Source: Holder et al. [29].

[a]Fractional amount of solute partitioning into the nonpolar phase of an equivolume immiscible binary solvent system.

Table 3.26. Analysis of 1- and 2-naphthylamine and their hydro-chloride salts in admixture by using simultaneous equations

Added (µg/ml)		Found (calculated µg/ml)	
1-Naphthylamine	2-Naphthylamine	1-Naphthylamine	2-Naphthylamine
Free Amines[a]			
0.50	0.50	0.49	0.50
0.50	0.10	0.49	0.11
1.00	0.10	1.00	0.09
2.00	0.10	1.90	0.08
0.50	0.01	0.48	0.02
Hydrochloride Salts[b]			
1.00	1.00	1.00	0.97
0.50	0.10	0.48	0.11
1.00	0.10	1.00	0.09
2.00	0.10	1.90	0.08
5.00	0.10	4.70	0.06

Source: Holder et al. [29].

[a]In methanol.

[b]In 0.01 N aqueous HCl.

partition the amines (as their HCl salts) into the aqueous phase; however, the use of 5.0 N HCl increased the partitioning efficiency and yielded p-values no higher than 0.03.

Since 1-naphthylamine has been of commercial importance and it has been known to be contaminated with the carcinogen 2-naphthylamine, we investigated the possibility of assaying mixtures of the free amines or their salts via SPF using simultaneous equations. Results obtained for various mixtures of the compounds are presented in Table 3.26. At approximately equal concentrations, the results are quite good and are acceptable up to a ratio of 20:1 of the 1- and 2-substituted isomers; one part of 2-naphthylamine was detectable in 50 parts of 1-naphthylamine, but it could not be accurately quantified at that level.

III   ESTROGENS

A. Diethylstilbestrol [39]

1. *General Description of Method*

An analytical method is described for determining residues of the synthetic estrogen diethylstilbestrol (DES) in animal chow at levels as low as 1 ppb. A methanol extract of the chow is subjected to a three-step cleanup procedure including a Sephadex LH-20 column, liquid-liquid partitioning at pH 14 and 10.2, and a silica gel column. Residues of DES in the cleaned-up extract are analyzed directly by high-pressure liquid chromatography (HPLC) or derivatized to PFP-DES and assayed by EC-GC. Tests with $[^{14}C]DES$ were used to develop and validate the procedure. Ancillary data concerning extraction efficiencies of various solvents, comparisons of various derivatizing reagents, rates of trans-cis isomerization in two solvents, p-values of DES in various solvent systems, and TLC behavior in nine solvent systems are also presented.

2. *Introduction*

The synthetic estrogen DES, administered either as a surgical implant in pellet form or as a feed additive, has been used extensively as a growth-promoting agent in the raising and fattening of livestock and poultry. However, residues of DES in foods are prohibited because of possible estrogenic and carcinogenic effects. (The formula of DES is shown in Figure 3.20.) The possibility that such residues might occur has stimulated much controversy and may well result in a complete, permanent ban on the use of DES in the production of meat for human consumption. Several methods [40-42] have consequently been reported for the assay of animal tissues for DES residues at levels as low as 1 ppb.

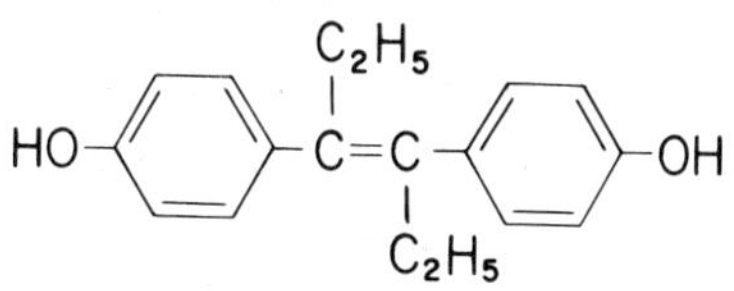

Figure 3.20. Formula of DES.
(From King et al. [39].)

Gass et al. [43] reported a significant increase in the incidence of mammary tumors and decline in time to the incidence of tumors
of C3H mice fed DES at levels of 6.25-25 ppb in feed. Studies to
document this result and to better establish the lower end of the dose-
response curve have been initiated by using feed containing as little
as 2.5 ppb of DES. Therefore, analytical methodology was needed to
assay animal chow containing DES at this and higher levels to verify
the accuracy and homogeneity of the spiked chow as well as the stability of DES in the mixture.

Donoho et al. [44] reported a method for the assay of DES in
animal feed at levels down to 2.2 ppm by using EC-GC. The method
consisted of extraction of the feed with 7% (v/v) ethanol in chloroform, cleanup of the extract with carbonate buffer (pH 10.5), partitioning the DES into 1 N NaOH, and reacting the DES in base with
dichloroacetyl chloride to form an ester which was partitioned into
chloroform and subsequently quantitated by EC-GC. A slight modification of this procedure is reported to give a precision of ±15% for
95% confidence limits at the 2 g/ton (2.2 ppm) level.

Colorimetric methods [45] for the assay of DES at the low ppm
level have been reported in which DES is either reacted with antimony
pentachloride or irradiated with ultraviolet light to produce a
colored compound. Jeffus and Kenner [46] improved the irradiation
method to quantitate down to 0.55 ppm and developed a TLC procedure
capable of detecting as little as 0.07 ppm.

Although none of the reported methods were sensitive enough for
our use, several were quite valuable in formulating our approach to
the problem and in the development of the following procedure.

3. Experimental

a. *Materials*   The DES (No. D-4628, Sigma Chemical Co., St. Louis,
Mo.) was used as received since it contained no extraneous peaks in
assays by HPLC or temperature-programmed GC with flame-ionization
detection. It was found to contain essentially 100% trans isomer as
determined by HPLC. The diethylstilbestrol monoglucuronide (No.

16444-5) was also used as received from Aldrich Chemical Co., Milwaukee, Wis.

The radiolabeled DES (monoethyl-1-^{14}C) obtained from Amersham/ Searle (Arlington Heights, Ill.) had a specific activity of 8.79 µCi/mg as determined by parallel HPLC and liquid scintillation radio-assays. All radioassays were performed with a Mark II instrument equipped with a Model PDS/3 Data Reduction System (Nuclear Chicago Corp., Houston, Tex.) by adding an appropriate amount of unknown to a scintillation vial containing PCS solubilizer (Amersham/Searle Corp.) and counting for an appropriate length of time.

Silica gel (No. 3405, J. T. Baker Chemical Co., Phillipsburg, N.J.) was heated overnight in an oven at 130°C and stored in a desiccator prior to use. The silica gel was then partially deactivated with 3% water for use in the analytical procedure by adding 32.3 g of the dry material to a glass-stoppered bottle containing 1.0 ml of water dispersed on its inner surface; the contents were mixed well and allowed to stand for 24 hr with occasional shaking prior to use. The Sephadex LH-20 was obtained from Pharmacia Fine Chemicals, Inc., Piscataway, N.J.

Trifluoracetic anhydride (No. 270084), PFP anhydride (No. 640110), and HFB (No. 270085) were obtained from Regis Chemical Co., Morton Grove, Ill. The 5-g septumed vials were individually nestled in beds of anhydrous silica gel contained in 150-ml beakers which were then stored in a desiccator. A 50-µl Hamilton syringe was used to withdraw the derivatizing agent from the vial and deliver it into the reaction vessel. Dichloroacetylchloride (No. 1390) and TMA hydrochloride (No. 265) were purchased from the Eastman-Kodak Co., Rochester, N.Y.

Trimethylamine reagent was prepared by dissolving 2.0 g of the hydrochloride salt in 5 ml of 5 N NaOH and extracting the free amine with four 5-ml portions of benzene which were successively percolated through a plug of sodium sulfate (ca. 25 mm diameter x 20 mm thick); the volume of the combined extracts was adjusted to 20 ml with benzene. This stock solution (ca. 1 M) was stored at 5°C; portions were diluted 10-fold with benzene immediately prior to use.

The buffer solution (pH 6.0) was prepared by dissolving 136.1 g of potassium monobasic phosphate in 900 ml of distilled water and adjusting the pH to exactly 6.0 with 10 N sodium hydroxide by using a pH meter; the volume was then adjusted to exactly 1 liter.

All solvents were pesticide grade and all reagents were CP grade.

The animal chow was type 5010C (Ralston Purina Co., St. Louis, Mo.).

b. Preparation of gravity-flow cleanup columns

(1) Sephadex LH-20. Five grams of the dry Sephadex powder were added to a glass column (15 mm i.d., No. K420280-022, Kontes Glass Co., Vineland, N.J.) equipped with a 250-ml reservoir and a Teflon stopcock and containing 60 ml of methanol. Additional methanol was used as needed to wash down the sides of the column. After 30 min, the methanol was allowed to percolate through the column and the Sephadex was then washed with four additional 10-ml portions of methanol followed by four 10-ml portions of benzene-10% methanol. The column was ready for use in the cleanup procedure after it had equilibrated with benzene-10% methanol for at least 1 hr. Each Sephadex column must be initially evaluated to provide assurance that trans and cis DES elutes as indicated in the analytical procedure. The column was regenerated after each use by washing it with four 10-ml portions of methanol followed by four 10-ml portions of benzene-10% methanol as described. Occasional evaluation of column performance indicated that the column could be used indefinitely. (Note: The top of the Sephadex column should not be allowed to dry out. When the column is not in use, the stopcock should be turned off and the Sephadex bed covered by at least 1 cm of solvent.)

(2) Silica gel. Columns (12 mm i.d., Kontes, No. 420,000) equipped with a 50-ml reservoir were prepared by successively adding a plug of glass wool, 2 g of sodium sulfate, 1 g of silica gel (3% water), and 2 g of sodium sulfate. The columns were prepared immediately prior to use and washed with 10 ml of benzene which was discarded. (Note: The silica gel must be evaluated prior to use to provide

assurance that trans and cis DES elute as indicated in the analytical
procedure. The container should be kept tightly sealed to avoid
changes in moisture content.)

c. Extraction and cleanup of animal chow   A 20-g portion of the
animal chow was weighed into a 250-ml glass-stoppered flask, 100 ml
of methanol were added, and the sample was mechanically extracted for
2 hr on a reciprocating shaker at a rate of 200 excursions per minute.
The extract was filtered through a plug of glass wool and a 50-ml
portion (10 g equivalents of chow) transferred to a 180-ml culture
tube containing 100 ml of distilled water and 6 g of sodium chloride.
(Note: All culture tubes were equipped with Teflon-lined screw caps.)
The mixture was extracted three times with 20-ml portions of benzene
which were successively withdrawn by using a syringe and cannula,
percolated through a plug of sodium sulfate (ca. 7 g in a 45 mm
diameter funnel), and collected in a 100-ml round-bottom flask. The
combined extracts were then evaporated to dryness by using a 60°C
water bath and water pump vacuum.

The residue was transferred to the Sephadex LH-20 column, prepared as described, by using five successive 2-ml portions of benzene-
10% methanol, allowing each portion to percolate into the bed; the
column was then eluted with an additional 30 ml of the solvent and
the eluate discarded. Finally, the column was eluted with a 20-ml
portion of benzene-10% methanol and the eluate collected in a 30-ml
culture tube (this eluate contains the DES residue). Eight milliliters of 1 N sodium hydroxide were added to the culture tube, the
contents shaken thoroughly, and centrifuged for 5 min at 2000 rpm.
The benzene layer was withdrawn and discarded and the aqueous layer
was extracted in the same manner with two additional 20-ml portions
of benzene which were also discarded. (Note: Care must be taken
not to remove any of the aqueous phase or the emulsified interface.)
Ten milliliters of 1 M sodium bicarbonate were added to the aqueous
layer and the mixture was extracted three times with 10-ml portions
of benzene which were successively percolated through a plug of
sodium sulfate and collected in a 100-ml round-bottom flask as

described. (Note: The 1 M sodium bicarbonate must be freshly prepared daily and the pH confirmed at about 8.0. Also the pH of the
mixture containing 8 ml of 1 N sodium hydroxide and 10 ml of 1 M
sodium bicarbonate must be confirmed within the pH range of 10.2 to
10.5 prior to using these solutions.) The combined extracts were
evaporated to dryness as described and the residue transferred to a
silica gel column, prepared as previously described, by using five
2-ml portions of benzene, and the eluate was discarded. The column
was then eluted with 20 ml of benzene-4% acetone; this eluate, containing the DES residue, was collected in a 50-ml round-bottom flask,
evaporated to dryness as described, and reserved for assay via HPLC
or EC-GC.

d. *High-pressure liquid chromatographic assays*   A Waters Associates,
Inc. (Milford, Mass.) liquid chromatograph equipped with a Model 6000A
solvent delivery system, a Model U6K septumless injector, a Model 440
multiple wavelength detector operated at 254 nm, and a 4 mm i.d. x
30 cm μ-Porasil column (Waters, No. 27477) was used. The mobile
phase (chloroform-2% methanol) flowed at the rate of 1 ml/min with a
pressure of 550 pounds per square inch (psi). Under these conditions
the t_R values of the trans and cis isomers of DES were 5.30 and 9.75
min, respectively. Responses (peak height or area) were linear up to
at least 2 μg of DES per injection. The minimum detectable amount of
the trans isomer was about 0.2 ng per 10-μl injection, based on twice
noise. Residues of DES per se in the cleaned-up extracts were quantitated on the basis of the sum of the peak heights of the trans isomer
and the cis isomer [expressed as trans (cis x 1.82 = trans)] as related
to standards of DES injected in the same volume of solvent and calculated in the same manner. A Hewlett-Packard (Palo Alto, Calif.) Model
3380A integrator was used in both the HPLC and EC-GC assays to measure
peak areas in order to calculate factors for expressing the peak height
of the cis isomer in terms of the trans isomer. For samples expected
to contain less than 50 ppb of DES, the dry residue in the flask from
the silica gel cleanup was carefully transferred to a 3-ml conical
tube by using four 0.5-ml portions of chloroform. The solvent was

then carefully evaporated to dryness by using a gentle stream of dry nitrogen; the residue was dissolved in 100-250 μl of chloroform-2% methanol, and 50 μl (1-5 g equivalents of chow) was injected into the liquid chromatograph. For samples expected to contain 50 ppb or more of DES, the dry residue from the silica gel cleanup was dissolved in an appropriate volume of chloroform-2% methanol (e.g., 1 ml or more) and aliquots for injection (5-50 μl) were withdrawn directly from the flask.

e. Gas chromatographic assays

(1) Electron-capture detection. A Hewlett-Packard Model 5750 instrument equipped with a ^{63}Ni EC detector (Tracor, Inc., Austin, Tex.) and a 100-cm glass column (4 mm i.d.) containing 5% OV-101 on Gas Chrom Q (80-100 mesh), conditioned at 275°C overnight prior to use, was operated isothermally at 185°C (unless otherwise specified) in the DC mode with a nitrogen carrier gas flow of 160 ml/min. The detector was 300°C and the injection port was set 20°C higher than the column oven. Under these conditions the t_R values of the PFP derivatives of cis and trans DES were 1.70 and 2.65 min, respectively. Derivatized samples of unknown DES residue content were quantified by relating the sum of the heights of the cis and trans peaks expressed as the trans isomer (cis x 0.722 = trans) to known amounts of PFP-DES calculated in the same manner. All injections were made in 5 μl of benzene. Heptachlor epoxide was employed as a reference standard to monitor the performance of the EC-GC system.

(2) Flame ionization detection. A Hewlett-Packard Model 7620A instrument, equipped with a FID and a column identical to that used for EC-GC except that it contained 10% OV-101, was operated either isothermally at 230°C or temperature-programmed from 100 to 260°C at a rate of 10°C/min and held at 260°C for 15 minutes. The helium carrier gas flowed at 100 ml/min, and the injection port and detector temperatures were 250 and 280°C, respectively. Isothermal operation was employed for p-value determinations, and under these conditions the t_R of DES was 3.70 min. Temperature-programmed operation was

used to test for contaminants in the unlabeled DES standard. All
injections were made in 5 µl of chloroform, and the isomers of DES
per se were not resolved under these conditions.

f. Derivatization of DES for EC-GC assays

(1) Preparation of various derivatives for EC-GC evaluation. The
PFP, HFB, and TFA derivatives of DES were prepared by our modification
of the procedure described by Ehrsson et al. [31]. Exactly 0.5 ml of
benzene was added to a 50-ml round-bottom flask containing a dry residue of DES (500 ng or less), followed by 100 µl of 0.1 M TMA and 10 µl
of the appropriate fluorinated anhydride reagent. The flask was immediately sealed with a glass stopper, the contents mixed by gentle
swirling, and allowed to stand at ambient temperature for 20 min.
The reaction was terminated by the addition of 1 ml of 1 M phosphate
buffer (pH 6.0), and the contents were mixed with moderate shaking for
about 30 sec. Exactly 1.4 ml of benzene was added to the flask (total
benzene = 2.0 ml) and, after gentle swirling, the entire contents were
transferred to an 8-ml culture tube. After the phases had separated,
the aqueous layer (bottom) was withdrawn and discarded. The benzene
layer was again shaken for about 30 sec with an additional 1-ml portion of the 1 M phosphate buffer; after the phases had separated, the
benzene layer (top) was carefully transferred to a dry 8-ml culture
tube containing 1 g of sodium sulfate. Finally, the tube was shaken
for about 30 sec and the benzene phase containing the derivatized DES
was injected either directly into the gas chromatograph or after
appropriate dilution with benzene.

The dichloroacetyl derivatives of DES were prepared by a modification of the method described by Donoho et al. [42]. Ten milliliters
of 1 N NaOH containing DES (500 ng or less) was added to a 20-ml culture tube containing 7 ml of benzene; 25 µl of dichloroacetylchloride
was rapidly dispensed into the tube and the contents were vigorously
shaken for 30 sec. The benzene layer was withdrawn and percolated
through a plug of sodium sulfate. Benzene and dichloroacetylchloride
were again added to the tube as described and the process was repeated.
The combined benzene extracts containing the dichloroacetyl derivatives

of DES were then evaporated to dryness by using a 60°C water bath and water pump vacuum; the dry residue was dissolved in an appropriate volume of benzene for injection into the instrument.

(2) Derivatization of DES residue in chow extracts for EC-GC assays. An appropriate portion of the cleaned-up chow extract from the silica gel column, contained in 0.5 ml of benzene, was subjected to derivatization with PFP anhydride as described. For assays of chow containing amounts in the order of 1, 5, or 50 ppb or more of DES residues, 5, 1, and 0.1 g equivalents, respectively, of the cleaned-up chow were derivatized. The 2-ml solution containing the PFP derivatives was either analyzed directly or appropriately diluted prior to analysis.

g. Isomerization experiment Fifty-milliliter amounts of the trans isomer were prepared at concentrations of 10, 300, and 1000 µg/ml in 95% ethyl alcohol and 10 and 300 µg/ml in chloroform and stored in glass-stoppered flasks in a light-free cabinet at ambient temperature. Samples of each solution were taken immediately and at various intervals thereafter to determine the extent of isomerization to the cis form. Analyses were performed by using HPLC; 5-µl amounts of the chloroform solutions were withdrawn from the flasks and injected directly. For analysis of the 95% ethyl alcohol solutions, 1-ml aliquots were withdrawn immediately, evaporated under vacuum at ambient temperature, dissolved in an appropriate amount of chloroform (e.g., 1-5 ml), and a 5-µl portion was injected for HPLC.

h. Solubility, p-value, and TLC determinations A saturated aqueous solution of DES was prepared at 25 ± 2°C by the procedure described by Bowman and King [1]. The solubility of DES in water at that temperature was then determined by evaporating 50 µl of the solution to dryness with a stream of dry nitrogen and assaying the residue as the PFP derivative by EC-GC as described.

Partition values for DES were determined in several solvent systems by FID-GC in the manner described by Bowman and Beroza [13].

The TLC determinations were made by using a Gelman Model 51325-1 apparatus (Ann Arbor, Mich.); the glass plates (silica gel GF, No. 6-601A, Fisher Scientific Co., Pittsburgh, Pa.) were activated at

120°C for 1 hr and cooled in a desiccator prior to use. The plates
were spotted with 5 µl (5 µg) of methanol solution of DES (20% cis
isomer) and the monoglucuronide, and after the developing solvent had
ascended 13 cm above the spotting line (ca. 30 min) the plates were
removed and the solvent allowed to evaporate. The spots were made
visible by viewing them under ultraviolet light (254 nm) and the R_f
values were calculated. All solvent systems except benzene-methanol
and chloroform-methanol (9/1, v/v) were those used by Stoloff [47]
for mycotoxins. Although the analysis of the DES monoglucuronide is
beyond the scope of this study, the compound was available to us and
is therefore included in the TLC evaluations to provide ancillary
information.

i. Extraction and recovery experiments with DES in animal chow   The
efficiency of removing DES residues at the low ppb level from chow
was investigated by using several extraction systems. Culture tubes
(50 ml), each containing 5 g of chow, were spiked at the 50-ppb level
by adding 1 ml of the appropriate solvent containing 250 ng of the
[^{14}C]DES. After the spiked samples had stood for about an hour, 25 ml
of acetone, methanol, acetonitrile, or chloroform-10% methanol were
added and the contents mechanically shaken for 2 hr as described.
Additional samples were extracted in an identical manner after the
addition of 5 ml of either distilled water or 0.1 N HCl to the spiked
chow. The percentage of DES recovered by using the various extraction
systems was determined by radioassays of portions of the extracts.
The amount of extraneous material removed from the chow was determined
by evaporating 10 ml of the extract (equivalent to 2 g of chow) at
110°C and weighing the residue.

Samples (20 g) of chow spiked with 50 ppb of DES were extracted
with and without the addition of 20 ml of distilled water by using a
Soxhlet apparatus containing 150 ml of chloroform-10% methanol operated at a rate of about 10 solvent exchanges per hour. The reflux
flask containing fresh solvent was replaced at 2-hr intervals, and
the percentage of total DES extracted during each interval was determined.

Quadruplicate 20-g samples of chow were spiked with 0, 1.0, 5.0,
50, or 500 ppb of DES or [^{14}C]DES by adding an appropriate amount of
the chemical in 1 ml of methanol. After 1 hr, an additional 99-ml
portion of methanol was added and the samples were extracted, cleaned-
up, and assayed as described either radiometrically or by HPLC or
EC-GC to determine the accuracy and precision of the procedure.

4. Results and Discussion

In preliminary experiments, chow was spiked with 50 ppb of [^{14}C]DES
and mechanically shaken with a variety of solvents, or Soxhlet-
extracted to determine the most efficient means of removing the DES
residue with only minimal amounts of coextractives and in a solvent
that could be easily interfaced with subsequent cleanup procedures.
Deactivation of the spiked chow by the addition of water or dilute
HCl was also tested as a means of enhancing the efficiency of extraction. Soxhlet extraction of the chow with and without deactivation
with water yielded a recovery of about 65% of the DES. Deactivation
slightly increased the recovery of DES via Soxhlet extraction, and
most of the recoverable residue was removed during the first 2 hr;
however, the Soxhlet extraction was abandoned because of the low
recoveries and the presence of large amounts of coextractives.
Results from the extraction experiments employing mechanical shaking
are presented in Table 3.27. All recoveries were 79% or better;
methanol with no deactivation, acetonitrile with acid deactivation,
and acetone with either deactivation all gave at least 98% recovery.
Methanol was selected for use in our analytical procedure because no
deactivation of the sample was required, the amount of coextractives
was fairly low, and methanol extracts interfaced well with subsequent
cleanup steps.

Major cleanup steps that were evaluated for the separation of
DES residues from the coextractives were (1) solvent partitioning,
(2) Sephadex LH-20, and (3) silica gel. It was found that no single
step or combination of any two were sufficient to permit HPLC or
EC-GC analysis at the low ppb level; however, the assays could be
performed by using all three cleanup steps.

Table 3.27. Residues and coextractives from animal chow spiked with [^{14}C]DES (50 ppb) after mechanical extraction under various conditions[a]

Solvent	Deactivation[b]	Milligrams of extractive per gram of sample	[^{14}C]DES recovered (%)
Chloroform-10% methanol	None	66	88.5
	Water	63	79.0
	Acid	61	78.6
Methanol	None	41	98.0
	Water	102	94.4
	Acid	112	87.5
Acetonitrile	None	19	95.6
	Water	29	96.5
	Acid	32	98.0
Acetone	None	44	94.0
	Water	56	99.8
	Acid	60	99.7

Source: King et al. [39].

[a]Five-gram samples were extracted with 25 ml of solvent on a recipro-cating shaker at 200 excursions per minute for 2 hr.

[b]Samples were extracted either directly with solvent or after deactivation by the addition of 5 ml of distilled water or 0.1 N HCl.

The p-values of DES in benzene versus aqueous phases of various pH values are presented in Figure 3.21; at a glance, the analyst can easily determine in which phase the DES resides under the various conditions. One extraction of a benzene solution with 1 N NaOH (pH 14), was sufficient to remove essentially all of the DES, whereas three extractions of a sodium bicarbonate buffered solution (pH 10.2-10.5) with benzene were required to obtain an equivalent extraction. Other p-values that were determined for DES were 0.002 for hexane-acetonitrile and 1.0 for chloroform-water or benzene-water.

Elution profiles of DES from the cleanup columns of Sephadex LH-20 and silica gel are presented in Figure 3.22. No apparent separation of the cis and trans isomers was obtained on Sephadex. How-

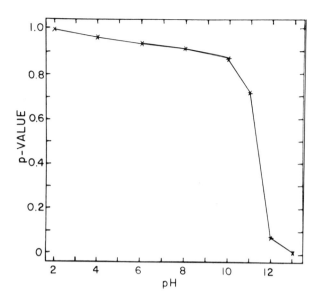

Figure 3.21. Partition values of DES in benzene versus various aqueous buffer solutions. (From King et al. [39].)

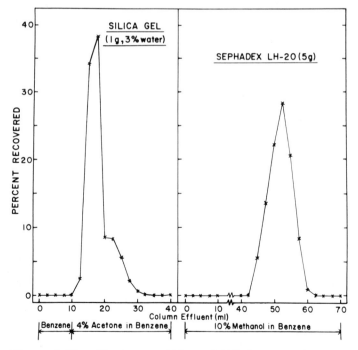

Figure 3.22. Elution profiles of DES from gravity-flow cleanup columns of silica gel and Sephadex LH-20. (From King et al. [39].)

Table 3.28. Analyses of DES residues in animal chow spiked with various amounts of [14C]DES or unlabeled DES as determined by three methods

Analytical method	DES added[a]		Milligram equivalents of chow used per analysis	DES recovered ($\bar{x}$ ± SE)[b]		
	μg	ppb		μg	ppb	%
EC-GC						
	0.0	0.0	12.5	<0.001[c]	<0.05[c]	--
	0.020	1.0	12.5	0.017 ± 0.002	0.86 ± 0.08	86 ± 8
	0.100	5.0	2.5	0.084 ± 0.003	4.22 ± 0.16	84 ± 3
	1.00	50.0	0.25	0.864 ± 0.02	43.2 ± 1.0	86.4 ± 2.0
	10.0	500	0.025	8.79 ± 0.25	439 ± 12	87.9 ± 2.5
HPLC						
	0.0	0.0	2500	<0.004[c]	<0.2[c]	--
	0.100	5.0	2500	0.087 ± 0.002	4.34 ± 0.12	87 ± 2
	1.00	50.0	1000	0.883 ± 0.013	44.2 ± 0.6	88.3 ± 1.3
	10.0	500	500	9.02 ± 0.31	451 ± 15	90.2 ± 3.1
Radioassay						
	0.0	0.0	1000	<0.0001[c]	<0.005[c]	--
	0.020	1.0	1000	0.0176 ± 0.0005	0.882 ± 0.026	88.2 ± 2.6
	0.100	5.0	1000	0.0890 ± 0.0027	4.45 ± 0.14	89.0 ± 2.8
	1.00	50.0	1000	0.902 ± 0.010	45.1 ± 0.5	90.2 ± 1.0
	10.0	500	100	9.25 ± 0.22	462 ± 11	92.5 ± 2.2

Source: King et al. [39].

[a]Per 20 g of chow.

[b]Per 20 g of chow. Mean and standard error from quadruplicate assays; corrected for apparent DES content of unspiked sample.

[c]Based on twice background.

ever, the column provided excellent cleanup because a high proportion
of the coextractives moved with the solvent front and could be
discarded prior to the elution of DES which began after about eight
column volumes. The elution profile of the silica gel column indi-
cates a partial separation of the cis and trans isomers with the
trans form emerging first; however, complete separation of the isomers was not attempted since excellent separation is obtained in the
determinative steps. The silica gel column removed the last traces
of colored coextractives, and the dry residue for analysis (10 g
equivalents of chow) contained no visible residue.

Results from quadruplicate samples of chow spiked at 0, 1.0,
5.0, 50, and 500 ppb with [^{14}C]DES or unlabeled DES are presented
in Table 3.28. Data obtained by using the three determinative procedures were in excellent agreement; all recoveries were 84 ± 8% or
better, and averaged 88.2 ± 2.8%.

Typical HPLC chromatograms of 50- and 12.5-ng standards of DES
and of 1.0 and 2.5 g equivalents of cleaned-up chow alone and spiked
with 50 and 5 ppb of DES are presented in Figures 3.23 and 3.24.
Electron-capture gas chromatograms of the various derivatives of DES,
a heptachlor epoxide reference standard, and underivatized DES are
shown in Figure 3.25. Typical EC chromatograms of 2.5 and 0.25 mg
equivalents of cleaned-up chow alone and spiked with PFP derivatives
equivalent to 5 and 50 ppb of DES are presented in Figure 3.26. The
EC-GC assays proved to be more sensitive than HPLC and less susceptible to interferences from coextractives in the cleaned-up extract;
however, the additional derivatization steps were required. The
EC-GC assay is therefore the method of choice, especially for levels
of 50 ppb or less.

With HPLC, the efficiency of cleanup varied from lot to lot of
chow and apparently decreased with the age of the sample. These
factors coupled with differences in the efficiency of supposedly
identical μ-Porasil columns preclude a general statement concerning
the general sensitivity of the HPLC method. Background interference
varied from 0.1 to several ppb, although, backgrounds of less than
1 ppb were usually achieved. For assays at low ppb levels, a smaller
portion (12 ml) of benzene-4% acetone may be used to elute DES from

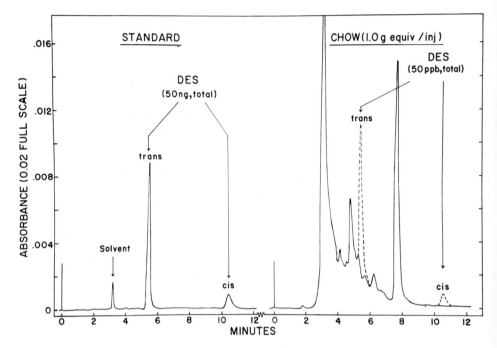

Figure 3.23. High-pressure liquid chromatograms
of DES. Left, 50 ng of DES (ca. 16% cis isomer)
injected in 10 µl of chloroform-2% methanol; right,
extract equivalent to 1 g of chow spiked with 50 ng
(50 ppb) of DES injected in 10 µl of chloroform-
2% methanol. (From King et al. [39].)

the silica gel column to greatly reduce interferences with only a
small additional loss of DES. The peak that interferes most with
the trans DES peak, although reproducible in replicate samples,
varies from being completely absent to somewhat larger than the
ones shown (Figures 3.23 and 3.24), depending on the lot and age of
the chow. The interfering peaks were also observed to shift if
cleaned-up extracts were allowed to stand (at 5°C) for more than
2 days. Therefore, assays should be performed immediately after
the silica gel clean-up.

Diethylstilbestrol which has been through the cleanup procedure
was found to consist of approximately 80% and 20% of the trans and
cis isomers, respectively, regardless of the original isomeric

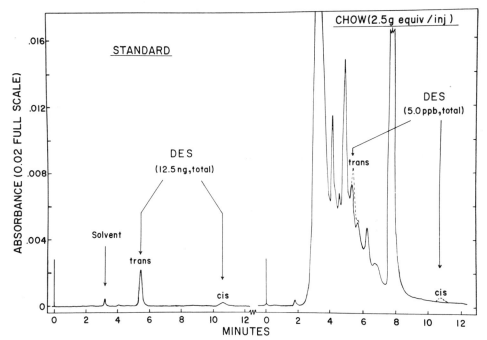

Figure 3.24. High-pressure liquid chromatograms
of DES. Left, 12.5 ng of DES (ca. 16% cis isomer)
injected in 25 μl of chloroform-2% methanol; right,
extract equivalent to 2.5 g of chow spiked with
12.5 ng (5 ppb) of DES injected in 25 μl of
chloroform-2% methanol. (From King et al. [39].)

composition, and in order to calculate the total amount of DES by

HPLC it was necessary to determine the detector response at 254 nm

for each isomer since the ultraviolet absorption spectra are differ-

ent. This was accomplished by injecting 2 μg of DES, previously

equilibrated in chloroform for 2 days, into the liquid chromatograph,

collecting the isomers in individual fractions, and assaying each

fraction by FID-GC, which gives identical t_R values for the two

isomers. The area of the HPLC peak for each isomer was found to be

proportional to the amount of that isomer and, therefore, the sum of

the peak areas was proportional to the total amount of DES injected.

This proportionality was further verified by the separation of the

geometrical isomers of [14C]DES by HPLC, collection of the fractions

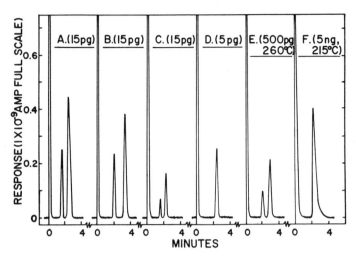

Figure 3.25. Electron-capture gas chromatograms.
A, B, C, and D are the PFP, HFB, and TFA derivatives of DES and the heptachlor epoxide reference
standard, respectively, at 185°C; E is the dichloroacetyl derivative of DES; and F is DES per se. All
injections are in 5 μl of benzene. The derivative
of the cis isomer emerges first. (From King et al.
[39].)

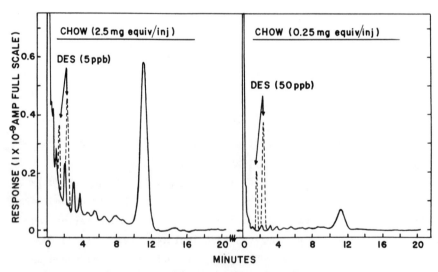

Figure 3.26. Electron-capture gas chromatograms
of cleaned-up chow extract spiked with DES then
derivatized to PFP-DES. Left, injection of 5 μl
of benzene containing extract equivalent to 2.5 mg
of chow and 12.5 pg (5 ppb) of DES; right, injection
of 5 μl of benzene containing extract equivalent to
0.25 mg of chow and 12.5 pg (50 ppb) of DES. (From
King et al. [39].)

containing each isomer, and assay of each fraction radiometrically.
In assays of chow extracts for DES it was necessary to use peak
heights instead of areas because of background interferences. The
peak height of the cis isomer was multiplied by a factor of 1.82 to
express it as an identical amount of trans isomer. This same factor
(i.e., 1.82) was also obtained by simply dividing the t_R of the cis
isomer by that of the trans isomer and this should be a suitable
method to use if an integrator is not available. As a further check
on the applicability of the sum of the peak heights [i.e., H_{trans}
+ 1.82 H_{cis} = H_{total} (expressed as trans)] the HPLC chromatogram of
1 μg of freshly prepared 100% trans DES was compared to that of 1 μg
of equilibrated DES (18.0 cis, 82.0 trans), and the calculation was
found to be valid.

Although DES per se responds to EC-GC, its sensitivity is not
sufficient for our requirements, therefore a variety of derivatizing
agents were evaluated for possible use in our procedure (Figure 3.25).
Gas chromatography conditions, retention times, and minimum detectable amounts of the various derivatives, a heptachlor epoxide
reference standard, and underivatized DES are presented in Table 3.29.
The geometrical isomers of all DES derivatives are well separated
with the cis isomer emerging first but the isomers of underivatized
DES are not. The PFP derivative exhibited the greatest response of
the four tested and, once the optimum conditions for the derivatization reaction were established, the reaction was reproducible, and
a total residue of 0.5 ng of DES per derivatization could be detected.
The use of the PFP derivative was therefore adopted for the procedure.

The rate of isomerization of the cis and trans isomers to reach
an equilibrium ratio has been studied in various solvents [48]. However, further data were needed to establish the stability of the
trans isomer at various concentrations in stock solutions of 95%
ethyl alcohol at ambient temperatures as well as its short-term
stability in chloroform solutions. Results of these tests as performed via HPLC are presented in Chapter 1 (Tables 1.1 and 1.2).
The compound isomerized rapidly in chloroform with more than 17% cis
isomer formed in 28 hr. In 95% ethyl alcohol the isomerization pro-
ceeded at a much slower rate with only 3% cis formed at 144 hr. In

Table 3.29. Electron-capture GC responses for various derivatives of DES, DES per se, and heptachlor epoxide[a]

Compound	Isomer	Oven temperature (°C)	Retention time (min)	Minimum detectable quantity (pg)[b]
PFP-DES	Cis	185	1.70	0.20
	Trans		2.65	0.30
HFB-DES	Cis	185	2.00	0.25
	Trans		3.40	0.35
TFA-DES	Cis	185	1.65	0.60
	Trans		2.30	0.90
Dichloroacetyl-DES	Cis	260	2.20	16
	Trans		3.10	22
DES, per se	--[c]	215	2.25	95
Heptachlor epoxide (reference standard)		185	2.50	0.25

Source: King et al. [39].

[a]The 100-cm glass column (4 mm i.d.) was packed with 5% OV-101 on Gas Chrom Q.

[b]Based on twice noise.

[c]Underivatized isomers are not resolved.

both solvents the rate of isomerization was slightly faster in the more concentrated solutions.

Results of the TLC determinations are presented in Table 3.30. The isomers of DES were separated well with chloroform-95% ethyl alcohol (19:1, v/v) benzene-methanol-acetic acid (18:1:1) and benzene-acetic acid (9:1). The only solvent systems that moved the DES mono-glucuronide from the origin were those containing toluene-ethyl acetate-90% formic acid.

The solubility of DES in water at 25 ± 2°C as determined by EC-GC was found to be 11.0 µg/ml.

Procedures for determining residues of DES in wastewater and human urine via EC-GC of PFP-DES are described in Chapter 4.

Table 3.30. Thin-layer chromatographic R_f values of DES and its
monoglucuronide in nine solvent systems

Solvent systems (v/v)	R_f values (x 100) of compound indicated		
	cis DES	trans DES	DES mono-glucuronide
Benzene-methanol (9:1)	31	35	0
Chloroform-methanol (9:1)	61	64	0
Chloroform-95% ethanol[a] (19:1)	34	56	0
Benzene-methanol-acetic acid[a] (18:1:1)	44	53	0
Hexane-acetone-acetic acid[a] (18:2:1)	16	16	0
Toluene-ethyl acetate-90% formic acid[a] (5:4:1)	85	85	33
Toluene-ethyl acetate-90% formic acid (6:3:1)	67	67	16
Benzene-methanol-acetic acid (24:2:1)	39	41	0
Benzene-acetic acid (9:1)	17	31	0

Source: King et al. [39].

[a]Solvent systems were used in unsaturated tanks.

B. Estradiol [49]

1. *General Description of Method*

A gas chromatographic method is described for trace analysis of the
natural steroidal hormone estradiol in animal chow at levels as low
as 3 ppb. Salient elements of the method include extraction of the
estradiol with methanol, an initial cleanup on a column of Sephadex
LH-20, liquid-liquid partitioning at pH 14 and 10.2, additional
cleanup on a silica gel column, conversion of the estradiol to the
PFP derivative and analysis by EC-GC on a column of OV-25. Samples
containing less than 100 ppb of estradiol are subjected to further
cleanup on silica gel after derivatization and prior to analysis.

   2. Introduction

Since the discovery of estradiol [estra-1,3,5(10)-triene-3,17β-diol]
in 1935, extensive research has been conducted concerning the chemistry, biological mechanisms, and therapeutic uses of this naturally
occurring steroidal hormone. This female estrogen is currently used
primarily in hormone replacement therapy of postmenopausal symptoms.

   Because estradiol is a natural steroidal hormone, it was selected
as a reference or model compound in tests against synthetic hormones
such as DES in long-term chronic feeding studies with large numbers
of mice at our laboratory. Analytical methodology was therefore
required to verify proper dosages, uniformity, and chemical stability
of the compound administered in the animal's diet at low ppb levels.

   Analytical methods for estradiol reported in the literature
include colorimetry and spectrophotometry [50-52], fluorometry [53-
55], TLC [56-57], high-resolution liquid chromatography [58], radio-
immunoassays [59-62], GC without derivatization of the estrogen [63],
GC-mass spectrometric assays [64-65], and GC assays after the preparation of various derivatives of estradiol [66-72]. A recent review
article [73] summarized chromatographic analysis of hormone residues
in food. All of these procedures dealt with samples such as urine,
plasma, dosage forms, and various biological material; methodology
for determining low ppb levels of estradiol in a substrate such as
animal chow could not be found. Therefore, a method was developed
for the analysis of trace amounts of estradiol in animal chow based
on modifications of our procedure for DES residues in chow [39].

   Formulas of estradiol and its PFP derivative are presented in
Figure 3.27.

   3. Experimental

a. *Materials*   The β-estradiol (No. 8875, Sigma Chemical Co.,
St. Louis, Mo.) was used as received since no extraneous responses
were obtained in assays by HPLC, TLC, or temperature-programmed
GC-FID. Materials volatile in a vacuum overnight at 60°C were 0.06%.

   Silica gel (No. 3405, J. T. Baker Chemical Co., Phillipsburg,
N.J.) was heated overnight in an oven at 130°C and stored in a

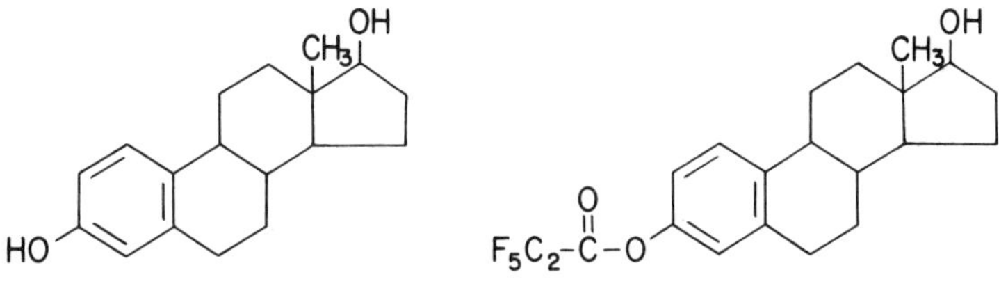

Figure 3.27. Formulas of estradiol (I) and its
PFP derivative (II). (From Bowman and Nony [49].)

desiccator prior to use. The silica gel was then partially deactivated with either 3% or 20% water for use in the analytical procedure
by adding 29.1 or 24.0 g of the dry material to a glass-stoppered
bottle containing 0.9 or 6.0 ml of water; the contents were mixed
well and allowed to stand for 24 hr with occasional shaking prior
to use. The Sephadex LH-20 was obtained from Pharmacia Fine Chemicals, Inc., Piscataway, N.J.

Pentafluoropropionic anhydride (No. 65193) was obtained from
Pierce Chemical Co., Rockford, Ill. All solvents were pesticide
grade and all reagents were CP grade. The TMA reagent (0.1 M in
benzene), buffer solution (potassium monobasic phosphate, pH 6),
sodium hydroxide (1 N) and sodium bicarbonate (1 M) solutions, and
the animal chow (type 5010C, Ralston Purina Co., St. Louis, Mo.)
were described by King et al. [39].

b. Gravity-flow cleanup columns

(1) Sephadex LH-20. Columns (15 mm i.d.) containing 5 g of dry
Sephadex powder were prepared, operated, and regenerated exactly
as described by King et al. [39] for DES.

(2) Silica gel for estradiol (underivatized). Columns (12 mm i.d.,
No. 420,000, Kontes Glass Co., Vineland, N.J.) equipped with a 50-ml
reservoir prepared immediately prior to use by successively adding
a plug of glass wool, 2 g of sodium sulfate, 1 g of silica gel (3%
water), and 2 g of sodium sulfate, were washed with 5 ml of benzene
which was discarded.

(3) Silica gel for PFP-estradiol. Columns were prepared as
described above except that 2 g of silica gel (20% water) were used
and the columns were washed with 20 ml of benzene which was discarded.

c. Extraction and cleanup of animal chow   The sample (20 g) was
extracted with methanol and a portion of the extract (10 g equivalents
of chow) was diluted with aqueous sodium chloride solution, extracted
with benzene, and the combined benzene extracts evaporated to dryness
exactly as described by King et al. [39]. The subsequent three-step
cleanup procedure was also performed as described for DES [39] with
the following modifications.

The residue was transferred to a Sephadex LH-20 column by using
a 5-, 3-, and 2-ml portion of benzene-10% methanol and allowing each
portion to percolate into the bed; the column was then eluted with an
additional 20 ml of the solvent and the eluate discarded. Finally,
the column was eluted with a 25-ml portion of benzene-10% methanol
and the eluate collected in a 100-ml round-bottom flask and evaporated
to dryness.

The residue (which contains the estradiol) was then dissolved
in 5 ml of benzene and transferred to a 20-ml culture tube containing
4 ml of 1 N NaOH. The contents of the tube were shaken, centrifuged
for 5 min at 1200 rpm, and the benzene layer was transferred to a
30-ml culture tube also containing 4 ml of 1 N NaOH; the contents of
the second tube were then shaken and centrifuged as described and the
benzene layer discarded. The flask and aqueous NaOH phases in both
tubes were again sequentially washed and extracted in the same manner
by using two additional 5-ml portions of benzene which were also discarded. The contents of the 20-ml tube were then transferred to the
30-ml tube and 10 ml of 1 M sodium bicarbonate, used to wash the 20-ml
tube, was also added to the mixture. The mixture was then extracted
three times with 10-ml portions of benzene which were successively
percolated through a plug of sodium sulfate and collected in a 100-ml
round-bottom flask.

The combined extracts were evaporated to dryness and the residue
transferred to a silica gel column (3% water) by sequentially using

a 5-, 3-, and 2-ml portion of benzene; the eluate was discarded. The
column was then eluted with 30 ml of benzene-4% acetone; this eluate
(which contains the estradiol residue) was collected in a 50-ml round-
bottom flask, carefully evaporated to dryness, and reserved for subsequent derivatization and assay via EC-GC.

d. *Gas chromatographic assays*   A Hewlett-Packard (Avondale, Pa.)
Model 5750B instrument equipped with a ^{63}Ni EC detector (Tracor, Inc.,
Austin, Tex.) and a 300-cm glass column (4 mm i.d.) containing 5%
OV-25 (a phenyl-methyl silicone, 75% phenyl) on Gas Chrom Q (80-100
mesh), conditioned overnight at 270°C prior to use, was operated
isothermally at 235°C in the DC mode with a nitrogen carrier gas flow
of 160 ml/min. The detector and injection port temperatures were 275
and 255°C, respectively. Under these conditions the t_R of PFP-
estradiol was 2.95 min. Derivatized samples of unknown estradiol
residue content were quantified by relating the peak heights to known
amounts of PFP-estradiol; all injections were in 5 μl of benzene.
Heptachlor epoxide, employed as a reference standard to monitor the
performance of the EC-GC system, had a t_R of 3.75 min.

e. *Derivatization of estradiol for EC-GC assays*   The PFP derivative
of estradiol was prepared, washed with buffer, and dried with sodium
sulfate exactly as described for DES [39] except that 200 μl of 0.1 M
TMA and 20 μl of PFP anhydride were used. Also, 1.3 ml of benzene
was added to adjust the final volume of the benzene phase to exactly
2.0 ml. The benzene solution (containing the PFP-estradiol) was
either reserved for subsequent cleanup (for levels less than 100 ppb)
on silica gel (20% water) or appropriately diluted with benzene and
assayed directly by EC-GC.

For assays of chow containing residues in the order of 0 to 100,
1000, and 10,000 ppb of estradiol, 10, 1.0, and 0.10 g equivalents,
respectively, of the cleaned-up sample were derivatized. The 2-ml
solution containing the PFP derivative was appropriately diluted with
benzene prior to analysis. [Note: In cases where only a portion of
the cleaned-up sample is to be derivatized, the residue (10 g equivalents) is dissolved in a known volume of benzene-methanol (1:1)

because of the low solubility of estradiol in benzene. An appropriate
aliquot is then transferred to another flask where the solvent is
evaporated and the derivatization performed as described.]

f. Cleanup of PFP-estradiol   Samples of chow containing about 100
ppb or less of estradiol required an additional cleanup on silica gel
prior to injecting the PFP derivative into the gas chromatograph in
order to diminish the magnitude of nearby peaks that interfered with
the assay. A known volume (1 ml or less) of the derivatized material
(2 ml) was added to a silica gel column (20% water) prepared as
described; the column was then eluted with an additional 8 ml of
benzene and the entire eluate collected in a 10-ml calibrated tube.
Gentle pressure was applied to the top of the column to obtain sufficient eluate to adjust the volume of the eluate in the tube to exactly
10 ml. The contents were mixed and either analyzed directly or appropriately diluted prior to analysis.

g. Recovery experiment with estradiol in animal chow   Quadruplicate
20-g samples of chow were spiked with 0, 10, 100, 1000, and 10,000 ppb
of estradiol by adding an appropriate amount of the chemical in 1 ml
of methanol. After standing for 1 hr, the solvent had evaporated from
the open flask; the sample was then mixed, 100 ml of methanol was
added, and the samples were extracted, cleaned up, derivatized, and
assayed as described to determine the accuracy and precision of the
procedure.

   4. Results and Discussion
The behavior of estradiol carried through the various cleanup steps
described for DES [39] was carefully evaluated and elution profiles
of the chemical from the columns of Sephadex LH-20 and silica gel
(3% water) were used to modify the DES procedure for use with estradiol to assure optimum cleanup and recovery. A major revision of the
DES procedure was required for the liquid-liquid partitioning step
when it was discovered that the p-value (fraction of solute partitioning into the nonpolar phase of an equivolume immiscible binary
solvent system) of estradiol in benzene versus aqueous NaOH (1 N) is
0.044 instead of 0.00 obtained with DES; almost 30% of the estradiol

residue would be lost in the partitioning cleanup described for DES.
The loss was limited to less than 2% by incorporating a solvent
evaporation step and a sequential partitioning procedure employing
two extraction tubes.

Several procedures based on the derivatization of estradiol to
electron-capturing products are reported in the literature. Those
employing HFB or diheptafluorobutyrate [67,68,70,71] derivatives permitted measurements of residues as low as 200 pg [71]. Mead et al.
[66] detected 80 pg of pure estradiol as the pentafluorophenylhydra-
zone after oxidation of estradiol-3 methyl ether to the corresponding estrone derivative, while Knorr et al. [69] employed the 3-methyl
ether-17-hexadecafluoronanoyl derivative to detect 100-pg levels.
We prepared both the PFP and the HFB derivatives as described by
King et al. [39] for DES; although both products gave about the same
response via EC-GC, the PFP derivative was adopted because its reagent
blank was essentially free of interfering peaks. The spectrum of the
PFP derivative of estradiol from a GC-mass spectrometer indicated the
presence of one PFP group, most likely at the 3 position (see formula
II, Figure 3.27); this was consistent with the molecular weight of
418. Typical EC-GC responses of 25 pg of estradiol as the PFP derivative and 10 pg of the heptachlor epoxide reference standard are presented in Figure 3.28 (chromatogram A). It is interesting to note
that under the conditions of our procedure, the minimum detectable
amount of PFP-estradiol is about 1 pg per 5-μl injection (based on
twice background); this sensitivity is superior to any previously
reported, even for the diheptafluorobutyrate. Therefore, no attempt
was made to prepare the disubstituted derivative since background
interference of the derivatized sample extract was the primary factor
that limited the sensitivity of the assays.

Results from the quadruplicate samples of chow spiked with 0,
10, 100, 1000 and 10,000 ppb of estradiol are presented in Table 3.31.
Recoveries averaged about 80 ± 3%; recoveries from samples spiked with
10 and 100 ppb or more were about 70 and 84%, respectively. Background interference from unspiked chow was about 1.75 ppb or less and
the limit of sensitivity of the method (based on twice background) is

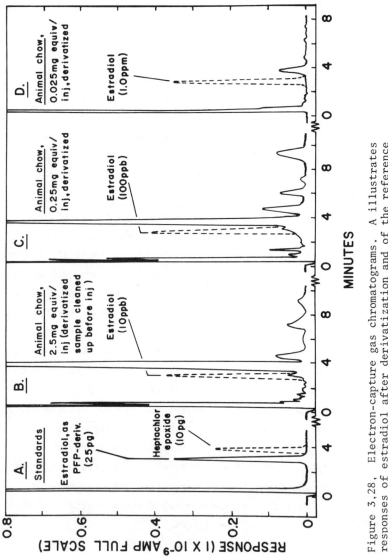

Figure 3.28. Electron-capture gas chromatograms. A illustrates responses of estradiol after derivatization and of the reference standard of heptachlor epoxide. In B, C, and D, solid lines are derivatized extracts of untreated samples and broken lines illustrate responses of residues spiked into the extracts. In B the derivatized sample was cleaned up prior to injection; in C and D it was not. (From Bowman and Nony [49].)

Table 3.31. Analysis of estradiol in animal chow spiked at various levels as determined by EC-GC

Estradiol added[a]		Milligram equivalents of chow used per analysis	Estradiol recovered ($\overline{x} \pm$ SE)[b]		
μg	ppb		μg	ppb	%
0.0	0	2.5	<0.035 ± 0.003	<1.75 ± 0.15	--
0.20	10	2.5	0.139 ± 0.010	6.95 ± 0.50	69.5 ± 5.0
2.00	100	0.25	1.73 ± 0.026	86.5 ± 1.30	86.5 ± 1.3
20.0	1000	0.025	16.8 ± 0.319	840 ± 16.0	84.0 ± 1.6
200	10,000	0.0025	167 ± 6.21	8350 ± 310	83.5 ± 3.1

Source: Bowman and Nony [49].

[a]Per 20 g of chow.

[b]Mean and standard error from quadruplicate assays; spiked samples are corrected for background of unspiked samples.

about 3 ppb. Apropos of this point, further tests indicated that estradiol could in fact be detected in chow which was spiked at the 3-ppb level and carried through the procedure.

Electron-capture gas chromatograms of 2.5, 0.25, and 0.025 mg equivalents of unspiked chow, after cleanup and derivatization, injected alone and spiked with the PFP derivative equivalent to 10, 100, and 1000 ppb of estradiol are presented in Figure 3.28. It should be noted that the sample containing a 2.5 mg equivalent of chow was subjected to further cleanup on a column of silica gel (20% water) prior to injection (chromatogram B); this was required in order to diminish the magnitude of the major interfering peak (t_R = 3.80 min) to a level that permitted assays of 10-ppb amounts of PFP-estradiol. In preliminary tests concerning the selection of an appropriate liquid phase for the GC assays, 180-cm columns containing 5% of AN-600, OV-101, Dexsil 300, or OV-17 failed to resolve the PFP-estradiol from the interfering peak. It was observed, however, that on OV-17 (50% methyl, 50% phenyl silicone) PFP-estradiol emerged earlier than the interfering peak and on OV-101 (methyl silicone) it emerged later. A longer column (300 cm) containing 5% OV-25 (25% methyl, 75% phenyl silicone), which was found to sufficiently resolve the peaks and allow quantitative measurements of PFP-estradiol, was therefore selected for the procedure.

Assays of production batches (45 kg) of chow spiked with 0, 25, and 12,800 ppb of estradiol, which represent a control and the lowest and highest levels of the chemical to be administered in large-scale studies with mice, indicated that homogeneity of mixing had been achieved and the chemical was essentially stable at these levels for at least 43 days when stored in a sealed stainless steel container at ambient temperature.

The solubility of estradiol in water at 25 ± 2°C was approximated by preparing a saturated solution in the manner described by Bowman and King [1] and assaying for estradiol as the PFP derivative by EC-GC; it was found to be 1.8 ppm.

C. Zearalenone and Zearalanol [74]

1. General Description of Method

An analytical method is described for determining residues of the estrogens zearalenone and/or zearalanol in animal chow at levels as low as 10 ppb. The chow is extracted with methanol and cleaned up by a three-step procedure employing a Sephadex LH-20 column, liquid-liquid partitioning at pH 13 and 8.3, and a silica gel column. Residues of the two compounds, separated on silica gel, are assayed by using HPLC with ultraviolet detection. Additional data are also included concerning p-values of the compounds in several solvent systems, solubilities in three solvents, and a procedure for preparing their PFP derivatives for analysis by EC-GC.

2. Introduction

Zearalenone [6-(10-hydroxy-6-oxo-trans-1-undecenyl)-β-resorcylic acid lactone], also known as F-2, is a potent estrogenic mycotoxin, and has been reported to be an inducer of uterotropic and anabolic responses in rats, mice, turkeys, and guinea pigs [75-78]. The compound is also suspected of causing infertility in dairy cattle and swine [79,80] and this effect may occur in nature when animals ingest moldy wheat, barley, maize, and especially corn. Mirocha et al. [81] reported that at least five naturally occurring metabolites of zearalenone exhibited biological activity. Zearalanol [6-(6,10-dihydroxyundecyl)-β-resorcylic acid lactone], synthesized from zearalenone, is a relatively new growth-promoting agent that could be important to the livestock industry and to the consumer. The formulas of zearalenone and zearalanol are presented in Figure 3.29.

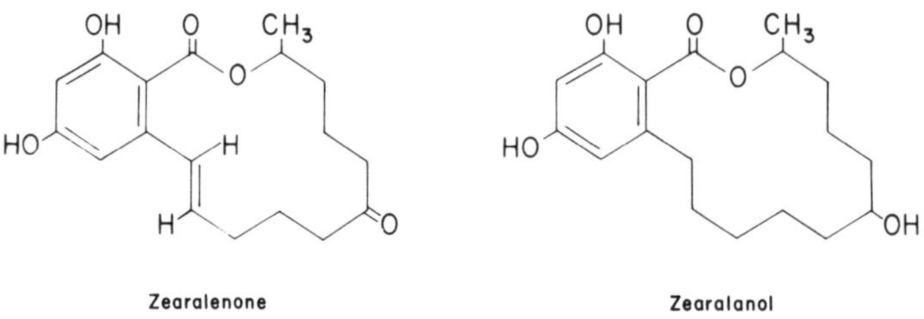

Zearalenone   Zearalanol

Figure 3.29. Formulas of zearalenone and zearalanol. (From Holder et al. [74].)

Since both compounds are potentially hazardous to a variety of animals, extensive research is required to properly evaluate the limits for their safe use. Short-term effects of zearalanol in sheep and steers have been reported [82,83]; however, information concerning long-term chronic effects is not available. Before such studies could be initiated, analytical methodology was needed to assay animal chow containing either or both compounds at the ppb level to verify the accuracy and homogeneity of spiked chow as well as the stability of the compounds in the mixture.

Eppley [84] reported rapid screening methods for zearalenone via TLC, and Stoloff et al. [85] also reported methods for a variety of toxicant residues in feed. Later, Mirocha et al. [86] employed solvent partitioning with an optional TLC technique for cleaning up extracts and assayed zearalenone residues as trimethylsilyl derivatives by using gas-liquid chromatography (GLC) with FID. Recently, Steele et al. [87] used a similar procedure in conjunction with a mass spectrometer to study zearalenone and six congeners in *Fusarium roseum* cultures. Since none of these procedures possessed the sensitivity, specificity, and/or utility required for our studies, the following procedure was developed.

3. *Experimental*

a. *Materials*   Zearalenone (No. E2-23-2) and zearalanol (Lot C3172) were obtained from Commercial Solvents Corp. (Terre Haute, Ind.). Both materials were used as received because assays by HPLC, GLC-FID, and TLC revealed no extraneous responses.

The buffer solution used for the liquid-liquid partitioning cleanup was prepared by dissolving boric acid (3.36 g) in distilled water and the volume adjusted to 100 ml. The solution was freshly prepared daily and the pH adjusted to exactly 4.0. Buffers (pH 1-12) used for the p-value determinations were purchased from Fisher Scientific Co., Pittsburgh, Pa.

Packings for the gravity-flow cleanup columns [silica gel (3% water) and Sephadex LH-20], animal chow, reagents, solvents, and derivatizing agents were identical to those described for DES [39].

Prepare the gravity-flow cleanup columns of silica gel and
Sephadex LH-20 exactly as described for DES [39]. Evaluate each
Sephadex LH-20 column and the silica gel to ensure that zearalenone
and zearalanol elute as indicated in the analytical procedure.

b. *Extraction and cleanup of animal chow*   Weigh 20 g of animal chow
into a 250-ml glass-stoppered flask, add 100 ml of methanol, and
mechanically extract the sample for 2 hr in a reciprocating shaker
at the rate of 200 excursions per minute. Filter the extract through
a plug of glass wool and transfer 50 ml (10 g equivalents of chow)
to a 180-ml culture tube containing 100 ml of water and 6 g of NaCl.
(Note: All culture tubes are equipped with Teflon-lined screw caps.)
Extract the mixture five times with 20-ml portions of benzene by using
a syringe and cannula, and successively percolate each portion through
a plug of anhydrous sodium sulfate (ca. 18 mm diameter x 20 mm thick)
into a 250-ml round-bottom flask (total extraction with benzene = 100
ml). Centrifuge to separate the phases (e.g., 500 rpm for 10 min).
Evaporate the combined extracts to dryness by using a 60°C water bath
and water pump vacuum, and reserve the residue for subsequent Sephadex
cleanup. When only residues of zearalenone are sought, three 20-ml
portions of benzene are adequate for extraction.

Transfer the residues to a Sephadex LH-20 column, prepared as
described, by using five successive 2-ml portions of benzene, allowing
each portion to percolate into the bed; then elute the column with an
additional 40 ml of benzene. Discard the first 40 ml of column eluate,
then begin collection in a 100-ml round-bottom flask. Finally, elute
the column with 60 ml of benzene-methanol (9:1), and evaporate the
eluate to dryness as described. When only residues of zearalenone
are sought, 50 ml of benzene-methanol (9:1) is sufficient.

Transfer the dry residue from the Sephadex column to a 30-ml
culture tube containing 10 ml of 0.1 N NaOH (pH 13) by using 10 ml
of benzene; thoroughly shake the contents and centrifuge for 5 min
at 1000 rpm. Withdraw and discard the benzene layer, then extract
the aqueous layer in the same manner with two additional 10-ml portions of benzene which should also be discarded. (Note: Take care
not to remove any aqueous phase or emulsified interface.)

Add 8 ml of boric acid buffer (pH 4) to the aqueous layer and extract three times with 10-ml portions of benzene; then successively percolate each portion through a plug of sodium sulfate into a 100-ml round-bottom flask as described. (Note: Prepare boric acid solution fresh daily and confirm the pH at 4.0. Also confirm that the mixture containing 10 ml of 0.1 N NaOH and 8 ml of boric acid buffer is pH 8.2-8.5 before using the solutions.) Evaporate the combined extract to dryness as described and transfer the residue to a silica gel column, prepared as previously described, by using five 2-ml portions of benzene followed by 10 ml of benzene; discard the eluate. Elute residues of zearalenone from the column by using 50 ml of benzene-acetone (49:1) and then change the receiver and elute the column with 60 ml benzene-acetone (47:3) to remove any residues of zearalanol. Evaporate the separate eluates to dryness as described and reserve them for subsequent analysis.

For HPLC assays, rinse the walls of the flask with 1 ml of methanol and again evaporate the contents to dryness as described to remove traces of benzene, and then dissolve the dry residues of separate fractions in 1 ml (or more) of methanol-water (65:35) for direct injection into the liquid chromatograph. Make all injections in 50 µl of methanol-water (65:35) and quantitate residues of zearalenone and zearalanol by relating their peak heights to those of standards.

c. *High-pressure liquid chromatography*   A Waters Associates, Inc. (Milford, Mass.) liquid chromatograph equipped with a Model 6000A solvent delivery system, a Model U6K septumless injector, an ultraviolet detector (254 nm), and a 4 mm i.d. x 30 cm column of µ-Bondapak C_{18} (reverse phase) was used. The mobile phase (methanol-35% water) flowed at the rate of 1 ml/min with a pressure of about 1400 psi. Under these conditions, t_R values for zearalanol and zearalenone were 9.30 and 10.80 min, respectively. Responses (peak height or area) were linear up to at least 2 µg per 50-µl injection; the minimum detectable amount of each compound was about 5 ng per 50-µl injection, based on twice noise.

d. Gas chromatography

(1) Electron-capture detection. A Hewlett-Packard (Palo Alto, Calif.) Model 5750 instrument equipped with a ^{63}Ni EC detector (Tracor, Inc., Austin, Tex.) and a 100-cm glass column (4 mm i.d.) containing 5% Dexsil 300 on Gas Chrom Q (80-100 mesh), conditioned at 275°C overnight prior to use, was operated isothermally at 220°C in the DC mode with a nitrogen carrier gas flow of 160 ml/min. The injection port and detector were set at 240 and 270°C, respectively. Under these conditions, t_R values of PFP derivatives of zearalanol and zearalenone were 2.05 and 4.05 min, respectively. All injections were made in 5 µl of benzene and heptachlor epoxide (t_R = 1.50 min) was used as a reference standard to monitor the performance of the GC system. Samples were quantitated by relating peak heights of unknowns to known amounts of PFP derivatives.

(2) Flame ionization detection. A Hewlett-Packard Model 7620A instrument equipped with FID and a 100-cm glass column (4 mm i.d.) containing 10% OV-101 on Gas Chrom Q (80-100 mesh) was operated either isothermally at 260°C or temperature-programmed from 100 to 260°C at a rate of 20°C/min then held at 260°C for 10 min. The helium carrier gas flowed at a rate of 100 ml/min and the injection port and detector were set at 280°C. Under these conditions, t_R values for zearalenone and zearalanol were 5.50 and 5.70 min isothermally and 13.30 and 13.50 min programmed, respectively. All injections were made in 5 µl of chloroform; the test substances were examined for contaminants by using both modes of operation.

e. Derivatization for GC Successively add exactly 0.5 ml of benzene, 1 ml of 0.1 M TMA, and 100 µl of PFP anhydride to a 50-ml round-bottom flask containing the dry residue of zearalenone and/or zearalanol (500 ng or less). Seal the flask immediately with a glass stopper, mix the contents gently by swirling, and allow to stand at ambient temperature for 20 min. Terminate the reaction by adding 1 ml of 1 M phosphate buffer (pH 4.2) and mix the contents with moderate shaking for 30 sec. Add exactly 0.5 ml of benzene (total benzene = 2.0 ml),

swirl gently, and transfer the entire contents to an 8-ml culture
tube. After the phases separate, withdraw and discard the aqueous
layer (bottom). Add an additional 1 ml of 1 M phosphate buffer, and
shake the contents for 30 sec; after the phases separate, carefully
transfer the benzene layer (top) to a dry 8-ml culture tube containing
1 g of anhydrous sodium sulfate. Shake for 30 sec, immediately separate the benzene layer containing derivatized compounds from the
sodium sulfate, and store in another tube for subsequent analysis.
Inject 5-μl portions of PFP derivatives either directly into the GC
apparatus or after appropriate dilution with benzene. Derivatize and
analyze portions of dry residue (5 g equivalents) from separate fractions of cleaned-up chow in the same manner.

f. *Recovery experiments* Prepare quadruplicate 20-g samples of chow
spiked with 0, 0.10, 1.0, and 10 ppm each of zearalenone and zearalanol
by adding appropriate amounts of chemicals in 1 ml of methanol. Seal
the containers with glass stoppers, mix the contents by shaking for
1 min, and let the spiked samples stand for 1 hr. Add additional
99-ml portions of methanol, and then analyze the samples by HPLC as
described to determine the accuracy and precision of the procedure.

g. *Thin-layer chromatographic, p-value, and solubility determinations*
Make the TLC determination by using a Gelman Model 51325-1 apparatus
(Ann Arbor, Mich.) and glass plates (silica gel GF, No. 6-601A, Fisher
Scientific Co., Pittsburgh, Pa.) activated for 1 hr at 120°C and
cooled in a desiccator before use. Spot the plates with 5 μl of
methanol containing 0.05-5.0 μg of individual compounds and in admixture. Remove the plates after the developing solvent has ascended
13 cm above the spotting line (ca. 30 min) and allow the solvent to
evaporate. View the spots under ultraviolet light (254 nm) and calculate the R_f values. All solvent systems except benzene- and
chloroform-methanol (9:1) are those used by Stoloff [88] for mycotoxins.

        Determine the p-values for the two compounds in several solvent
systems as described by Bowman and Beroza [13]; use HPLC for analysis.

Determine the solubilities of the two compounds at 25 ± 2°C in water, methanol, and 95% ethanol by preparing saturated solutions as described by Bowman and King [1]. Analyze solutions both by HPLC as described and by ultraviolet absorption spectrophotometry at 218 nm for zearalanol and 235 nm for zearalenone. For HPLC assays, dilute methanol and 95% ethanol solutions appropriately with methanol-35% water for injection into the instrument; inject aqueous solution directly.

4. Results and Discussion

A comprehensive study concerning the trace analysis of the synthetic estrogen DES in animal chow, which was previously conducted at our laboratory, used [^{14}C]DES to evaluate the efficiency of various extraction systems for removing low ppb levels of the compound. In the procedure that was chosen, the compound was extracted by mechanically shaking the substrate for 2 hr in methanol [39]. Since zearalenone and zearalanol both have analytical chemical properties similar to those of DES, the mechanical extraction with methanol was used and a cleanup procedure similar to that for DES was also developed.

All three of the major cleanup steps (Sephadex LH-20, solvent partitioning, and silica gel) were required for assays of the two compounds at levels as low as 10 ppb. Also, a peak that interfered with zearalenone eluted with zearalanol; therefore, it was necessary to collect the separate fractions from the silica gel column in order to analyze for both compounds via HPLC.

Elution profiles of zearalenone and zearalanol from the Sephadex LH-20 column are presented in Figure 3.30. Partial separation of the compounds on the column is apparent with zearalenone emerging first; however, complete separation was not attempted because excellent separation is obtained during the silica gel cleanup step. Sephadex provided an effective preliminary cleanup because a high proportion of the coextractives moved with the solvent front and could be discarded prior to the elution of the compounds which began to occur at an appreciable rate after elution with about 50 ml of benzene (about 10 solvent exchanges of the column).

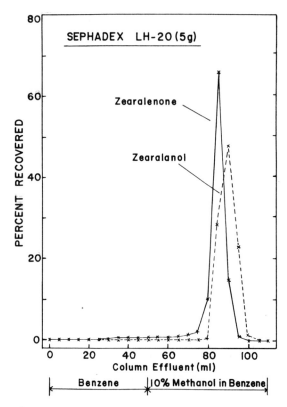

Figure 3.30. Elution profiles of zearalenone and zearalanol from gravity-flow cleanup column of Sephadex LH-20. (From Holder et al. [74].)

The p-values of zearalenone and zearalanol in benzene versus aqueous solutions of various pH values are presented in Figure 3.31. A cursory inspection of this figure provides information concerning the phase in which each compound resides under various conditions of pH. One extraction of a benzene solution with 0.1 N NaOH (pH 13) removes essentially all of both compounds; on the other hand, three extractions of the boric acid buffered solution (pH 8.3) are required to remove the zearalenone and especially the more polar zearalanol. Data presented in Figure 3.31 provided the basis for the development of the liquid-liquid partitioning procedure (pH 13 and 8.3) which serves as the intermediate cleanup step.

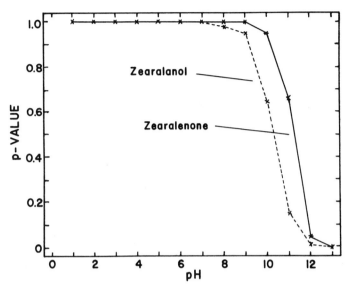

Figure 3.31. Partition values of zearalenone and
zearalanol in benzene versus various aqueous buffer
solutions. (From Holder et al. [74].)

The elution profiles of the two compounds on the silica gel
cleanup column are presented in Figure 3.32. Zearalenone is eluted
from the column first by using benzene-acetone (49:1); zearalanol is
then eluted by the addition of benzene-acetone (47:3). Separation
of the compounds is essentially complete. The fractions are collected
separately for analysis via HPLC because of the extraneous material
in the zearalanol that interferes with the analysis of zearalenone.

Results from quadruplicate samples of chow spiked with 0, 0.10,
1.0, and 10 ppm each of the two compounds in admixture are presented
in Table 3.32. Recoveries were 76-86% and precision was good. No
residues of zearalenone or zearalanol were detected in the unspiked
chow and the background was about 5 and 4 ppb, respectively. Minimum
detectable levels of about 10 and 8 ppb for zearalenone and zearalanol
in chow (based on twice background) would therefore be expected.
Apropos of this point, samples of chow were spiked with 0, 10, and
20 ppb of each compound and carried through the analytical procedure;
peaks for both compounds were clearly distinguished above background

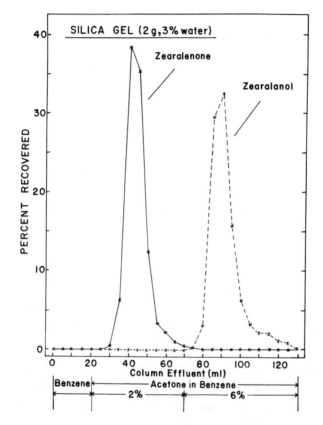

Figure 3.32. Elution profiles of zearalenone and
zearalanol from gravity-flow cleanup column of
silica gel (From Holder et al. [74].)

Table 3.32. High-pressure liquid chromatographic analysis of animal chow spiked at various levels with zearalenone and zearalanol

Trial	Compound	Added[a]		Milligram equivalents of chow used per analysis	Recovery ($\bar{x}$ ± SE)[b]		
		μg	ppm		μg	ppm	%
1	Zearalenone	0.0	0.0	500	<0.10 ± 0.00	<0.005 ± 0.000	--
	Zearalanol	0.0	0.0	500	<0.08 ± 0.00	<0.004 ± 0.000	--
2	Zearalenone	2.0	0.1	500	1.52 ± 0.10	0.076 ± 0.005	76 ± 5
	Zearalanol	2.0	0.1	500	1.52 ± 0.08	0.076 ± 0.004	76 ± 4
3	Zearalenone	20.0	1.0	250	16.1 ± 1.20	0.806 ± 0.060	80.6 ± 6.0
	Zearalanol	20.0	1.0	250	16.0 ± 0.18	0.798 ± 0.009	79.8 ± 0.9
4	Zearalenone	200.0	10.0	50	162 ± 2.0	8.12 ± 0.10	81.2 ± 1.0
	Zearalanol	200.0	10.0	50	173 ± 1.8	8.65 ± 0.09	86.5 ± 0.9

Source: Holder et al. [74].

[a]Per 20 g of chow.

[b]Per 20 g of chow. Mean and standard error from quadruplicate assays; unspiked chow contained no detectable residues of either compound.

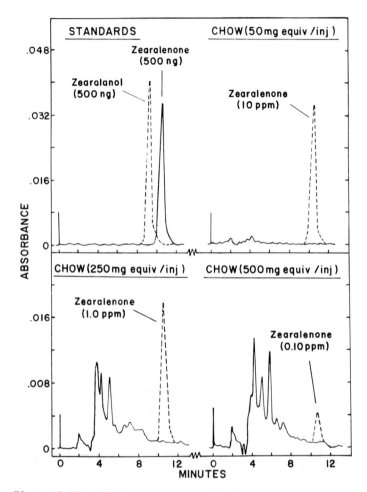

Figure 3.33. High-pressure liquid chromatograms of standards of zearalenone and zearalanol and of chow extracts spiked with 0.10, 1.0, or 10 ppm zearalenone; 50-µl injections in methanol-35% water. (From Holder et al. [74].)

and the residues were estimated at 10 or 20 ± 5 ppb. The use of an
improved ultraviolet detector (Waters Associates, Model 440) increased
the minimum detectable level of both compounds at least 10-fold; however, this added sensitivity offered no advantage in the analysis of
chow because the background of cleaned-up samples was enhanced by
about the same amount. Typical HPLC chromatograms of 500-ng amounts
of standards of the two compounds and 50, 250, and 500 mg equivalents
of the cleaned-up fraction of chow alone and spiked with 0.10, 1.0,
and 10.0 ppm are presented in Figures 3.33 and 3.34.

Derivatization of the two compounds and subsequent analysis via
EC-GC was sought as an alternative method of analysis. Chromatograms
of their PFP derivatives are presented along with a heptachlor epoxide
reference standard in Figure 3.35. Unfortunately, the cleaned-up
fractions from the silica gel column contained extraneous materials
that on derivatization precluded the analysis of residues of either
compound at levels below 1.0 ppm (based on twice background). It
was possible but not advantageous to collect the zearalenone or
zearalanol fractions from the HPLC assays of chow, derivatize them,
and assay via EC-GC with the same sensitivity obtained from the HPLC
analysis. The GC procedure is therefore reported for confirmatory
use pending the development of a more sophisticated cleanup procedure
for either the parent compounds or their PFP derivatives.

Results from the ancillary TLC determinations which may be useful
for confirmatory purposes are presented in Table 3.33. The two compounds were completely separated in all instances with the less polar
zearalenone exhibiting a higher R_f value than zearalanol in each of
the nine solvent systems. Minimum amounts of zearalenone and zearalanol detectable on the developed plates were about 100 and 200 ng,
respectively.

The solubilities of the two compounds in three solvents at
25 ± 2°C as determined by both HPLC and ultraviolet spectrophotometry
were essentially identical. Both compounds were about equally soluble
in water (1.0 µg/ml); the solubilities (milligrams per milliliter) of
zearalenone and zearalanol in 95% ethanol were 108 and 52, and in
methanol, 150 and 106, respectively.

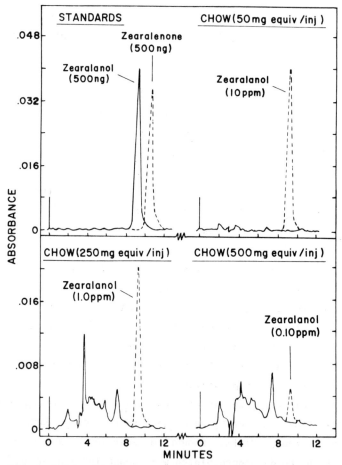

Figure 3.34. High-pressure liquid chromatograms of standards of zearalenone and zearalanol and of chow extracts spiked with 0.10, 1.0, or 10 ppm zearalenone; 50-μl injections in methanol-35% water. (From Holder et al. [74].)

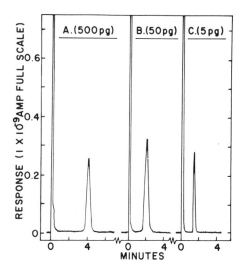

Figure 3.35. Electron-capture gas chromatograms.
A and B, PFP derivatives of zearalenone (500 pg)
and zearalanol (50 pg), respectively; C, heptachlor
epoxide reference standard (5 pg); 5-μl injections
in benzene. (From Holder et al. [74].)

Table 3.33. Thin-layer chromatographic R_f values of zearalenone
and zearalanol in nine solvent systems

Solvent system (v/v)	R_f values (x 100)	
	Zearalenone	Zearalanol
Benzene-methanol (9:1)	53	25
Chloroform-methanol (9:1)	87	64
Chloroform-95% ethanol[a] (19:1)	86	34
Benzene-methanol-glacial acetic acid[a] (18:1:1)	66	40
Hexane-acetone-glacial acetic acid[a] (18:2:1)	19	6
Toluene-ethyl acetate-90% formic acid[a] (5:4:1)	86	78
Toluene-ethyl acetate-90% formic acid[a] (6:3:1)	62	54
Benzene-methanol-glacial acetic acid (24:2:1)	49	29
Benzene-glacial acetic acid (9:1)	32	15

Source: Holder et al. [74].
[a]Solvents were used in unsaturated tanks.

IV   PESTICIDES

A.   2,4,5-Trichlorophenoxyacetic Acid and Its Glycineamide [89]

1. *General Description of Method*

Chemical methods are described for the trace analysis of the herbicide 2,4,5-trichlorophenoxyacetic acid (2,4,5-T), its glycineamide, and their alkaline hydrolyzable conjugates in mouse blood, urine, and feces. The salient elements of the methods are extraction of the free acids with benzene, methylation, cleanup on a silica gel column, and quantification via EC-GC. Any unextracted conjugates remaining in the substrates are then subjected to alkaline hydrolysis, and the liberated 2,4,5-T is assayed. Data are presented concerning recoveries of the compounds from the three spiked substrates. The utility of the procedures is illustrated by a preliminary pharmacokinetic study employing parallel EC-GC and radioassays of the substrates from mice injected with a single intravenous dose of $[^{14}C]$2,4,5-T. Gas chromatographic characteristics and p-values of the compounds and hydrolysis of the glycineamide under various conditions are also discussed.

2. *Introduction*

In 1971, the Panel on Herbicides of the President's Science Advisory Committee [90] indicated that additional information was needed to understand the effects of 2,4,5-T in humans and animals; therefore, further research on this compound was initiated. The major objective of studies with 2,4,5-T in our laboratory was to ascertain any potential relationships between embryonic and/or fetal exposure to the chemical and the abnormalities. To obtain a pharmacokinetic profile of the chemical in relation to its teratogenic effects, pharmacokinetic data must be available on the unbred female and at various intervals during the gestation period. Therefore, chemical methodology was required for the trace analysis of 2,4,5-T and its glycineamide (a known conjugate produced under certain conditions in the liver of most mammalian systems), and other possible conjugates in mouse blood, urine, and feces. Formulas of 2,4,5-T and its glycineamide are presented in Figure 3.36.

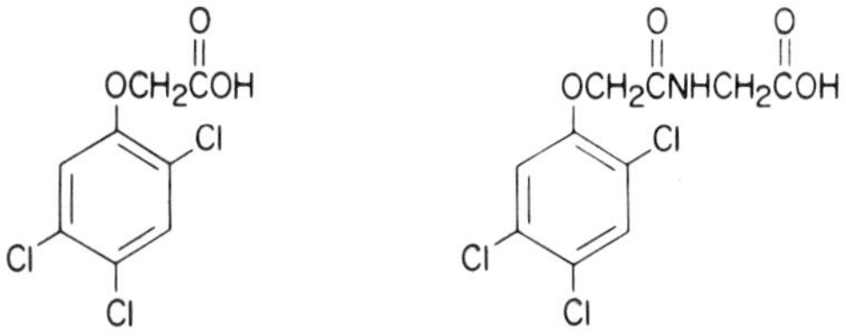

2,4,5-T   2,4,5-T Glycineamide

Figure 3.36. Formulas of 2,4,5-T and its glycineamide. (From Nony et al. [89].)

Pharmacokinetic studies have been conducted using rats, dogs, and humans and single doses of [^{14}C-carboxy]2,4,5-T [91] and analytical grade 2,4,5-T [92]. Also, the absorption, elimination, and metabolism of 2,4,5-T were studied in rats, pigs, calves, and chickens [93,94]. A method was reported for determining 2,4,5-T, 2-4-dichlorophenoxyacetic acid, and related compounds in rat urine based on ethylation, cleanup on silica gel, and analysis of the derivative by EC-GC [95]. The liquid-liquid extraction properties of phenoxy acid herbicides from water were also investigated [96]. None of these procedures, however, met the high sensitivity requirements (low nanogram level) of our study. The following procedures were therefore developed and tested in a preliminary pharmacokinetic study with mice.

3. Experimental

a. Materials Benzene and hexane, pesticide grade, were redistilled in glass and screened for interfering EC-GC peaks by analyzing 5 µl of a 25-fold concentrate. Solvent concentrates having responses less than 1 and 5 pg equivalents of the methyl esters of 2,4,5-T and its glycineamide (per 5-µl injection), respectively, were considered satisfactory.

Diazomethane reagent was prepared from N-methyl-N-nitroso-p-toluenesulfonamide (Diazald, No. D2800-0, Aldrich Chemical Co., Milwaukee, Wis.) by using the reagent, kit, and instructions provided by the manufacturer. The ethereal diazomethane was then dried by percolation through a plug of anhydrous sodium sulfate, redistilled,

and stored at -10°C until used. A hexane solution of diazoethane
also was prepared from N-ethyl-N,N'-dinitroguanidine (Aldrich, No.
E4160-5) for ethylating 2,4,5-T and its glycineamide.

Silica gel (No. 3405, J. T. Baker Chemical Co., Phillipsburg,
N.J.), oven dried at 110°C, was deactivated with 2% buffer (No.
50-B-108, Fisher Scientific Co., Pittsburg, Pa.; 0.05 M monobasic
potassium phosphate-sodium hydroxide, pH 7). The appropriate amount
of buffer was dispersed on the inner surface of a dry, glass-stoppered
bottle, and dry silica gel was added. The contents were then mixed
by mechanically rolling the bottle for 1 hr. The adsorbent was freshly prepared daily.

The $[^{14}C]$2,4,5-T (Mallinckrodt Chemical Works, St. Louis, Mo.),
uniformly ring-labeled (1.92 µCi/mg), was assayed as the methyl ester
by EC-GC and was essentially identical to the unlabeled standard and
free of extraneous GC peaks.

b. *Radioassays*   Radiolabeled samples were counted with a liquid
scintillation instrument equipped with a data reduction system
(Mark II instrument with Model PDS/3 data reduction system, Nuclear-
Chicago Corp., Houston, Tex.). A one-tenth aliquot (0.5-1.0 ml) from
each sample assayed by EC-GC was added to a vial containing 12 ml of
PCS solubilizer (Amersham/Searle Corp., Arlington Heights, Ill.) and
counted for 20 min. Residual samples (e.g., after hydrolysis and
extraction) and the adsorbent from the cleanup column were combusted
by using a Model JA 101 Oxymat (Teledyne, Inc., Westwood, N.J.), and
any ^{14}C-labeled carbon dioxide was assayed by liquid scintillation.

c. *Gas chromatography*   A gas chromatograph (Hewlett-Packard, Model
5750; Palo Alto, Calif.) equipped with a ^{63}Ni EC detector (Tracor,
Inc., Austin, Tex.) and a 100-cm glass column (4 mm i.d.) containing
10% OV-101 on Gas Chrom Q (80-100 mesh), conditioned overnight at
275°C prior to use, was operated isothermally at 200°C in the DC
mode. The nitrogen carrier gas flow rate was 160 ml/min. Temperatures of the injection port and detector were 240 and 280°C, respectively. Under these conditions, t_R values of the methyl esters of
2,4,5-T and its glycineamide were 1.40 and 8.00 min, respectively.

Samples of unknown residue content were quantified by relating their peak heights to dilutions of standards of the two esters prepared by methylating 1-mg amounts of the free acids. Samples for injection contained up to 25 and 160 pg of the methyl esters of 2,4,5-T and its glycineamide, respectively, in 5 µl of benzene or hexane-20% benzene.

Where more rapid and sensitive analysis of only the methyl ester of the glycineamide was sought, the instrument was operated isothermally at 240°C. Under this condition, the t_R was 2.25 min and the response was linear up to about 70 pg per injection.

d. *Animal chamber*   A special sampling chamber for an individual mouse was fabricated from a 2-liter beaker by reshaping the bottom to form a cone (50 mm deep) and attaching a glass drain tube (6 mm i.d. x 10 mm long). A disk of stainless steel screen (2 x 2 mm square openings), approximately the same diameter as the beaker, rested on the bottom of the vessel; a 30-ml culture tube with a Teflon-lined screw cap was placed under the drain tip. This arrangement allowed urine to be collected in the tube while feces were retained on the screen. The animal was supported by a heavier disk of larger mesh (8 x 25 mm diamond-shaped openings, measured from opposite corners) equipped with metal legs, which suspended the animal about 25 mm above the bottom screen.

Several animal chambers of this type were used to collect urine and feces from untreated mice for use in developing the analytical methodology via EC-GC; they were also used in preliminary pharmcokinetic and other studies with the [14C]2,4,5-T. Composites of samples collected for use in developing the analytical methodology were stored at -10°C prior to use; all others were extracted immediately after collection.

e. *Hydrolysis studies*   Samples (100 ng) of the methyl and ethyl esters of the glycineamide were subjected to alkaline hydrolysis (1 N NaOH) for 2 hr at 85°C to determine the completeness of cleaving the compound and of recovering the 2,4,5-T reaction product. The hydrolysates were acidified, extracted with benzene, methylated, and assayed by EC-GC. One hundred nanograms of glycineamide was also subjected to aqueous acid and alkali treatments at three different temperatures for various periods to determine its stability during extraction and analysis.

f. Animal experiments   Unbred female CD-1 mice, 32-33 g, were individually confined in the special sampling chambers. The mice were allowed free access to food and water throughout the experiment, and control samples of urine and feces were collected for 24 hr preceding the injection of radiolabeled 2,4,5-T. The control sample of blood was withdrawn from each mouse just prior to an intravenous injection of 1.86 mg of $[^{14}C]$2,4,5-T (contained in 100 μl of water-60% ethanol) into the tail vein of the animal; this dosage was equivalent to about 57 mg of 2,4,5-T per kilogram. In the pharmacokinetic studies, samples of blood (5 or 20 μl), urine, and feces were collected at various intervals and assayed.

In experiments prior to the pharmacokinetic studies, mice injected with the $[^{14}C]$2,4,5-T were confined overnight. Various solvents in different combinations were used to determine the most efficient means of recovering the radioactive urine deposits from the inner surface of the chamber.

g. Analysis of blood   An accurately measured sample of mouse blood was withdrawn from the tip of the animal's tail and immediately delivered into an 8-ml culture tube, containing 0.5 ml of distilled water, by using either a 5- or 20-μl micropipet (Drummond Wiretrol, Bolab, Inc., Derry, N.H.). Serial samples were taken from the same three animals throughout the experiment. The tube was sealed with a Teflon-lined screw cap, subjected to vortex mixing for a few seconds until the blood was uniformly dispersed, acidified by adding 0.5 ml of 2N HCl, and again subjected to vortex mixing. Then 5 ml of benzene was added, and the tube was vigorously shaken for 1 min and centrifuged at 2000 rpm for 5 min.

The benzene layer was carefully transferred to a 50-ml glass-stoppered flask with a syringe and cannula, and the aqueous layer in the tube was extracted with an additional 5-ml portion of benzene in

an identical manner. [Note: Care was taken to withdraw as much of
the benzene layer as possible (4.75 ml) with each extraction; however,
none of the aqueous phase should ever be withdrawn into the cannula
or syringe. Anhydrous sodium sulfate was shown to absorb nanogram
amounts of 2,4,5-T from benzene solutions. Therefore, it cannot be
used to remove water from the benzene extracts in these procedures.]

The aqueous phase was reserved for subsequent alkaline hydrolysis
of possible conjugates. One milliliter of keeper solution (100 μg of
paraffin oil per milliliter of benzene) and a boiling bead were added
to the flask containing the combined benzene extracts (2,4,5-T and
its glycineamide), and the contents were evaporated just to dryness
by using water pump vacuum and a 60°C water bath. Residues of the
free acids were then converted to their methyl esters by the addition
of 2 ml of an ethereal solution of diazomethane. After 15 min, the
diazomethane solution was evaporated under water pump vacuum at
ambient temperature, and the residue was dissolved in 5 ml of hexane-
20% benzene for the subsequent column cleanup or in an appropriate
volume of benzene (1 ml or more) for direct injection into the gas
chromatograph.

The aqueous phase was subjected to alkaline hydrolysis by adding
0.5 ml of 4 N NaOH and heating the sealed tube at 85°C for 2 hr with
occasional shaking. After the tube had cooled, 1 ml of 4 N HCl was
added; any 2,4,5-T or glycineamide freed from the conjugates by the
digestion was extracted as 2,4,5-T, methylated, and analyzed as previously described. (Any conjugate of the glycineamide freed by the
hydrolysis would also be further hydrolyzed to 2,4,5-T.) Gas chromatographic analysis of the methylated extracts without column chromatographic cleanup was performed whenever possible, because the recovery
was higher and the time per analysis was shorter than analysis with
column cleanup. However, total residues of 10 ng or less of the
compounds, particularly after alkaline hydrolysis, must be subjected
to the cleanup because the high electron-capturing background pre-
cludes accurate quantitation at these low levels.

The chromatographic cleanup column (No. 420,000, Kontes Glass
Co., Vineland, N.J.) consisted of 0.5 g of the silica gel supported

by a small plug of glass wool; it was prewashed with 10 ml of hexane. The methylated extract from the free acid fraction or from the alkaline hydrolysis dissolved in 5 ml of hexane-20% benzene was added to the column and allowed to percolate into the adsorbent; then the flask and column were washed with two additional 1.5-ml portions of the solvent. The effluent was discarded, and the original 50-ml boiling flask was placed under the column to receive the subsequent eluate. The column was then eluted with 20 ml of hexane-40% benzene. This eluate, containing the methyl ester of 2,4,5-T, was evaporated just to dryness, and the residue was dissolved in an appropriate amount of benzene (1 ml or more) for injection.

When residues of the methyl ester of the glycineamide were also sought from the column, the adsorbent was deactivated by the addition of 1 ml of absolute methanol and eluted with 10 ml of benzene. The eluate was evaporated and reconstituted in benzene for GC analysis as described for the methyl ester of 2,4,5-T. (Note: If a column cleanup of the ethyl ester of 2,4,5-T is sought, the extract is added to the column with 15 ml of hexane-20% benzene and the eluate is discarded. The ethyl ester is then eluted from the column with 25 ml of hexane-40% benzene.)

h. Analysis of urine   The urine samples were collected in the 30-ml tube of the animal chamber. The animal and its metal support were removed, and any feces collected on the screen were reserved for separate analysis. The screen and walls of the chamber were then washed three times with 5-ml portions of 1 N HCl and twice with 5-ml portions of benzene. The 30-ml culture tube containing the urine and washings was removed, sealed, vigorously shaken for 1 min, and centrifuged at 2000 rpm for 5 min. The benzene layer was transferred to a 50-ml glass-stoppered flask, and the aqueous layer was extracted with two additional 10-ml portions of benzene; the combined extracts were evaporated, methylated, and analyzed as described for blood.

The aqueous phase was subjected to alkaline hydrolysis by adding 2.5 ml of 10 N NaOH and heating the sealed tube at 85°C for 2 hr with occasional shaking. After the tube had cooled, 2.5 ml of 12 N HCl was added, and the aqueous phase was extracted with three 10-ml portions of benzene. The combined extracts were then prepared and analyzed as described for blood. Column chromatographic cleanup of the samples was performed as described for blood. The cleanup was usually required for all samples containing residues of 10 ng or less.

i. *Analysis of feces*   The excrement obtained from the screen of the animal chamber was transferred to a 12-ml culture tube, and three glass beads (5 mm diameter) and 3 ml of 1 N HCl were added. The sealed tube was subjected to vigorous vortex mixing for 1 min. After the addition of 5 ml of benzene, the acidified sample was gently shaken for 1 min and centrifuged at 2000 rpm for 5 min; the benzene layer was transferred to a 50-ml glass-stoppered flask as described for blood. The extraction was repeated with two additional 5-ml portions of benzene, and the combined extracts were prepared and analyzed as described for blood.

The aqueous phase was subjected to alkaline hydrolysis as described for blood, except that 1 ml of 6 N NaOH was used. After hydrolysis, 1 ml of 8 N HCl was added; then the sample was extracted, prepared, and analyzed as described for blood. The column cleanup of fecal extracts on silica gel also was performed as described for blood; this cleanup was required for extracts containing residues of 100 ng or less.

j. *Recovery experiments*   Forty-four 24-hr collections of urine and feces from untreated mice in the sampling chambers yielded a mean volume of 0.48 ± 0.26 ml of urine and a mean weight of 0.19 ± 0.05 g of feces per animal per day. The urine was composited and diluted with distilled water to produce 0.48 ml of undiluted mouse urine per 3 ml of solution. The feces were composited and mixed by grinding with a mortar and pestle to ensure uniformity. Portions of these samples and fresh mouse blood (20 µl) were used as substrates in the development of analytical methodology based on EC-GC analysis.

Portions (0.5 ml) of distilled water, each containing the equivalent of 20 µl of whole mouse blood, were added to triplicate

8-ml culture tubes containing 0-, 10-, 100-, or 1000-ng amounts of 2,4,5-T or 0-, 10-, or 100-ng amounts of the glycineamide as dry residues. After vortex mixing, the samples were analyzed for free acids as described. After extraction, the aqueous samples were again spiked at the same levels by adding 50 μl of acetone containing the appropriate amount of acid or glycineamide. These samples were then subjected to alkaline hydrolysis and analyzed as described.

Triplicate 0.19-g portions of the composited feces in 12-ml culture tubes, or 3-ml portions of the diluted urine composite in 30-ml culture tubes, were spiked with 0, 10, 100, or 1000 ng of 2,4,5-T or 0, 25, or 250 ng of glycineamide in 50 μl of acetone. After vortex mixing, the samples were analyzed as described. The aqueous phases were then spiked again in an identical manner, hydrolyzed, and analyzed as described.

4. *Results and Discussion*

The analytical methods previously described were developed specifically for the mouse substrates to be assayed in pharmacokinetic studies with 2,4,5-T; the analytical scheme is presented in Figure 3.37. The binding of the free acids to proteins, especially in the whole blood, is considered to be relatively weak, since acidification with hydrochloric acid and extraction with benzene yielded good recoveries from samples spiked with both 2,4,5-T and the glycineamide.

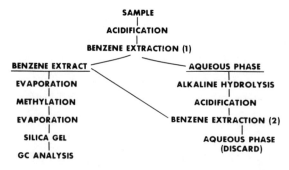

Figure 3.37. Analytical scheme for 2,4,5-T, its glycineamide, and alkaline hydrolyzable conjugates in mouse blood, urine, and feces. (From Nony et al. [89].)

Table 3.34. Gas chromatographic data for the quantification of 2,4,5-T and its glycineamide as their methyl and ethyl esters

Compound	Retention time (min)[a]		Upper limit of linearity (pg)[b]	
	200°C	240°C	200°C	200°C
2,4,5-T methyl ester	1.40	--[c]	25	--[c]
2,4,5-T ethyl ester	1.90	--[c]	44	--[c]
Glycineamide methyl ester	8.00	2.25	160	70
Glycineamide ethyl ester	8.80	2.52	250	125

Source: Nony et al. [89].

[a]Column oven operated isothermally at stated temperatures.

[b]Response was for 5-μl injection at about 5 x 10^{-10} amp.

[c]Solvent interference precluded determination.

Nevertheless, the acidification and extraction of free acids should be expedited and the residues should be methylated and stored as the esters to prevent losses due to the tendency of nanogram amounts of the free acids to become associated with various surfaces. The aqueous phase remaining after extraction of the free acids may be stored in a refrigerator pending alkaline hydrolysis.

Data concerning the EC-GC characteristics of the methyl and ethyl esters of 2,4,5-T and the glycineamide are presented in Table 3.34. Although ethylation of the compounds was not required in this study, information pertaining to the ethyl esters may be useful for assaying other substrates having background interferences at the t_R's of the methyl esters.

Typical chromatograms of standards of the methyl esters of 2,4,5-T and its glycineamide and extracts of untreated mouse blood before and after being spiked with the esters of the two compounds are presented in Figure 3.38. Similar chromatograms of mouse urine and feces are presented in Figure 3.39.

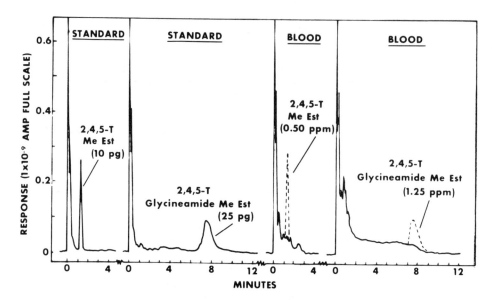

Figure 3.38. Gas chromatograms of methyl ester
(Me Est) standards of 2,4,5-T, its glycineamide,
and cleaned-up blood extracts in benzene spiked
with the standards (injection = 5 µl). (From
Nony et al. [89].)

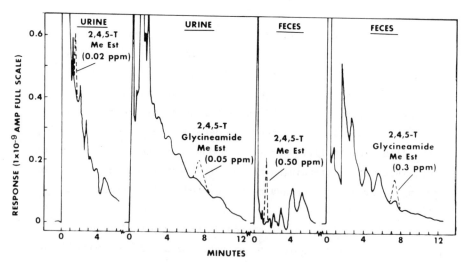

Figure 3.39. Gas chromatograms of cleaned-up
urine and feces extracts spiked with the methyl
esters (Me Est) of 2,4,5-T, and its glycineamide.
Extracts containing 10 and 25 pg of the methyl
esters of 2,4,5-T and its glycineamide, respectively, were injected in 5 µl of benzene.
(From Nony et al. [89].)

192

Table 3.35. Extraction p-values of the methyl and ethyl esters
of 2,4,5-T and its glycineamide

	2,4,5-T		Glycineamide	
Solvent system	Methyl ester	Ethyl ester	Methyl ester	Ethyl ester
Chloroform-water	1.00	1.00	1.00	1.00
Chloroform-60% methanol	1.00	1.00	1.00	1.00
Hexane-water	1.00	1.00	0.95	1.00
Hexane-acetonitrile	0.078	0.12	0.011	0.018
Isooctane-80% acetone	0.73	0.81	0.27	0.40
Isooctane-dimethylformamide	0.035	0.048	--[a]	--[a]
Isooctane-85% dimethylformamide	0.12	0.21	0.00	0.01
Heptane-90% ethanol	0.39	0.50	0.050	0.076
Benzene-water[b]	1.00	0.96	1.00	0.98

Source: Nony et al. [89].

[a]Solvent interference precluded determination.

[b]Detection was by EC-GC. All others were by FID-GC.

The p-values of the methyl and ethyl esters of 2,4,5-T and the
glycineamide, which are extremely useful in developing extraction and
cleanup methods and confirming identity at trace levels, are presented
in Table 3.35. The p-values for 2,4,5-T and the glycineamide in
chloroform-water or benzene-water (pH 0-2) were in line with those
reported [96] for 2,4,5-T (i.e., 0.96-1.0). The identity of trace
levels of 2,4,5-T and the glycineamide extracted from the blood and
excreta of animals dosed with 2,4,5-T in the present studies was
confirmed by using p-values.

In tests pertaining to the efficiency of hydrolyzing the methyl
and ethyl esters of the glycineamide with aqueous sodium hydroxide
at 85°C for 2 hr, recoveries of 2,4,5-T accounted for 98 and 97% of
the compounds, respectively. Since no trace of intact glycineamide
could be detected, these hydrolysis conditions were adopted for the
analytical procedure.

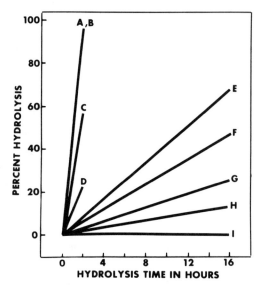

Figure 3.40. Percent hydrolysis of the
glycineamide of 2,4,5-T under various
conditions. Key: A, 1 N NaOH at 85°C;
B, 5 N HCl at 85°C; C, 1 N HCl at 85°C;
D, 0.5 N NaOH at 25°C; E, 5 N NaOH at 5°C;
F, 1 N NaOH at 5°C; G, 0.5 N NaOH at 5°C;
H, 0.1 N NaOH at 25°C; and I, 0.1 N NaOH
at 5°C or 0.1, 1, or 5 N HCl at 5 and 25°C.
(From Nony et al. [89].)

    The extent of hydrolysis of the glycineamide under various
conditions is illustrated in Figure 3.40. Aqueous sulfuric acid
(0.01, 0.05, 0.10, 0.50, and 1.0 N) failed to yield any detectable
hydrolysis at 25°C for 2 hr. Also, aqueous hydrochloric acid (0.1,
1.0, and 5.0 N) failed to hydrolyze the glycineamide at 5 or 25°C
over 16 hr. However, significant hydrolysis occurred with aqueous
sodium hydroxide (0.1-0.5 N) at 25°C. These data indicated that
residues of the glycineamide should not be mixed with sodium hydroxide
unless hydrolysis is intended. Therefore, samples containing the
glycineamide or conjugates were immediately acidified and extracted
to ensure the integrity of the analytical results.
    Results from blood, urine, and feces of untreated mice, spiked
and analyzed via EC-GC, are presented in Tables 3.36, 3.37, and 3.38,

Table 3.36. Electron-capture GC analysis of 2,4,5-T and its glycineamide from mouse blood before and after silica gel cleanup of free acid and hydrolyzed fractions

Compound	Added (ng)	Recovered ($\bar{x} \pm$ SE)[a]			
		Before cleanup		After cleanup	
		ng	%[b]	ng	%[b]
2,4,5-T[c]	0	1.2 ± 0.07	--	1.0 ± 0.44	--
	10	9.2 ± 0.70	80 ± 7	9.2 ± 1.05	82 ± 10
	100	96 ± 2.1	95 ± 2	66 ± 2.1	65 ± 2
	1000	987 ± 11.6	99 ± 1	718 ± 20.2	72 ± 2
2,4,5-T[d]	0	--[e]	--	0.9 ± 0.25	--
	10	--[e]	--	6.5 ± 0.91	54 ± 9
	100	99 ± 3.1	99 ± 3	75 ± 3.1	74 ± 3
	1000	1063 ± 63.5	106 ± 6	863 ± 35.9	86 ± 4
Glycineamide[f]	0	1.7 ± 0.25	--	1.4 ± 0.00	--
	10	7.6 ± 0.75[g]	59 ± 7[g]	9.9 ± 0.75	85 ± 8
	100	91 ± 3.8	89 ± 4	85 ± 7.9	84 ± 8
Glycineamide[h] (10 ng = 8.2 ng of 2,4,5-T)	0	--[e]	--	0.7 ± 0.16	--
	10	--[e]	--	5.4 ± 3.1	66 ± 4
	100	79 ± 1.2	96 ± 1	68 ± 3.2	83 ± 4

Source: Nony et al, [89].
[a]Mean and standard error from triplicate assays.
[b]Corrected for background interference in the unspiked sample.
[c]Analyzed as the methyl ester of 2,4,5-T.
[d]Respiked after extraction of 2,4,5-T and then hydrolyzed.
[e]High background interference precluded assay without column cleanup.
[f]Analyzed as the methyl ester of glycineamide.
[g]High background interference; quantitation is an estimate.
[h]Respiked after extraction of glycineamide and then hydrolyzed.

Table 3.37. Electron-capture GC analysis of 2,4,5-T and its glycineamide from mouse urine before and after silica gel cleanup of free acid and hydrolyzed fractions

Compound	Added ng	Recovered ($\bar{x} \pm SE$)[a]			
		Before cleanup		After cleanup	
		ng	%[b]	ng	%[b]
2,4,5-T[c]	0	35.3 ± 1.16	--	5.1 ± 0.00	--
	10	43.6 ± 0.00	83 ± 0	15.3 ± 1.01	102 ± 10
	100	147 ± 0.0	112 ± 0	113 ± 3.8	108 ± 4
	1000	1200 ± 10	116 ± 1	987 ± 130	98 ± 13
2,4,5-T[d]	0	15.0 ± 2.25	--	0.68 ± 0.13	--
	10	18.5 ± 0.17	35 ± 2	5.6 ± 0.14	49 ± 1
	100	97 ± 2.2	82 ± 2	110 ± 1.7	109 ± 2
	1000	1053 ± 13	104 ± 1	1043 ± 46	104 ± 5
Glycineamide[e]	0	12.3 ± 2.24	--	5.8 ± 0.70	--
	25	27.0 ± 1.07	59 ± 4	29.4 ± 1.34	94 ± 5
	250	246 ± 7.5	94 ± 3	259 ± 8.3	101 ± 3
Glycineamide[e,f] (25 ng = 20.4 ng of 2,4,5-T)	0	15.0 ± 2.25	--	0.7 ± 0.13	--
	25	26.3 ± 1.52	55 ± 7	20.3 ± 0.91	96 ± 4
	250	218 ± 7	100 ± 3	205 ± 18	100 ± 9

Source: Nony et al. [89].

[a]Mean and standard error from triplicate assays.
[b]Corrected for background interference in the unspiked sample.
[c]Analyzed as the methyl ester of 2,4,5-T.
[d]Respiked after extraction of 2,4,5-T and then hydrolyzed.
[e]Analyzed as the methyl ester of glycineamide.
[f]Respiked after extraction of glycineamide and then hydrolyzed.

Table 3.38. Electron-capture GC analysis of 2,4,5-T and its glycineamide from mouse feces before and after silica gel cleanup of free acid and hydrolyzed fractions

Compound	Added ng	Recovered ($\bar{x} \pm SE$)[a]			
		Before cleanup		After cleanup	
		ng	%[b]	ng	%[b]
2,4,5-T[c]	0	18[d]	--	1.0 ± 0.67	--
	10	26[d]	80	8.4 ± 0.79	74 ± 8
	100	128[d]	110	91 ± 3.8	90 ± 4
	1000	983 ± 10	96 ± 1	950 ± 23	95 ± 2
2,4,5-T[c,e]	0	34.3 ± 13.9	--	0.7 ± 0.29	--
	10	45.1 ± 1.0	108 ± 10	7.8 ± 0.10	71 ± 1
	100	116 ± 13	82 ± 13	104 ± 6	103 ± 6
	1000	1006 ± 1	97 ± 0	1013 ± 6	101 ± 1
Glycineamide[f]	0	71.4 ± 0.0	--	23.8 ± 4.0	--
	25	138 ± 6	266 ± 24	75.3 ± 2.9	105 ± 12
	250	297 ± 6[h]	90 ± 2	274 ± 2	100 ± 1
Glycineamide[c,g] (25 ng = 20.4 ng of 2,4,5-T)	0	--[h]	--	0.7 ± 0.29	--
	25	--[h]	--	18.5 ± 3.21	87 ± 16
	250	194 ± 26	95 ± 13	208 ± 3	102 ± 2

Source: Nony et al. [89].

[a] Mean and standard error from triplicate assays.
[b] Corrected for background interference in the unspiked sample.
[c] Analyzed as the methyl ester of 2,4,5-T.
[d] High background interference; quantitation is an estimate.
[e] Respiked after extraction of 2,4,5-T and then hydrolyzed.
[f] Analyzed as the methyl ester of glycineamide.
[g] Respiked after extraction of glycineamide and then hydrolyzed.
[h] High background interference precluded assay without column cleanup.

Table 3.39. Electron-capture GC and radiochemical analyses of 2,4,5-T, its glycineamide, and alkaline hydrolyzable conjugates in blood from mice injected with $[^{14}C]$2,4,5-T(nanograms per microliter of blood)[a]

Sampling time	Assay	2,4,5-T	Glycineamide	Alkaline hydrolyzable conjugates	Total as 2,4,5-T
Pretreatment	EC-GC	0.31 ± 0.06[b]	0.20 ± 0.03	0.26 ± 0.40	0.73
	Radiochemical	3.73 ± 1.61[b]	--	12.0 ± 1.6	15.7
5 min	EC-GC	950 ± 431	0.36 ± 0.12	0.41 ± 0.64	951
	Radiochemical	904 ± 410	--	23.0 ± 15.1	927
30 min	EC-GC	672 ± 101	0.41 ± 0.17	0.19 ± 0.32	673
	Radiochemical	690 ± 109[b]	--	3.53 ± 1.88	694
1 hr	EC-GC	450 ± 126	0.36 ± 0.08	<0.26 ± 0.40[c]	450
	Radiochemical	423 ± 125[b]	--	8.72 ± 2.60	432
2 hr	EC-GC	381 ± 111	0.73 ± 0.31	5.37 ± 3.12	387
	Radiochemical	355 ± 104[b]	--	6.18 ± 5.41	361
4 hr	EC-GC	489 ± 157	1.01 ± 0.14	11.8 ± 3.9	502
	Radiochemical	472 ± 157[b]	--	6.03 ± 4.41	478
8 hr	EC-GC	279 ± 65	1.05 ± 0.15	5.80 ± 3.63	286
	Radiochemical	266 ± 71[b]	--	26.6 ± 8.62	293
24 hr[d]	EC-GC	68.9	0.05	2.24	71.2
	Radiochemical	57.8[b]	--	<12.0[c]	69.8
48 hr[d]	EC-GC	60.1	0.13	1.46	61.7
	Radiochemical	50.4[b]	--	0.23	50.6
72 hr	EC-GC	47.5 ± 34.0	0.43 ± 0.55	2.95 ± 3.19	50.8
	Radiochemical	41.3 ± 30.8[b]	--	11.5 ± 1.5	52.8

Source: Nony et al. [89].
[a]Mean and standard error from three mice. Results are corrected for pretreatment sample background.
[b]The ^{14}C assay did not resolve the individual free acids; therefore, this result represents both.
[c]None detected above background.
[d]Data from a single and different mouse treated in the same manner. Physical condition of the other three animals precluded sampling at this interval.

respectively. Excellent recoveries were obtained from all three
substrates spiked with 100- and 1000-ng amounts of 2,4,5-T analyzed
both before and after the silica gel cleanup. Results from the
aqueous sample residues respiked prior to hydrolysis indicated that
the previous extractions had efficiently removed 2,4,5-T and that
the additional 2,4,5-T was recovered from the hydrolysis procedure.
Samples of blood or urine containing 100 ng or more of 2,4,5-T should
be analyzed without utilizing the silica gel cleanup to obtain higher
recoveries and to speed the analysis. The background interference in
urine was reduced from about 35.3 to 5.1 ng equivalents of 2,4,5-T by
utilizing a silica gel column; therefore, the cleanup is required
where low levels of residues are sought. Feces should be cleaned up
at all residue levels below 1000 ng.

Good recoveries were obtained for the glycineamide from the
three substrates spiked at all levels and especially after the extracts were cleaned up on silica gel. Results from the analysis of
the residual aqueous substrates respiked with glycineamide prior to
hydrolysis and assayed as 2,4,5-T demonstrated that the previous
extraction of glycineamide was complete and that hydrolysis of
glycineamide and recovery of the 2,4,5-T moiety were accomplished.

Rinses of the animal chambers with various amounts, combinations,
and sequences of aqueous sodium hydroxide (1 N), hydrochloric acid
(1 N), benzene, methanol, acetone, ether, and aqueous (ethylenedi-
nitrilo)tetraacetate (1 mg/ml) were performed to determine the most
efficient means of conveniently recovering the radioactivity depos-
ited by the urine from mice injected with [^{14}C]2,4,5-T. The use of
aqueous sodium hydroxide followed by benzene yielded a slightly
better recovery (99.4%) of the total radioactivity than did aqueous
hydrochloric acid followed by benzene (97.3%). Nevertheless, the use
of hydrochloric acid was adopted to prevent any possible hydrolysis
of the glycineamide or conjugates by the alkali during the rinsing
process.

Results of the preliminary pharmacokinetic studies with mice
injected with [^{14}C]2,4,5-T, as determined by parallel EC-GC and radioassays, are presented for blood, urine, and feces in Tables 3.39,

Table 3.40. Electron-capture GC and radiochemical analyses of 2,4,5-T, its glycineamide, and alkaline hydrolyzable conjugates in urine from mice injected with [14C]2,4,5-T (micrograms per sampling interval)a

Sampling interval (hr)	Assay	2,4,5-T	Glycineamide	Alkaline hydrolyzable conjugates	Total as 2,4,5-T
Pretreatment	EC-GC	0.01 ± 0.00	0.06 ± 0.05	<0.01 ± 0.00b	0.07
	Radiochemical	0.02 ± 0.01c	--	0.03 ± 0.02	0.05
0-6	EC-GC	1.86 ± 1.45	<0.06 ± 0.05b	<0.01 ± 0.00b	1.92
	Radiochemical	1.83 ± 1.41c	--	0.05 ± 0.02b	1.88
6-24	EC-GC	13.7 ± 5.0	11.7 ± 6.25	<0.01 ± 0.00b	23.3
	Radiochemical	29.8 ± 11.5c	--	2.16 ± 0.98	32.0
24-30	EC-GC	7.10 ± 4.86	3.61 ± 4.18	<0.01 ± 0.00	10.1
	Radiochemical	9.16 ± 5.70c	--	1.03 ± 1.05	10.2
30-48	EC-GC	61.7 ± 76.6	28.3 ± 25.7	38.1 ± 39.9	123
	Radiochemical	83.8 ± 92.2c	--	39.8 ± 41.5	124
48-52	EC-GC	35.8 ± 54.6	7.28 ± 8.94	13.6 ± 2.9	55.4
	Radiochemical	39.5 ± 56.7c	--	14.2 ± 2.4	53.7
52-72	EC-GC	40.0 ± 32.4	22.0 ± 17.2	36.5 ± 12.8	94.5
	Radiochemical	59.4 ± 46.7c	--	37.1 ± 13.9	96.5

Source: Nony et al. [89].
aMean and standard error from three mice. Results are corrected for pretreatment sample background.
bNone detected above background.
cThe 14C assay did not resolve the individual free acids; therefore, this result represents both.

Table 3.41. Electron-capture GC and radiochemical analyses of 2,4,5-T, its glycineamide, and alkaline hydrolyzable conjugates in feces from mice injected with [14C]2,4,5-T (micrograms per sampling interval)[a]

Sampling interval (hr)	Mean sample weight (mg, mean ± SE)	Assay	2,4,5-T	Glycineamide	Alkaline hydrolyzable conjugates	Total as 2,4,5-T
Pretreatment	538 ± 108	EC-GC	0.01 ± 0.00	0.04 ± 0.03	0.01 ± 0.00	0.05 ± 0.02
		Radiochemical	0.02 ± 0.01[b]	--	0.02 ± 0.01	0.04 ± 0.01
0-6	43.6 ± 42.1	EC-GC	1.44 ± 1.07[b]	<0.06 ± 0.01[c]	0.10 ± 0.07	1.54 ± 1.14
		Radiochemical	1.52 ± 1.05[b]	--	0.10 ± 0.06	1.62 ± 1.11
6-24	89.0 ± 7.4	EC-GC	4.62 ± 0.78[b]	<0.04 ± 0.02[c]	0.89 ± 0.61	5.51 ± 0.71
		Radiochemical	5.56 ± 0.82[b]	--	1.01 ± 0.60	6.57 ± 0.48
24-30	57.7 ± 29.1	EC-GC	2.07 ± 1.14	<0.04 ± 0.03[c]	0.73 ± 0.42	2.80 ± 1.56
		Radiochemical	2.75 ± 1.55[b]	--	0.85 ± 0.53	3.60 ± 2.08
30-48	262 ± 203	EC-GC	16.9 ± 11.8	1.47 ± 1.96	7.10 ± 9.23	25.2 ± 21.7
		Radiochemical	19.4 ± 13.8[b]	--	7.30 ± 9.32	26.7 ± 22.4
48-52	25.8 ± 14.8	EC-GC	0.99 ± 0.44	<0.05 ± 0.01[c]	0.11 ± 0.06	1.12 ± 0.45
		Radiochemical	1.09 ± 0.52[b]	--	0.10 ± 0.06	1.19 ± 0.54
52-72	363 ± 265	EC-GC	7.30 ± 6.70[b]	0.12 ± 0.10	2.56 ± 2.40	9.95 ± 9.07
		Radiochemical	7.96 ± 7.86[b]	--	2.50 ± 2.39	10.5 ± 10.2

Source: Nony et al. [89].

[a]Mean and standard error from three mice. Results are corrected for pretreatment sample background.

[b]The ^{14}C assay did not resolve the individual free acids; therefore, this result represents both.

[c]None detected above background.

3.40, and 3.41, respectively. No results are reported for the
glycineamide via radioassay; since the radioassay did not resolve
2,4,5-T and the glycineamide, the value reported for 2,4,5-T
includes both compounds. The concentration of 2,4,5-T and its
products found in the blood was highest (>900 ng/μl) at the first
sampling period (5 min after injection) and declined to about 50
ng/μl during the 72-hr test period, as expected after intravenous
injection. Residues of the glycineamide and the alkaline hydrolyzable conjugates accounted for only a small percentage of radioactivity
of the material present, which existed primarily as 2,4,5-T.

   Results from the urine assays indicated that only trace amounts
of 2,4,5-T and its products were excreted during the 6-hr period
immediately after injection. However, during the 6 to 24-hr interval
and thereafter, appreciable amounts of 2,4,5-T, the glycineamide, and
conjugates were excreted. Low levels of 2,4,5-T and lesser amounts
of conjugates were found in the mouse feces at all intervals of sampling. No significant amount of the glycineamide was obtained from
the feces.

   Radioassay results from the blood, urine, and feces generally
correlated well with those from the EC-GC procedure. Radioassays
of the residual substrates (after hydrolysis and extraction), column
adsorbents, and discarded solvents indicated that essentially all
radioactivity had been extracted from the samples and that losses
during the analytical procedure were negligible.

   B.   Rotenone and Degradation Products [97]

   1. General Description of Methods
A procedure is described for determining residues of rotenone,
rotenolone, dehydrorotenone, and rotenonone in admixture in animal
chow and tissues. The methanol or diethyl ether extracts from
samples of chow and tissues, respectively, are subjected to a
liquid-liquid partitioning cleanup with hexane-acetonitrile, further
cleanup on a column of silica gel, and subsequent analysis by HPLC
by using an ultraviolet absorption detector set at 295 nm. Data are

presented concerning rates of decomposition of rotenone in spiked
chow and on glass surfaces under various conditions of exposure.
Information is also presented concerning transplacental activity of
rotenone in mice as well as the stability of the compound within the
gastrointestinal (GI) gract of the test animal.

   2. *Introduction*

Rotenone {1,2,12,12a-tetrahydro-8,9-dimethoxy-2-(1-methylethenyl)-
[1]benzopyrano[3,4-b]furo[2,3-h][1]benzopyran-6(6H)-one}, a principal
insecticidal constituent of derris root, was first isolated in 1895
by Geoffrey [98]; its structure was established by LaForge et al. in
1933 [99]. Derris resins have been approved for use on a variety of
crops and for controlling pests including mosquitos [100]. Recently,
however, rotenone was shown to be tumorigenic in rats [101,102] and
the U. S. Environmental Protection Agency has scheduled a reevalua-
tion of its possible hazards to humans and the environment [103].
The possibility that this extremely useful insecticide may be banned
prompted Haley [102] to review the chemistry, toxicology, and carcinogenic effects of the compound to ascertain whether a problem actually
exists. Haley [102] concluded that additional lifetime studies with
large groups of rodents fed rotenone at low levels (50 ppm or less)
in the diet would be required to solve the dilemma. Because of the
instability of rotenone and its degradation to a multitude of rotenoid-
type products of unknown carcinogenic properties, Haley [102] also
placed special emphasis on the need for assaying the purity of the
rotenone employed as well as on dietary analysis for its stability
under the experimental conditions. Since these tests were to be conducted at the NCTR, an analytical procedure capable of satisfying
these requirements was sought. The analysis of tissues from rodents
(e.g., GI tracts and fetuses) was also sought to determine the stability of rotenone in the digestive system of the test animals and
to signal possible transplacental activity of the compound.

   Most of the early analytical methods for rotenone were based on
colorimetry [104-107], infrared spectrometry [108-110], gravimetric
analysis [111], and paper chromatography [112-115]. Later, several

procedures employing TLC appeared [116-118] and during this period, data concerning the photodecomposition of rotenone was also reported [119,120]. Delfel developed a GC procedure for rotenone and deguelin employing FID [121] and also reported on the effect of rotenoids on the ultraviolet and infrared analysis of rotenone [122].

Recently, procedures were reported for determining rotenone and several rotenoids in admixture via HPLC [123-125]; however, only pesticide formulations or pure compounds were analyzed. None of the procedures described in the literature appeared amenable to the analysis of low ppm levels of rotenone and its common degradation products in substrates such as animal chow and tissues. The following procedures were therefore developed for use in our toxicological tests. Formulas of rotenone and three degradation products are shown in Figure 3.41.

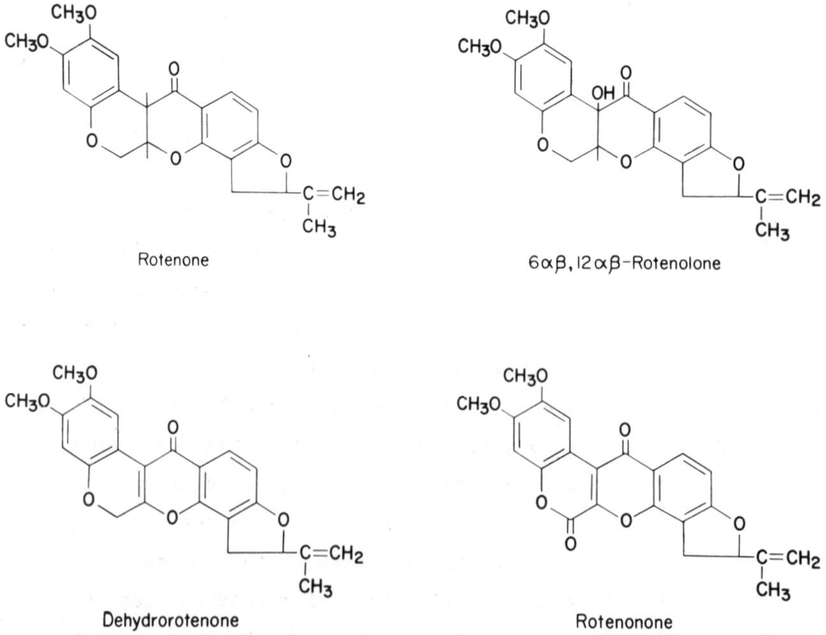

Rotenone

6αβ,12αβ-Rotenolone

Dehydrorotenone

Rotenonone

Figure 3.41. Formulas of rotenone and three of its degradation products. (From Bowman et al. [97].)

3. Experimental

a. Materials

(1) Test chemicals. The rotenone, obtained from Battelle Laboratories, Columbus, Ohio, contained no extraneous responses via HPLC
and was therefore considered essentially pure. The three degradation
products of rotenone, kindly furnished by N. E. Delfel, Northern
Regional Research Center, U. S. Department of Agriculture, Peoria,
Ill., were analyzed by HPLC and the results were as follows:
rotenolone also contained 4.8% of rotenone, dehydrorotenone also
contained 1.4% of rotenone and 4.2% rotenonone, and the rotenonone
contained 5.5% of dehydrorotenone and 5.5% of an unknown product
(calculated as rotenone) having a t_R value 1.23 times that of
rotenonone. The presence of these impurities was considered in the
preparation of individual standard solutions and of mixtures.

(2) Silica gel cleanup columns. Heat silica gel (No. 3405, J. T.
Baker Chemical Co., Phillipsburg, N.J.) overnight at 130°C and store
in a desiccator. Partially deactivate by adding 97 g of the dry
material to a glass-stoppered bottle containing 3 ml of water dispersed on its inner surface. Mix the contents well and allow to
stand for 24 hr with occasional shaking prior to use.

Prepare columns (12 mm i.d., No. 420,000, Kontes Glass Co.,
Vineland, N.J.), equipped with a 50-ml reservoir, immediately prior
to use by successively adding a plug of glass wool, 5 g of sodium
sulfate, 5 g of silica gel (3% water), and 5 g of sodium sulfate;
wash with 20 ml of benzene and discard the eluate.

(3) Solvents and reagents. All solvents were pesticide grade and
all reagents were CP grade; the sodium sulfate was anhydrous.

(4) Solvents for partition cleanup. The hexane and acetonitrile
were equilibrated with each other immediately prior to use.

(5) Test animals and chow. The mice, females about 10 weeks old,
of either CD-1 or C3H strains were reared at the NCTR. The chow was
type 5010C (Ralston Purina Co., St. Louis, Mo.).

b. High-pressure liquid chromatography A Waters Associates, Inc., instrument (Milford, Mass.) equipped with a Model 6000 solvent delivery system, a Model U6K septumless injector, a Model 970 variable wavelength detector (Tracor, Inc., Austin, Tex.) set at 295 nm, and a 30 cm x 4 mm i.d. column of μ-Bondapak C_{18} (reverse phase, Waters, No. 27324) was operated with the mobile phase (methanol-water, 75:25) flowing at the rate of 1 ml/min at 1300 psi. Under these conditions, t_R values of the compounds in minutes were as follows: rotenolone, 5.90; rotenone, 6.80; dehydrorotenone, 12.70; and rotenonone, 14.80. All injections were 5 μl, responses (peak height or area) were linear, and samples were quantified by relating their peak height to those of known amounts of standards.

c. Extraction and cleanup of animal chow Weigh 20 g of animal chow into a 250-ml glass-stoppered flask, add 20 ml of distilled water to wet the sample, then add 100 ml of benzene. Extract the sample for 2 hr in a reciprocating shaker at a rate of 200 excursions per minute. Filter the extract through a plug of anhydrous sodium sulfate (ca. 27 mm diameter x 30 mm thick), transfer 50 ml of the filtrate (10 g equivalents of chow) to a 100-ml round-bottom flask, and evaporate the extract to dryness by using a 60°C water bath and water pump vacuum. Transfer the residue to a 13-ml culture tube (Note: All culture tubes are equipped with Teflon-lined screw caps) by using 5 ml each of hexane and acetonitrile; shake the contents for 1 min, then centrifuge for 5 min at 1500 rpm. Carefully transfer the hexane layer to another 12-ml culture tube containing 5 ml of acetonitrile by using a syringe and cannula. Shake and centrifuge the contents of the second tube as described; discard the hexane layer. Use two additional 5-ml portions of hexane to sequentially rinse the flask and extract the acetonitrile layers in the two tubes as described. Transfer the acetonitrile phases to a 100-ml round-bottom flask by using 10 ml of benzene to wash the tubes; evaporate the contents to dryness at 60°C under reduced pressure as described and reserve the dry residue for subsequent cleanup on silica gel.

Transfer the residue to a silica gel column prepared as described
by using 5 ml of benzene then wash the flask and column with five
additional 5-ml portions of benzene allowing each portion to percolate
into the adsorbent; discard the eluate. Elute the rotenoids by using
70 ml of benzene-acetone (97:3), and collect the eluate in a 100-ml
round-bottom flask and evaporate it to dryness at 60°C under water
pump vacuum as described. Dissolve the residue in an appropriate
amount of methanol (0.5 ml or more) for injection (5 μl) into the
liquid chromatograph.

d. Extraction and cleanup of animal tissues   Transfer the sample
(ca. 2.5-5 g) of fetuses or GI tracts from mice to a tube (150 mm x
22 mm diameter), add 10 g of sodium sulfate and 20 ml of diethyl
ether, then thoroughly grind and extract the sample by using a glass
rod. Decant the supernatant solvent through a plug of sodium sulfate
(2 g) suspended in a small funnel by a plug of glass wool. Repeat
the extraction process with two additional 20-ml portions of diethyl
ether and evaporate the combined extracts to dryness as described.
Transfer the residue to a 13-ml culture tube by using 5 ml each of
hexane and acetonitrile and proceed with the analyses as described
for animal chow.

e. Recovery experiments

(1) Animal chow. Prepare triplicate 20-g samples of chow spiked
with 0, 5.0, and 50 ppm of rotenone or 0.50 ppm each of the four
compounds in admixture by adding the appropriate amount of chemical
in 1 ml of methanol. Allow the solvent to evaporate from the sample
by storing the open flask in a light-free cabinet for 1 hr, then mix
the sample and extract and analyze it as described.

(2) Tissues from mice. Prepare a homogeneous composite of fetuses
taken from untreated mice on the 19th day of pregnancy by blending
them in a Waring blender for about 1 min. Use individual GI tracts
(stomach and small intestine) from untreated mice. Prepare triplicate samples of fetuses (5 g) and GI tracts (ca. 2.5 g) spiked with
0 and about 0.50 ppm each of the four compounds in admixture by

adding the appropriate amount of the chemicals in 0.5 ml of methanol.
Mix the sample with a stirring rod and allow it to stand in a light-
free cabinet for 1 hr prior to extraction and analysis as described.

f. *Stability tests with rotenone*

(1) Animal chow. Prepare 1-kg batches of dosed chow at levels of
0, 5.0, and 50 ppm of rotenone by using a Model LV Twin-Shell Lab
Blender (Patterson-Kelley Co., Inc., East Stroudsburg, Pa.). Add
the appropriate amount of chemical dissolved in 50 ml of 95% ethyl
alcohol to the chow and use an additional 25-ml portion of the solvent
as a rinse. Operate the shell of the mixer at 20 rpm during the 25-
min mixing process and the intensifier bar at 3300 rpm only during
the first 5 min of mixing. Transfer each batch to a stainless steel
pan and dry it in an autoclave at ambient temperature for 18 hr under
reduced pressure (ca. 0.11 atm); divide each batch into two 450-g
portions and a 100-g portion. Place one of the 450-g portions from
each batch in a crystallizing dish (ca. 10 cm x 29 cm diameter) and
allow to stand in the open vessel in a fume hood with incandescent
lighting at ambient temperature for 16 days. Collect duplicate
samples for analysis of the rotenoids immediately and 1, 2, 4, 8, 12,
and 16 days later. Transfer the other 450-g portion to an amber glass
bottle; seal and store in a light-free cabinet at ambient temperature.
Collect duplicate samples for analysis of rotenoids immediately and
1, 2, 3, 4, 8, and 20 weeks later. Store the 100-g portions in a
sealed container in a freezer (-15°C) and analyze for rotenoids after
1, 2, 4, and 8 weeks.

Prepare 1-kg batches of chow containing 1.0 and 100 ppm of
rotenone exactly as described except that the appropriate amount of
chemical is contained in 10 ml of corn oil; use several small portions of the chow from the blender to remove any oil and chemical
adhering to the container. Divide each batch into three portions
immediately after mixing and perform stability studies in a manner
similar to those previously described.

(2) Dry residues. Prepare 24 150-ml beakers containing dry residues
of rotenone (ca. 1 $\mu g/cm^2$) by adding 0.5 ml of methanol containing

25 µg of rotenone to each beaker and plating the chemical on the bottom of the vessel by using a gentle stream of dry nitrogen. Analyze the contents of two of the beakers immediately and store half of those remaining in either a fume hood or in a light-free cabinet as described for stability studies with chow. Analyze duplicate beakers from each location after 1, 2, 5, 12, and 16 days.

g. Animal studies

(1) Stability of rotenone in the GI tract of mice. Prepare chow containing about 50 ppm of rotenone by using the procedure employing ethyl alcohol as a solvent. Analyze the feed on the following day and place four mice on test with the dosed chow for either 1 day or 4 days. Sacrifice the animals at the end of each test and analyze the GI tracts (and contents) for rotenone and degradation products. Also, analyze the dosed chow remaining in the cages at the end of each test.

Prepare a formulation of rotenone in corn oil (2 mg/ml) and administer an oral daily dose of 20 or 30 mg/kg in duplicate to mice for four consecutive days by using a syringe with a ball-tipped needle. Sacrifice the animals at the end of the fourth day and analyze the GI tracts and contents for rotenone and degradation products.

(2) Transplacental transfer of rotenone. Prepare a formulation of rotenone in corn oil (1.5 mg/ml) and administer seven consecutive oral daily doses of 0, 10, 15, 20, or 25 mg/kg to 10 mice for each dose level beginning on the 12th day of pregnancy. Sacrifice the animals on the 19th day of pregnancy, combine the live and dead or resorbed fetuses into separate groups from each dose level. (Note: Take care not to disturb the GI tract or otherwise contaminate the fetuses with traces of rotenone.) Analyze the samples of fetuses for rotenone and degradation products.

4. Results and Discussion

High-pressure liquid chromatography was selected for use as the determinative step of the procedure to provide good resolution of

the compounds [123-125] and to minimize possible degradation of the
residues during the assays. Ultraviolet absorption spectra for
rotenone, rotenolone, dehydrorotenone, and rotenonone in methanol
yielded maxima of 295, 298, 280, and 270 nm, respectively; however,
the 295-nm maximum for rotenone was selected for use in the procedure
since assays for the parent compound were of primary interest. The
295-nm setting yielded responses for rotenolone, dehydrorotenone, and
rotenonone that were about 99, 55, and 72%, respectively, of those
that could be obtained at their absorption maxima.

Cleanup columns of Sephadex LH-20, silica gel, and alumina
placed in tandem beneath silica gel were evaluated for possible use
in cleaning up extractives for residue analysis. In experiments with
the four compounds on a column of Sephadex (5 g) using benzene as the
solvent, only rotenolone was retained by the packing and it also
began to emerge after an elution of about 30 ml. A 5-g column of
silica gel (3% water) employing benzene as the solvent completely
retained all four compounds during an 80-ml elution; then by using
benzene-acetone (97:3) as the solvent, rotenone, dehydrorotenone,
and rotenonone began to emerge after about 10 ml of elution and were
completely recovered in the 10- to 30-ml fraction. On the other
hand, rotenolone first appeared after 20 ml of elution and was completely recovered in the 20- to 50-ml fraction; hence an elution
with 70 ml of benzene-acetone (97:3) was used in the analytical procedure to ensure complete recovery of all four compounds from the
column. In a trial with a column of neutral alumina (5 g, 3% water)
placed beneath a silica gel column and eluted as described, rotenone
and dehydrorotenone were completely recovered in the 20- to 40-ml
fraction of the benzene-acetone (97:3) eluate. However, an additional
60-ml portion of the solvent followed by 100 ml of benzene-acetone
(95:5) failed to remove any of the rotenolone or rotenonone. Further
elution with 50 ml of acetone followed by an equal volume of methanol
yielded 61 and 39% of the rotenolone; no rotenonone was detected.
Subsequent deactivation of the alumina with 2 ml of water and elution
with an additional 50-ml portion of methanol also failed to yield any

detectable amount of rotenonone. The column of silica gel was therefore selected for use in the procedure; nevertheless, the information
obtained concerning alumina could be useful for substracting residues
of rotenolone and rotenonone from a mixture of rotenoids or for iso-
lating rotenolone.

Methanol and benzene were found to be equally effective in extracting residues of the rotenoids from chow spiked at the 0.50-ppm
level and yielded recoveries in excess of 90%; benzene was selected
because an aliquot of the extract (e.g., 50 ml) could be conveniently
evaporated directly to dryness for the subsequent cleanup steps.
Both methanol and benzene extracts of unspiked chow after cleanup on
silica gel contained substances that interfered with the analysis of
low levels of rotenone and rotenonone; however, a liquid-liquid partitioning step employing hexane-acetonitrile prior to the silica gel
cleanup was effective in removing the interferences. Extraction
p-values for rotenone, rotenolone, dehydrorotenone, and rotenonone
in the hexane-acetonitrile system were found to be 0.021, 0.013,
0.032, and 0.059, respectively. All four compounds were found to
have p-values of about 1.00 in systems of chloroform-water, benzene-
water, benzene-10% acetonitrile (90% water), benzene-20% acetonitrile
(80% water), and benzene-30% methanol (70% water, 3% sodium chloride).
Diethyl ether was employed for the extraction of animal tissues since
recoveries of the four rotenoids averaged about 51% as compared with
an average of 21% obtained with benzene.

Results from assays of chow spiked with 0 and 0.5 ppm of all
four compounds and with 5.0 and 50 ppm of rotenone are presented in
Table 3.42. Recoveries of all compounds at all levels averaged about
93%. Minimum amounts of rotenone, rotenolone, dehydrorotenone, and
rotenonone detectable in chow (based on twice background) are 0.32,
0.07, 0.10, and 0.03 ppm, respectively. Results from assays of
fetuses and GI tracts spiked with 0 and about 0.50 ppm of the four
compounds are also presented in Table 3.42. Recoveries from fetuses
and GI tracts averaged about 51 and 79%, respectively; minimum amounts
of the rotenoids detectable in the two substrates (based on twice

Table 3.42. Analysis of rotenone, rotenolone, dehydrorotenone, and rotenonone in animal chow, fetuses, and GI tracts

Trial	Compounds	Added		Recovered ($\bar{x}$ ± SE)[a]		
		µg	ppm	µg	ppm	%
Animal Chow[b]						
1	Rotenone	0.0	0.0	3.22 ± 0.36	0.161 ± 0.018	--
	Rotenolone	0.0	0.0	0.72 ± 0.12	0.036 ± 0.006	--
	Dehydrorotenone	0.0	0.0	1.00 ± 0.04	0.050 ± 0.002	--
	Rotenonone	0.0	0.0	0.30 ± 0.02	0.015 ± 0.001	--
2	Rotenone	10.0	0.50	9.52 ± 0.42	0.476 ± 0.021	95.2 ± 4.2
	Rotenolone	10.0	0.50	9.48 ± 0.42	0.474 ± 0.021	94.8 ± 4.2
	Dehydrorotenone	10.0	0.50	8.66 ± 0.70	0.433 ± 0.035	86.6 ± 7.0
	Rotenonone	10.0	0.50	9.26 ± 0.84	0.463 ± 0.042	92.6 ± 8.4
3	Rotenone	100.0	5.00	93.2 ± 2.4	4.66 ± 0.12	93.2 ± 2.4[c]
4	Rotenone	1000.0	50.0	938 ± 6.2	46.9 ± 0.31	93.8 ± 0.6[c]
Fetuses[d]						
1	Rotenone	0.0	0.0	0.100 ± 0.005	0.020 ± 0.001	--
	Rotenolone	0.0	0.0	0.025 ± 0.005	0.005 ± 0.001	--
	Dehydrorotenone	0.0	0.0	0.110 ± 0.010	0.022 ± 0.002	--
	Rotenonone	0.0	0.0	0.105 ± 0.010	0.021 ± 0.002	--

2	Rotenone	1.85	0.37	1.10 ± 0.155	0.220 ± 0.031	59.4 ± 8.4
	Rotenolone	2.90	0.58	1.42 ± 0.255	0.284 ± 0.045	49.0 ± 8.8
	Dehydrorotenone	2.50	0.50	1.06 ± 0.125	0.212 ± 0.025	42.4 ± 5.0
	Rotenonone	1.50	0.30	0.800 ± 0.160	0.160 ± 0.032	53.3 ± 10.7
GI Tracts[e]						
1	Rotenone	0.0	0.0	0.200 ± 0.008	0.080 ± 0.003	--
	Rotenolone	0.0	0.0	0.050 ± 0.002	0.020 ± 0.001	--
	Dehydrorotenone	0.0	0.0	0.218 ± 0.005	0.087 ± 0.002	--
	Rotenonone	0.0	0.0	0.210 ± 0.010	0.084 ± 0.004	--
2	Rotenone	0.50	0.20	0.468 ± 0.058	0.187 ± 0.023	93.6 ± 11.6
	Rotenolone	1.60	0.64	0.982 ± 0.030	0.393 ± 0.012	61.4 ± 1.8
	Dehydrorotenone	1.30	0.52	1.21 ± 0.078	0.483 ± 0.031	93.1 ± 6.0
	Rotenonone	0.80	0.32	0.532 ± 0.078	0.213 ± 0.031	66.5 ± 9.8

Source: Bowman et al. [97].

[a]Mean and standard error from triplicate assays; spiked samples are corrected for background of unspiked samples.

[b]Per 20 g of sample.

[c]None of the other rotenoids were detected.

[d]Per 5 g of sample.

[e]Per 2.5 g of sample.

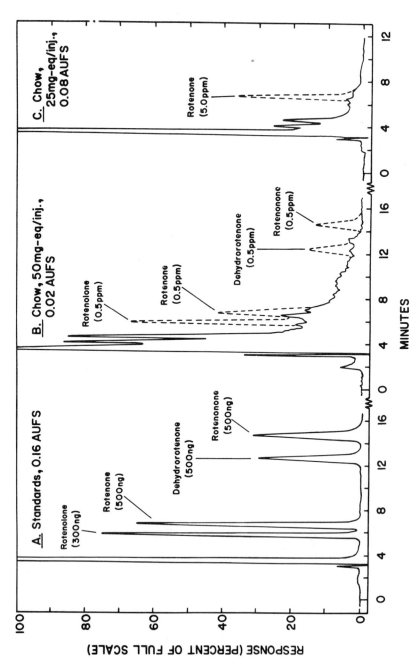

Figure 3.42. High pressure liquid chromatograms. A, analytical standards of the four rotenoids; in B and C, solid lines are cleaned-up extracts of unspiked chow, and broken lines (superimposed) represent 0.5 ppm of each compound or 5.0 ppm of rotenone, respectively. All injections were in 5 µl of methanol. (From Bowman et al, [97].)

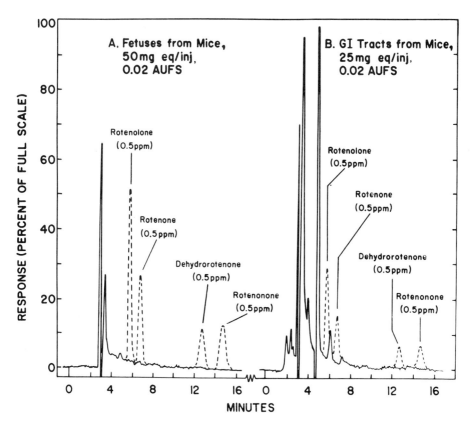

Figure 3.43. High-pressure liquid chromatograms.
In A and B solid lines are cleaned-up extracts of
fetuses and GI tracts, respectively; broken lines
(superimposed) represent 0.5 ppm of each compound.
All injections were in 5 µl of methanol. (From
Bowman et al. [97].)

background) are 0.04 and 0.16 ppm or better, respectively. There
was no evidence that any degradation of the residues occurred during
the analytical process.

Typical high-pressure liquid chromatograms for standards of the
rotenoids and for cleaned-up extracts of chow spiked with 0.5 ppm of
each compound or 5.0 ppm of rotenone are presented in Figure 3.42.
Similar chromatograms from cleaned-up extracts of fetuses and GI
tracts spiked with 0.50 ppm of the four rotenoids are presented in
Figure 3.43.

Table 3.43. Results from stability studies with rotenone in animal chow spiked at two levels by using ethyl alcohol

| Sampling interval | Rotenoids (ppm) recovered from preparation indicated[a] | | | | | |
| | 5 ppm | | | 50 ppm | | |
	Rotenone	Rotenolone	Total	Rotenone	Rotenolone	Total
Short-term Study (Ambient)[b]						
(days)						
0	4.07	0.34	4.41	38.5	3.2	41.7
1	3.75	0.52	4.27	35.5	5.0	40.5
2	3.45	0.67	4.12	31.2	6.3	37.5
4	2.79	0.86	3.65	24.5	8.2	32.7
8	2.45	1.22	3.67	20.4	11.1	31.5
12	2.09	1.42	3.51	16.4	12.4	28.8
16	1.78	1.54	3.32	15.0	14.2	29.2
Long-term Study (Ambient)[c]						
(weeks)						
0	4.07	0.34	4.41	38.5	3.2	41.7
1	2.97	0.89	3.86	25.6	9.4	35.0
2	2.24	1.24	3.48	19.6	12.4	32.0
4	1.50	1.55	3.05	13.9	14.6	28.5
8	1.48	1.85	3.33	11.8	16.0	27.8
20	1.14	1.68	2.82	10.8	16.1	26.9
Long-term Study (-15°C)[c]						
(weeks)						
0	4.86	0.13	4.99	43.9	1.0	44.9
1	4.90	0.09	4.99	44.2	1.4	45.6
2	4.95	0.16	5.11	43.6	1.3	44.9
4	4.50	0.25	4.75	43.4	2.2	45.6
8	4.35	0.34	4.69	43.2	2.0	45.2

Source: Bowman et al. [97].

[a]Average of duplicate assays corrected for background of 0.04 and 0.02 ppm of rotenone and rotenolone, respectively, in untreated chow.

[b]Open container, incandescent lighting.

[c]Sealed container, light-free storage.

Table 3.44. Results from stability studies with rotenone in animal chow spiked at two levels by using corn oil[a]

| Sampling interval (days) | Rotenoids (ppm) recovered from preparation indicated[b] | | | | | |
| | 1 ppm | | | 100 ppm | | |
	Rotenone	Rotenolone	Total	Rotenone	Rotenolone	Total
0	0.77	0.00	0.77	94.6	0.3	94.9
1	0.81	0.05	0.86	83.2	1.1	84.3
2	0.70	0.05	0.75	86.8	2.1	88.9
4	0.67	0.23	0.90	79.1	5.1	84.2
8	0.67	0.25	0.92	82.6	8.2	90.8
12	0.41	0.41	0.82	73.4	9.6	83.0
16	0.22	0.67	0.89	74.6	10.5	85.1
21	--[c]	--[c]	--[c]	66.0	10.3	76.3
25	--[c]	--[c]	--[c]	69.9	10.8	80.7
36	--[c]	--[c]	--[c]	61.7	10.5	72.2

Source: Bowman et al. [97].

[a]Exposed in open container under incandescent lighting.

[b]Average of duplicate assays corrected for background of 0.12 ppm of rotenone and rotenolone in untreated chow. No other rotenoids were detected.

[c]Background analysis of untreated chow precluded an accurate assay.

Results from the stability studies with rotenone spiked into chow by using alcohol or oil are presented in Tables 3.43-3.45; results concerning dry residues on glass surfaces are presented in Table 3.46. In all instances where rotenone was found to degrade, residues of rotenolone tended to increase; however, the sum of the two residues did not always account for the initial rotenone content. Since no residues of dehydrorotenone or rotenonone nor any extraneous chromatographic peaks were detected in the extracts we must conclude that appreciable levels of the degradated products cannot be detected by the present procedure. High-pressure liquid chromatographic assays of aged samples of spiked chow versus unspiked chow employing

Table 3.45. Residues of rotenoids in chow spiked with rotenone
(100 ppm) by using corn oil and assayed after various periods of
exposure in sealed containers at ambient temperature and -15°C

| Sampling interval (weeks) | Rotenoids (ppm) recovered[a] | | | | | |
| | Ambient | | | -15°C | | |
	Rotenone	Rotenolone	Total	Rotenone	Rotenolone	Total
0	94.6	0.3	94.9	94.6	0.3	94.9
1	85.2	6.5	91.7	98.3	0.7	99.0
2	75.8	9.7	85.5	100	0.8	101
4	70.4	12.6	83.0	85.2	1.2	86.4
8	61.5	12.9	74.4	96.0	1.5	97.5

Source: Bowman et al. [97].

[a]Average of duplicate assays corrected for background of 0.12 ppm of
rotenone and rotenolone. No other rotenoids were detected.

gradient elution (Waters Associates; Curve No. 3) were performed in
an attempt to discover the missing degradation products. In 30-min
assays (initial solvent composition, 65% methanol-35% water; final
solvent composition, 100% methanol) no differences could be detected
between spiked and unspiked chow except for the residues of rotenone
and rotenolone in the spiked sample.

Results from tests designed to determine the stability of
rotenone in the GI tract of mice are presented in Tables 3.47 and
3.48. In Table 3.47, the value for percent of rotenolone is used
to roughly approximate the percent of rotenone degraded. Hence,
after the spiked chow had stood for 0, 1, and 4 days in the feeders,
1.4, 4.6, and 9.3% of the rotenone, respectively, had degraded. On
the other hand, degradation in the GI tract at 1 and 4 days was found
to be about 6.0 and 13.0%, respectively. It is therefore concluded
that degradation of rotenone within the GI tract at 1 and 4 days
was about 1.4 and 3.7%, respectively.

Table 3.46. Results from stability studies with dry residues of
rotenone on glass surfaces[a]

Sampling interval (days)	Rotenoids (µg) recovered[b]		
	Rotenone	Rotenolone	Total
Exposed to Incandescent Light			
0	24.3	0.19	24.5
1	18.9	0.41	19.3
2	16.6	0.44	17.0
5	14.8	0.60	15.4
12	14.3	0.64	14.9
16	11.8	0.61	12.4
Stored in Light-free Cabinet			
0	24.3	0.19	24.5
1	25.2	0.23	25.4
2	23.8	0.21	24.0
5	23.1	0.35	23.5
12	25.1	0.36	25.4
16	24.1	0.66	24.8

Source: Bowman et al. [97].

[a]Open residues (25 µg, 1 µg/cm^2) were exposed to ambient temperature as indicated.

[b]Average of duplicate assays.

Table 3.47. Rotenoids recovered from GI tracts of mice fed chow
spiked with rotenone for 1 or 4 days

Sampling interval (days)	Rotenoids recovered (ppm)		
	Rotenone	Rotenolone	Percent Rotenolone[a]
GI Tracts			
1	4.9	0.34	6.5
	3.3	0.18	5.2
	2.5	0.16	6.0
	5.3	0.37	6.5
(Mean)	4.0	0.26	6.0
4	1.2	0.16	11.8
	1.6	0.21	11.6
	1.1	0.18	14.1
	2.9	0.49	14.5
(Mean)	1.7	0.26	13.0
Spiked Chow from Feeders			
0	50.8	0.73	1.4
1[b]	34.7	1.63	4.6
4	43.6	4.48	9.3

Source: Bowman et al. [97].

[a]Rotenolone content divided by the sum of rotenolone and rotenone
x 100.

[b]Assay values are low because the sample was contaminated with
animal bedding and feces.

Table 3.48. Rotenoids recovered from GI tracts of mice dosed with rotenone in oil by gavage for four consecutive days

Dose level (mg/kg)	Rotenoids recovered (μg)			
	Rotenone	Rotenolone	Dehydrorotenone	Total
20	459	6.2	5.7	471
	508	12.3	4.3	525
30	447	9.6	5.7	462
	910	22.2	5.7	938

Source: Bowman et al. [97].

Data from assays of GI tracts from mice subjected to four consecutive daily doses of rotenone in oil via gavage are presented in
Table 3.48. In addition to rotenone, small amounts of both rotenolone
and dehydrorotenone were also detected. However, the sum of the two
degradated products represents an average degradation of about 2.8%
of the total residue. The rotenone formulation in corn oil stored
in the dark at ambient temperature during the animal test was found
to be essentially stable.

In tests performed to detect any transplacental transfer of
rotenone or its products, no detectable amounts of the four compounds
could be found in fetuses from animals dosed for seven consecutive
days with rotenone at levels of 0 and 25 mg/kg.

V   OTHER COMPOUNDS

A.   4-Ethylsulfonylnaphthalene-1-sulfonamide [126]

1. General Description of Method

Procedures are described for the determination of 4-ethylsulfonyl-
naphthalene-1-sulfonamide (ENS) residues in laboratory chow by SPF
and by flame photometric GC (sulfur mode) after methylation. Relative efficiencies of several solvent extraction systems were evaluated. Spectrophotofluorimetric methods for trace analysis of ENS

in microbiological media, urine, blood, and wastewater are also presented. Solubility values for ENS in water and hexane and p-values
in 14 solvent systems are presented. The efficacy of the SPF method
is demonstrated by the analysis of urine from a dog dosed with
[14C]ENS. Ancillary data concerning the optimization of the methylation reaction of ENS with diazomethane are discussed.

   2. *Introduction*

4-Ethylsulfonylnaphthalene-1-sulfonamide (ENS or 4-ENS), a known
carcinogen, administered as a single dose induced epithelial hyperplasia of the bladder in mice [127]; prolonged dietary dosing with
ENS produced a greater degree of epithelial hyperplasia and frequently bladder tumors [128,129]. More recent investigations [130,
131] indicated that most of these effects resulted from an alteration
of urinary pH and irritation from calculi induced by ENS rather than
from direct action of the chemical on the bladder epithelium. Since
toxicological tests with this compound were planned at our laboratory
and no suitable procedure could be found in the literature, the
following procedures were developed to satisfy our requirements.
The formula of ENS is shown in Figure 3.44.

   3. *Experimental*

a. Materials   4-Ethylsulfonylnaphthalene-1-sulfonamide (mp 199-
200°C) from Pfaltz and Bauer Inc., Flushing, N.Y., was used as
received, since it contained no extraneous GC peaks and recrystallization failed to change its GC or SPF response.

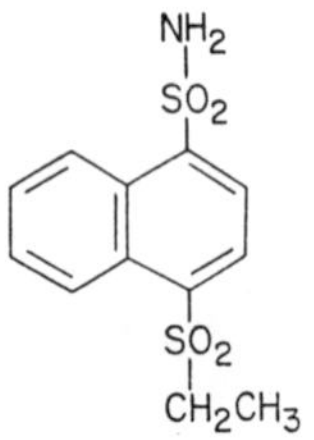

Figure 3.44. Formula of ENS.
(From King and Bowman [126].)

Adsorbents were silica gel (No. 3405, Baker Chemical Co.,
Phillipsburg, N.J.) and acid alumina, Brockman Activity I (No. A-948,
Fisher Scientific Co., Pittsburg, Pa.). The silica gel, used as
received, contained 3.7% moisture. The sodium sulfate was anhydrous.
All reagents were CP grade and solvents were pesticide grade. The
chow was type 5010C (Ralston Purina Co., St. Louis, Mo.). Ingredients
for the microbiological culture media (from Difco Laboratories,
Detroit, Mich.) were prepared in accordance with the directions supplied by the manufacturer. The ethereal diazomethane reagent was
prepared from Diazald by using the reagent, kit, and instructions
supplied by the manufacturer (Aldrich Chemical Co., Milwaukee, Wis.),
then stored at -10°C prior to use.

b. *Preparation of samples for analysis by SPF*

(1) Chow. Two extraction methods were employed to determine the
relative efficiencies of recovering residues of ENS. (a) A 20-g
portion of the sample was deactivated by the addition of 20 ml of
distilled water, then extracted with 100 ml of chloroform-methanol
(9:1, v/v) in a 250-ml glass-stoppered bottle by shaking for 2 hr
at 200 excursions per minute on a Eberbach shaker (Curtin Scientific
Co., No. 205-575). The supernatant was then percolated through a
plug of anhydrous sodium sulfate (25 mm diameter x 30 mm thick),
centrifuged at 2000 rpm for 10 min, carefully decanted through a
plug of glass wool, and stored in a tightly sealed container for
subsequent cleanup. (b) A 20-g sample was tightly wrapped in Whatman
No. 1 filter paper, placed in a Soxhlet apparatus (W. H. Curtin Co.,
No. 087-486) and extracted with 100 ml of chloroform-methanol (9:1,
v/v) for 2 hr at the rate of about 30 solvent exchanges per hour.
The extract was then quantitatively percolated through a plug of
sodium sulfate as described, the volume was adjusted to 100 ml, and
the extract stored for subsequent cleanup.

A 10-ml aliquot of the chow extract from the mechanical or
Soxhlet procedure was pipetted into a 30-ml culture tube containing
10 ml of 1 N NaOH, sealed with a Teflon-lined cap, shaken vigorously
for 2 min, then centrifuged at 1500 rpm for 10 min. The chloroform

layer (bottom) was withdrawn and discarded by using a 10-ml syringe
and cannula. The aqueous layer was extracted twice more with 10-ml
portions of chloroform which were also discarded. The aqueous phase
was then made strongly acid by the addition of 2 ml of concentrated
HCl and extracted three times with 10-ml portions of chloroform,
successively percolating them through a plug of anhydrous sodium
sulfate. The combined extracts were evaporated to dryness on a 60°C
water bath under water pump vacuum and reserved for subsequent column
cleanup.

Two glass columns (12 mm i.d., No. 420,000, Kontes Glass Co.,
Vineland, N.J.) were prepared by adding successively a plug of glass
wool, 5 g of sodium sulfate, the adsorbent, and 5 g of sodium sulfate.
In one column, the adsorbent was silica gel (2 g), as received, and
in the other acid alumina (1 g), Activity I. The columns were
arranged in tandem and prewashed by adding 10 ml of benzene-5% acetone
to the one on top, which contained the silica gel; the lower column
(alumina) was then removed. The dry extract from the solvent partitioning step was then dissolved in 5 ml of benzene-5% acetone and
added to the silica gel column. The container and column were washed
with three additional 5-ml portions of the same solvent and the eluate
discarded. The columns were again placed in tandem and 20 ml of
benzene-10% acetone was added to elute the ENS from the silica gel
column onto the alumina. The silica gel column and the effluent from
the alumina column were discarded. Finally, the alumina column was
eluted with 25 ml of chloroform-methanol (9:1, v/v). The effluent
was collected, evaporated to dryness as described, and the residue
dissolved in an appropriate volume of acetonitrile for SPF analysis.

(2) Microbiological media. Ten milliliters of the medium was added
to a 30-ml culture tube containing 1 g of NaCl; 0.2 ml of concentrated HCl and 10 ml of benzene were added, then the tube was sealed,
shaken, and centrifuged. The benzene layer was carefully withdrawn
by using a syringe and cannula and added to a dry acid alumina column
prepared as described for chow. The extraction was repeated with two
additional 10-ml portions of benzene and the eluate from the column

was discarded. The residue of ENS was eluted from the alumina column
by using 20 ml of chloroform-methanol (9:1, v/v). The column effluent
was evaporated to dryness and the residue dissolved in acetonitrile
for SPF analysis.

(3) Wastewater. Fifty milliliters of the sample was added to a 70-ml
culture tube containing 2 g of NaCl; 0.5 ml of concentrated HCl and
15 ml of benzene were then added and the tube was sealed, shaken, and
centrifuged. The benzene layer was removed, added to an alumina
column, and the extraction was repeated with two additional 15-ml
portions of benzene. The ENS on the alumina was then eluted, evaporated, and prepared for SPF analysis as described for media.

(4) Blood. Procedures employing no hydrolysis of the substrate prior
to the extraction of ENS residues as well as those involving acid or
alkaline hydrolysis were used. (a) No hydrolysis--6 ml of distilled
water, 1 ml of concentrated HCl, and 1 g of NaCl were added to a 20-ml
culture tube containing 1 ml of whole blood. The contents were mixed
and extracted twice with 10-ml portions of benzene, cleaned up on an
alumina column, and prepared for SPF analysis as described for media;
(b) Acid hydrolysis--samples were analyzed as for no hydrolysis except
that the mixture in the sealed tube was held in an 80°C heating block
for 2 hr with frequent shaking, then cooled prior to extraction with
benzene; (c) Alkaline hydrolysis--samples were analyzed as for no
hydrolysis except that 1 ml of 10 N NaOH was substituted for the HCl.
The mixture was then held at 80°C for 2 hr, cooled, and acidified
with 2 ml of concentrated HCl. The mixture was then extracted,
cleaned up, and prepared for SPF analysis as described.

(5) Urine. Procedures utilizing acid or alkaline hydrolysis prior
to extraction as well as those involving no hydrolysis were tested.
(a) No hydrolysis--analyses were performed exactly as described for
wastewater; (b) Acid hydrolysis--analyses were performed exactly as
described for wastewater, except that the acidified mixture was
heated at 80°C for 2 hr in a water bath, then cooled prior to the
extraction with benzene; (c) Alkaline hydrolysis--these analyses

were also performed as described for wastewater except that 0.5 ml
of 10 N NaOH was substituted for the HCl; the mixture was heated at
80°C for 2 hr, cooled, and acidified with 1 ml of concentrated HCl
prior to extraction with benzene.

c. *Preparation of samples for GC*   A 25-ml aliquot of the chow
extract from the mechanical or Soxhlet procedure was pipetted into
a 50-ml culture tube containing 10 ml of 1 N NaOH, tightly sealed
with a Teflon-lined cap, vigorously shaken for 2 min, and centrifuged
at 1500 rpm for 10 min. The chloroform layer was withdrawn and discarded, and the aqueous layer was extracted with two additional 10-ml
portions of chloroform which were also discarded. The aqueous phase
was acidified by adding 2 ml of concentrated HCl, then extracted with
three 10-ml portions of chloroform which were successively percolated
through a plug of sodium sulfate. The combined extracts were evaporated to dryness under water pump vacuum in a 60°C water bath. The
ENS was then methylated by adding 5 ml of ethereal diazomethane
reagent to the dry residue and allowing the mixture to stand tightly
sealed, overnight, in the dark at ambient temperature. The solvent
was then evaporated under water pump vacuum in a 60°C water bath and
the residue dissolved in an appropriate volume of chloroform for
injection into the GC.

d. *Spectrophotofluorimetric analysis*   An Aminco-Bowman instrument
(American Instrument Co., Silver Spring, Md.) equipped with a xenon
lamp and a 1P28 detector was used with 1-cm cells and a 2-2-2-mm
slit program to measure fluorescence. Excitation and emission maxima
for ENS were 308 nm and 380 nm, respectively. All dilutions were
made in acetonitrile. The instrument was frequently calibrated to
produce a RI of 5.0 with a dilution of 0.3 μg quinine sulfate per
milliliter of 0.1 N sulfuric acid (λ_{Ex} = 350 nm, λ_{Em} = 450 nm).
Readings were corrected for the solvent blank and RI was plotted
versus concentration of ENS on log-log paper to produce a standard
curve.

To ensure that the RI was within the linear range (ca. 0.3 μg/ml
or less) of the standard curve and thus unaffected by concentration

quenching, samples were diluted with an equal volume of solvent to
ascertain whether the RI was about half that of the undiluted solution. If it was not, dilution was continued until the RI was halved
by dilution. The RI of the untreated control sample was then subtracted from that of the unknown, and concentration in micrograms
per milliliter was determined from the standard curve.

e. *Gas chromatographic analysis*   A Hewlett-Packard (Palo Alto,
Calif.) Model 5750 gas chromatograph equipped with a flame photometric
detector (Tracor, Inc., Austin, Tex.) fitted with the water-cooled
adapter was operated in the sulfur mode (394 nm filter). The 100-cm
glass column (4 mm i.d.) contained 5% Dexsil 300 GC (w/w) on Gas
Chrom Q (80-100 mesh) and was operated isothermally at 280°C; it was
conditioned overnight at 350°C prior to use. Flow rates of the gases
in milliliters per minute were nitrogen (carrier), 160; hydrogen,
200; oxygen, 40. Temperatures of the injection port and detector
were 300 and 280°C, respectively. Under the stated conditions t_R
values for ENS, its monomethyl and its dimethyl derivatives were
2.25, 1.95, and 1.70 min, respectively. Two sulfur-containing pesticide reference compounds, coumaphos [O-(3-chloro-4-methyl-2-oxo-2H-1-
benzopyran-7-yl)O,O-diethylphosphorothioate] and Dition [2-(2,4-
dihydroxyphenyl)-1-cyclohexene-1-carboxylic acid-δ-lactone O,O-
diethylphosphorothioate] had t_R values of 1.40 and 2.55 min, respectively. All injections were made in 25 μl of chloroform.

f. *Derivativization, p-values, and solubility determinations*
Because of the unusually slow methylation reaction of ENS with
ethereal diazomethane (ca. 12 mg of diazomethane per milliliter of
reagent), rate studies at three temperatures were performed to optimize conditions of the reaction. Three flasks, each containing 120
μg of ENS and 30 ml of the diazomethane reagent, were stored either
in a freezer (-10°C), refrigerator (5°C), or in the dark at ambient
temperature (25°C). Samples (2 ml) were taken immediately and 0.25,
0.50, 0.75, 1, 2, 3, 4, 5, 6, 7, and 24 hr later at each temperature.
The diazomethane reagent was immediately evaporated under water pump
vacuum at ambient temperature to stop the reaction and the residue

was dissolved in 2 ml of chloroform for GC analysis. The percentages
of ENS derivatized as the monomethyl and dimethyl derivatives, and
the total of both, were plotted versus reaction time.

The water solubility of ENS at 25 ± 2°C was determined by SPF
as described by Bowman and King [1].

Extraction p-values for ENS were determined in several immiscible binary solvent systems by SPF in the manner described by Bowman
and Beroza [13].

g. Recovery experiments   Quadruplicate 20-g samples of chow for
the mechanical extraction procedure were separately spiked with 1 ml
of chloroform containing the appropriate amount of ENS to yield residues of 0, 1, 5, 10, and 20 ppm. After the addition of 20 ml of
water and 99 ml of chloroform-methanol (9:1, v/v), the samples were
extracted and analyzed in the usual manner. It should be noted that
some of the methanol from the mixed solvent remains in the water;
therefore, each 5-ml aliquot of the extract is equivalent to 1.088 g
of sample. This factor must be used in calculating the residue
results. Additional samples of chow were spiked with 10 ppm of ENS
and mechanically extracted with several other mixed solvent systems
to check the efficiency of extraction. Quadruplicate samples for
the Soxhlet extractions were also spiked as described for the mechanical procedure, except the solvent containing the ENS was pipetted
directly onto the chow on the filter paper; the sample was then
wrapped, inserted into the apparatus, and extracted as described.

Quintuplicate samples of both biological media were separately
spiked with 100 μl of methanol containing the appropriate amount of
ENS to produce residues of 0, 0.1, and 1.0 ppm. The samples were
allowed to stand in the refrigerator (5°C) overnight prior to extraction. Samples (1 ml) of whole rat blood were spiked in the same
manner at 0 and 10 ppm, held at 5°C overnight, and analyzed as described. Wastewater and urine samples (50 ml) were spiked at 0 and
20 ppb by adding 1 ml of methanol containing the appropriate amount
of ENS, held at 5°C overnight, and analyzed as described.

h. Assays of urine from a dog dosed with [^{14}C]ENS This experiment
was performed to determine the efficacy of our SPF assay of urine
from an animal dosed with ENS, since it is recognized that residues
resulting from the metabolic process may behave differently from
those spiked directly into the substrate.

The NCTR Division of Molecular Biology was engaged in metabolic
studies with an 11-month-old female beagle (10 kg). The animal was
given a single oral dose of 41.3 mg of [^{14}C]ENS (18.2 µCi/mg) and its
urine was subsequently collected at 24-hr intervals. Portions of
these samples previously assayed radiometrically (total equivalents
of ENS) were used to evaluate our procedure.

To determine free ENS by SPF, a 1-ml sample of urine, 9 ml of
water, 0.5 g of NaCl, and 0.1 ml of concentrated HCl were mixed in a
20-ml culture tube and extracted with three 5-ml portions of benzene.
The extraction and cleanup of free ENS and hydrolyzed conjugates were
carried out as described for media. The aqueous phase was then subjected, consecutively, first to alkaline and then to acid hydrolysis
at 80°C for 2 hr to evaluate the possibility of assaying conjugated
ENS. Tests were also made to determine the effect of reversing the
order of hydrolysis. The hydrolysis procedures were as follows.
(1) Alkaline hydrolysis followed by acid hydrolysis; the aqueous
phase was made alkaline by adding 0.2 ml of 10 N NaOH, heated,
cooled, acidified with 0.2 ml of concentrated HCl, and extracted.
(2) Acid hydrolysis followed by alkaline hydrolysis; the aqueous
phase, already acid, was heated, cooled, and extracted. Then after
the addition of 0.2 ml of 10 N NaOH, the sample was heated, cooled,
acidified with 0.2 ml of concentrated HCl, and extracted.

Samples of water and untreated urine, unspiked and spiked with
10 ppm of ENS, were carried through the entire SPF procedure.

4. Results and Discussion

In preliminary studies to select an efficient solvent system for
mechanically extracting residues of ENS from chow, samples were
spiked with 10 ppm and analyzed by GC. Samples of chow for the

Table 3.49. Results of preliminary studies of ENS recovery using
seven solvent systems

Solvent (v/v)	ENS recovered (%)
Chloroform-methanol (9:1)	84.9
Benzene	52.9
Benzene-methanol (9:1)	58.2
Acetone-water (2:1)	86.4
Acetone-water (5:1)	67.3
Acetonitrile-water (2:1)	59.5
Acetonitrile-water (5:1)	52.5

chloroform-methanol (9:1, v/v), benzene, and benzene-methanol (9:1,
v/v) extractions were deactivated with an equal weight of water prior
to extractions. Results of these tests are given in Table 3.49.

The mechanical extraction with chloroform-methanol (9:1, v/v)
was essentially as efficient as any solvent tested, and it was therefore adopted for use because the solvent was directly extractable
with aqueous alkali for the initial cleanup step. A Soxhlet extraction of chow spiked with 10 ppm of ENS employing chloroform-methanol
(9:1, v/v) yielded a recovery of 99.1%. Samples of chow were therefore spiked with ENS at several levels, extracted by using both
methods, and assayed by SPF and GC to evaluate the analytical procedure.

The SPF procedure is highly sensitive and it is the method of
choice, especially where ultra low residues of ENS are sought in the
presence of low-level interferences. Nevertheless, some type of
cleanup is usually necessary prior to SPF analysis of most substrates
and in the case of chow (high-level interferences) the extensive
multistep procedure previously described is required. The excitation
and emission spectra of ENS are shown in Figure 3.45 and a plot of
RI versus concentration of ENS is presented in Figure 3.46. Relative
fluorescent intensity is directly proportional to the concentration

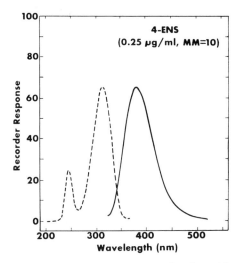

Figure 3.45. Excitation (broken line) and
emission (solid line) spectra of ENS in
acetonitrile. (From King and Bowman [126].)

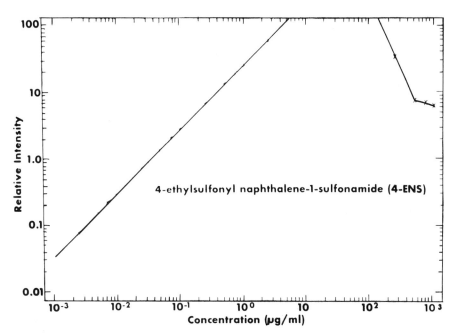

Figure 3.46. Standard curve for ENS in
acetonitrile. (From King and Bowman [126].)

of ENS within the range of about 2 ng to 3 μg per milliliter of acetonitrile.

The GC of microgram amounts of ENS per se was accomplished with difficulty and only after the column was conditioned with the compound by repeatedly injecting amounts of 5 μg or more. Reproducible GC of submicrogram amounts could not be accomplished, probably because the conditioned state of the column could not be maintained by injecting the smaller amounts. We therefore sought a means of derivatizing ENS to eliminate the conditioning requirements and permit analysis at the nanogram level. One milligram of ENS heated in a sealed tube overnight at 80°C with 1 ml of BSA reagent [N,O-bis(trimethylsilyl)acetamide, Pierce Chemical Co., Rockford, Ill.] failed to produce any trace of a trimethylsilyl derivative of the compound; however, tests with ethereal diazomethane at room temperature indicated a slow methylation reaction. Experiments were therefore initiated to optimize the process for use in quantitative determinations of ENS. Results of reaction rate studies with ENS and diazomethane at three temperatures are illustrated in Figure 3.47.

The reaction of ENS with diazomethane resulted in the formation of two compounds presumed to be its monomethyl (MM) and dimethyl (DM) derivatives. This assumption is based on the GC retention times of the compounds and the rates of their formation. If two consecutive reactions occur to produce the DM via MM, the overall reaction is of the form

$$A \xrightarrow{k_1} B \xrightarrow{k_2} C \tag{1}$$

where A is ENS, and B and C are the monomethyl and dimethyl derivatives of ENS, respectively. The applicable simultaneous differential rate equations are

$$\frac{-dx}{dt} = k_1 x \tag{2}$$

$$\frac{-dy}{dt} = -k_1 x + k_2 y \tag{3}$$

$$\frac{dz}{dt} = k_2 y \tag{4}$$

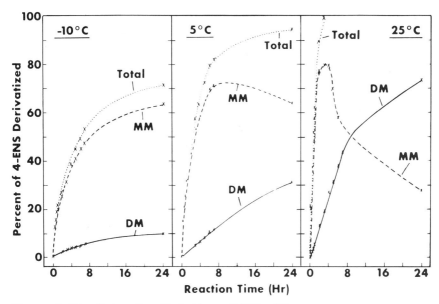

Figure 3.47. Rate of methylation of ENS with
diazomethane at three temperatures (MM and DM
denote monomethyl and dimethyl derivatives).
(From King and Bowman [126].)

where x, y, and z are the respective concentrations of A, B, and C;
t is the time; and k_1 and k_2 are the reaction rates of compounds A
and B, respectively. The solution of these equations, based on the
assumption that only irreversible first-order steps are involved, is
found in general textbooks [132]. The data indicate that this
assumption is valid for this reaction under the specified conditions.
Equation (2) can be integrated directly, giving

$$x = x_0 \exp(-k_1 t) \tag{5}$$

where x_0 is the initial concentration. Because of the large molar
excess of diazomethane to ENS (21,400:1) used in this work, the concentration of ENS declined exponentially with time, as occurs in any
first-order reaction, i.e., there was no apparent effect on rates
due to the competition of ENS and MM-ENS for diazomethane.

Plots of log x versus time for the first hour of reaction,
which exhibited excellent linearity at all three temperatures, were

extrapolated and the time τ at which the ENS concentration had decreased to one-half the original concentration was measured and used
to calculate the reaction rates by use of the relation [132]

$$k = \ln 2/\tau \tag{6}$$

The reaction rates were found to be 0.17, 0.38, and 0.95 $\mu g\ ml^{-1}\ hr^{-1}$
at -10, 5, and 25°C, respectively. Another observation of the agreement between theory and these experimental data is that the plot of
ln k versus the reciprocal of the absolute temperature gives a linear
relationship as predicted by the Arrhenius equation [132]

$$k = A \exp\ (-E_a/RT) \tag{7}$$

where E_a is the activation energy, R is the gas constant, T is the
absolute temperature, and A is a constant of integration.

At 25°C the reaction of ENS is essentially complete (>98%)
after 3 hr (Figure 3.47). As the concentration of ENS asymptotically
approaches 0 the formation of MM decreases and its conversion to DM
continues causing its net concentration to decrease. At 5 and 25°C
the concentration of MM reaches a maximum when its rate of formation
equals its rate of reaction. At -10°C, even after 24 hr, sufficient
unreacted ENS remained so that no maximum for MM was observed.

These data indicate that 4 hr at 25°C is adequate for essentially
complete conversion of ENS to MM and DM. Although at lower temperatures the diazomethane is more stable and available to react for a
longer period of time, the decrease in reaction rate negates these
advantages. We therefore adopted an overnight reaction (ca. 16 hr)
at ambient temperature in order to produce a higher proportion of DM
since its response (peak height) is 1.27 greater than that of MM.

Calculations of ENS residues via GC were accomplished in the
following manner. A standard sample of ENS was reacted with diazomethane at ambient temperature for 24 hr as previously described and
a series of dilutions were made to allow 25-μl injections containing
7.5-500 ng equivalents of ENS. The detector response of each peak
(MM and DM) was plotted on log-log paper versus nanogram equivalents
of ENS, and in both cases the plots were found to be linear with

identical slopes. The plots are represented by an equation of the
form

$$\log n = m \log R + k \tag{8}$$

where n = nanograms injected, R = detector response (amp), m = slope,
and k = arbitrary constant.

The slope for both lines was determined to be 0.524 compared to
0.5 which would be expected from previous studies of the flame photometric detector operated in the sulfur mode [133], i.e., the plot of
amount injected versus the square root of the detector response would
be linear.

Gas chromatography responses from samples, methylated at 25°C
for 4 hr (mostly MM) and 24 hr (mostly DM) as illustrated in Figure
3.48, were used to set up simultaneous equations to determine the

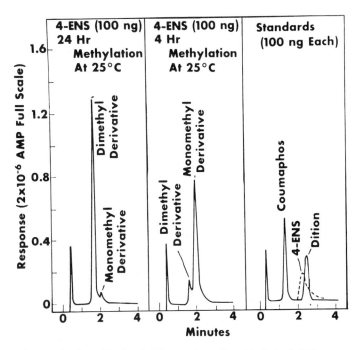

Figure 3.48. Typical GC curves of methylated ENS,
reference compounds, and ENS per se injected in
25 μl of chloroform. (From King and Bowman [126].)

relative response for each derivative of ENS. Each peak height was
first converted to an arbitrary concentration, using values from
the MM curve already described, in order to obtain values linearly
related to concentration. These linear values, M and D, were then
employed in the following equations:

$$aM_1 + bD_1 = 100 \text{ ng ENS} \tag{9}$$

$$aM_2 + bD_2 = 100 \text{ ng ENS} \tag{10}$$

where a and b are constants which are the detector response factors
of the two derivatives. By equating the sum to 100 ng ENS, actual
concentrations in nanogram equivalents of ENS are calculated for
each derivative. The ratio of the DM to MM response (b/a) was found
to be 1.27. These results were then used to calculate actual response
curves of the MM and DM derivatives (Figure 3.49). Calculations performed on samples intermediate to those at 4 and 24 hr confirmed the
validity of this method of calculation, since the sum of MM and DM
remained constant. Total residues of ENS in all samples were obtained
by summing the nanogram equivalents of the two derivatives.

Dition can be used as a stable reference standard for the
detector response but, since the slope of its curve is 0.482, the
same amount should always be injected.

Results from assays of chow spiked with ENS at various levels,
extracted by two procedures, and assayed both by SPF and GC are presented in Table 3.50. Soxhlet extractions yielded higher recoveries
of ENS residues in all instances; however, the SPF background of
untreated control samples was also higher due to the more rigorous
extraction. Recoveries from the GC method were also superior to
those via SPF because of the minimal cleanup required for GC. Most
of the losses of ENS in the SPF procedure occurred at the alumina
absorption step. Both methods are of about equal sensitivity and
require about the same amount of time, but, less labor is required
for the GC method. On the other hand, the GC procedure has the
disadvantage of requiring regular preparation of diazomethane. Any

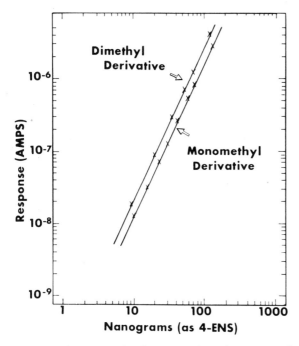

Figure 3.49. Standard curves for the monomethyl
and dimethyl derivatives of ENS with the flame
photometric detector (394 nm filter). (From
King and Bowman [126].)

combination of the two extraction and analytical procedures are
considered acceptable for the analysis. In cases where maximum
recovery, sensitivity, and specificity are required, the Soxhlet-GC
procedure is recommended. It should also be noted that even after
the rigorous cleanup for SPF analysis some concentration-quenching
occurs in the untreated controls; therefore, for the purpose of
correcting SPF readings both the spiked and unspiked samples must
be diluted identically.

Results from SPF assays of biological media are presented in
Table 3.51. Limits of sensitivity (twice background) for the 10-ml
samples were about 1 and 4 ppb for trypticase soy dextrose and brain

Table 3.50. Spectrophotofluorimetric and GC analyses of extracts of laboratory chow spiked with ENS and extracted by two procedures

Extraction procedure	Added ppm	Added μg[a]	Milligram equivalents of chow used per analysis[b]	Recovered ($\bar{x}$ ± SE)[c] ppm	Recovered ($\bar{x}$ ± SE)[c] %
SPF Analysis					
Mechanical	0	0	40	0.278 ± 0.005	--
	0	0	20	0.328 ± 0.026	--
	0	0	10	0.341 ± 0.010	--
	0	0	5	0.426 ± 0.015	--
	1.0	20	40	0.686 ± 0.026	68.6 ± 2.6
	5.0	100	20	3.91 ± 0.13	78.2 ± 2.6
	10.0	200	10	7.46 ± 0.07	74.6 ± 0.7
	20.0	400	5	15.7 ± 0.1	78.5 ± 0.5
Soxhlet	0	0	40	0.739 ± 0.041	--
	0	0	20	0.790 ± 0.026	--
	0	0	10	0.909 ± 0.043	--
	0	0	5	0.938 ± 0.044	--
	1.0	20	40	0.783 ± 0.004	78.3 ± 4.4
	5.0	100	20	4.22 ± 0.21	84.4 ± 4.2
	10.0	200	10	8.25 ± 0.66	82.5 ± 6.6
	20.0	400	5	16.9 ± 0.6	84.5 ± 3.3
GC Analysis					
Mechanical	0	0	125	<0.15	--
	1.0	20	125	0.864 ± 0.040	86.4 ± 4.0
	5.0	100	25	4.05 ± 0.19	81.0 ± 3.8
	10.0	200	12.5	8.70 ± 0.13	87.0 ± 1.3
	20.0	400	6.25	17.1 ± 0.3	85.5 ± 1.5
Soxhlet	0	0	125	<0.15	--
	1.0	20	125	1.00 ± 0.023	100 ± 2.3
	5.0	100	25	4.48 ± 0.03	89.6 ± 0.6
	10.0	200	12.5	8.50 ± 0.33	85.0 ± 3.3
	20.0	400	6.25	17.7 ± 0.4	88.5 ± 2.0

Source: King and Bowman [126].

[a] Per 20 g of chow.

[b] Per milliliter for SPF readings or per 25-μl injection for GC.

[c] Mean and standard error of four samples.

Table 3.51. Spectrophotofluorimetric analysis of extracts of
biological media spiked with ENS

Biological medium	Added		Milligram equivalents of medium used per analysis[b]	Recovered ($\bar{x} \pm$ SE)[c]	
	ppm	μg[b]		ppm	%
Brain heart infusion	0	0	1000	0.0380 ± 0.0018	--
	0.10	1.0	1000	0.0912 ± 0.0015	91.2 ± 1.5
	1.00	10.0	200	0.908 ± 0.011	90.8 ± 1.1
Trypticase soy dextrose	0	0	1000	0.0138 ± 0.0004	--
	0.10	1.0	1000	0.0998 ± 0.0019	99.8 ± 1.9
	1.00	10.0	200	0.863 ± 0.027	86.3 ± 2.7

Source: King and Bowman [126].

[a]Per 10 ml of medium.

[b]Per milliliter for SPF readings.

[c]Mean and standard error of five samples.

heart infusion media, respectively. Recoveries at 0.10 and 1.0 ppm
and precision were excellent.

Table 3.52 lists the results of SPF assays of urine, wastewater,
and blood. Urine spiked with 20 ppb of ENS (no hydrolysis) yielded
98% recoveries and a control background of about 18 ppb; with alkaline
hydrolysis the recovery dropped to 76% with a background of 38 ppb.
Assays of urine after acid hydrolysis could not be accomplished because
a purple-colored interference was produced by the reaction of the acid
with the unspiked substrate. Wastewater spiked with 20 ppb of ENS
gave recoveries of 80% while the control background was about 1 ppb.
Sensitivity could easily be increased by extracting larger samples.
Recoveries of ENS from blood spiked at 10 ppm were 31, 51, and 81% by
procedures employing no hydrolysis, alkaline hydrolysis, and acid
hydrolysis, respectively. The acid hydrolysis procedure with its
control background of 38 ppb is therefore the preferred method. The
development of analytical methodology for metabolites of ENS was not

Table 3.52. Spectrophotofluorimetric analysis of extracts of urine, wastewater, and whole rat blood spiked with ENS

Added		Type of hydrolysis	Milligram equivalents of substrate used per analysis[b]	Recovered[c]	
ppm	μg[a]			ppm	%
Urine					
0	0	None	5000	0.0184	--
0.020	1.0	None	5000	0.0196	98
0	0	Alkaline	5000	0.0380	--
0.020	1.0	Alkaline	5000	0.0152	76
0	0	Acid	5000	--[d]	--[d]
0.020	1.0	Acid	5000	--[d]	--[d]
0.200	10.0	Acid	5000	--[d]	--[d]
Wastewater					
0	0	None	5000	0.0010	--
0.020	1.0	None	5000	0.0160	80
Whole Rat Blood					
0	0	None	200	0.022	--
10.0	10.0	None	20	3.14	31
0	0	Alkaline	200	0.051	--
10.0	10.0	Alkaline	20	5.10	51
0	0	Acid	200	0.038 ± 0.0031	--
10.0	10.0	Acid	20	8.13 ± 0.17	81.3 ± 1.7

Source: King and Bowman [126].

[a]Per 50 ml of urine and wastewater; per milliliter of rat blood.

[b]Per milliliter for SPF reading

[c]Mean of duplicate samples except for rat blood (acid hydrolysis) where values are means and standard errors of four samples.

[d]Development of purple-colored product upon acid hydrolysis of unapiked urine prevented the assay via SPF.

Table 3.53. Spectrophotofluorimetric and radiometric analyses of urine taken at various intervals from a dog treated with [^{14}C]ENS

Sample	Total equivalents (ppm), radiometric assay	ENS recovered (ppm), SPF assays Free (no hydrolysis)	After hydrolysis[a] Alkaline	Acid	Total
Water[b] (control)	--	0.10	0.08 (0.06)	0.06 (0.13)	0.24
Water (spiked at 10 ppm)	--	9.32	0.51 (0.001)	0.02 (0.44)	9.85
Urine[b] (control)	--	0.18	0.15 (0.12)	0.21 (0.36)	0.54
Urine[c] (spiked at 10 ppm)	--	8.62	0.67 (0.01)	0.12 (0.79)	9.41
Treated urine[c]	41.57	15.5	8.23 (6.02)	1.08 (1.72)	24.8
Treated urine[c] (1-2 days)	30.25	11.5	5.73 (5.19)	0.60 (1.49)	17.8
Treated urine[c] (2-3 days)	5.19	2.70	0.29 (0.00)	0.00 (0.13)	2.99
Treated urine[c] (3-4 days)	10.15	4.79	0.87 (0.16)	0.16 (.078)	6.00

Source: King and Bowman [126].

[a]Alkaline hydrolysis performed prior to acid hydrolysis. Data for alkaline hydrolysis subsequent to acid hydrolysis are given in parentheses.

[b]Excitation and emission maxima did not correspond to those of ENS.

[c]Appropriate control has been subtracted for SPF data.

undertaken because metabolism studies employing [^{14}C]ENS were incomplete and analytical standards were not available.

The results of SPF and radiometric assays of untreated urine and urine from the dog dosed with [^{14}C]ENS are presented in Table 3.53. Recoveries via SPF of unlabeled ENS from water and untreated urine spiked with 10 ppm of ENS were 98.5 and 94.1%, respectively. Recovery of ENS, even from a sample of urine spiked directly with the compound and extracted within the hour, was enhanced by hydrolysis, which indicated that some conjugation had already occurred.

The total recovery of ENS (free + conjugated) from treated urine by the SPF method was 58.8 ± 1.2% of that indicated by radiometric assays at all sampling intervals. On the other hand, free ENS (no hydrolysis) varied from 37 to 52%, which indicated that hydrolysis is necessary for higher and more consistent results. Radiometric and SPF assays of the free and hydrolyzed fractions from the SPF procedure were essentially identical. About 41% of the radioactivity in the treated urine was not extractable as free ENS or after alkaline and acid hydrolysis under the rather mild conditions employed. Although the order in which the alkaline and acid hydrolyses were performed had little effect on the total hydrolyzable residues recovered, both types of hydrolyses were required for optimum recovery. The nature of the unextractable radioactive material and whether a more rigorous hydrolysis will increase the recovery are not known but are currently being investigated. Nevertheless, the results of this study demonstrate the usefulness of the SPF procedure for determining traces of unlabeled ENS in a biological substrate.

Partition values for ENS are presented in Table 3.54. The following systems all gave p-values of 0.00: hexane-water, hexane-acetonitrile, hexane-80% acetone (20% water), isooctane-dimethyl sulfoxide (DMSO), isooctane-90% DMSO (10% water), isooctane-dimethyl-formamide (DMF), isooctane-85% DMF (15% water), and heptane-90% ethanol (10% water). The solubilities of ENS at 25 ± 2°C in water and hexane were found to be 113 and 0.031 ppm, respectively.

Table 3.54. Partition values for ENS in six solvent systems

Solvent system	Partition value
Benzene-water	0.62
Chloroform-water	0.94
Chloroform-60% methanol (40% water)	0.80
Chloroform-aqueous Na_2CO_3 (saturated)	0.18
Chloroform-aqueous $NaHCO_3$ (saturated)	0.94
Chloroform-aqueous NaOH (1 or 4 N)	0.00

B. Sodium Phenobarbital

1. General Description of Method

A procedure is described for determining residues of sodium phenobarbital in animal chow at levels as low as 0.14 ppm. The methanol
extract is subjected to a liquid-liquid cleanup at pH 13 and 1,
further cleaned up on a silica gel column, and assayed by HPLC by
using an ultraviolet absorption detector at 210 nm. Data concerning
extraction efficiency, p-values, and stability of the chemical in
animal chow are also presented.

2. Introduction

An experiment designed to better understand the role of injury as a
possible mechanism for carcinogenesis was to be initiated at our
laboratory. Sodium phenobarbital [5-ethyl-5-phenyl-2,4,6-(1H,3H,5H)
pyrimidinetrione monosodium salt], a compound thought to induce liver
tumors only in mice, was to be administered at graded dose levels via
the animal's diet to determine whether liver cell injury is a pre-
requisite for the development of liver neoplasms. Analytical methodology was therefore required to verify that accurate dosages were
administered and that the chemical was stable and uniformly distrib-
uted in the spiked diet.

More than a hundred analytical procedures for determining phenobarbital in various substrates have been reported during the past

five years. Most of these procedures utilized GC or TLC; however,
a variety of other methods were also described. A few of the more
recent GC procedures for phenobarbital were described by Joern [136]
in blood serum, Kumps and Mardens [137] in serum and plasma, Friel
and Troupin [138] in serum, cerebrospinal fluids, or saliva after
flash-heater ethylation, and Davis et al. [139] in human serum after
on-column methylation. Brachet-Liermain and Ferrus [140] employed a
thermionic detector which was 40-fold more sensitive than a FID in
determining a mixture of 11 methylated barbituates in blood. Pranitis
et al. [141] cleaned up samples of urine and blood on Amberlite XAD-2
resin and assayed for phenobarbital by using GC or ultraviolet spectrometry. Methods using TLC were described by Kaistha [142] in urine,
Kohsaka [143] in serum, and Hishida et al. [144] in stomach contents,
cadavers, blood, urine, and organs from experimental animals. A
radioimmunoassay technique was described by Booker and Darcey [145]
and compared with a GC procedure for analysis of serum; Horning et al.
[146] developed a sensitive GC-mass spectrometry-computer method for
phenobarbital in human breast milk. Methods employing HPLC were reported by Honigberg et al. [147] for phenobarbital in admixture with
other drugs, by Atwell et al. [148] for phenobarbital in plasma,
Quercia et al. [149] in water and urine, and Evans [150] in blood
serum. However, methodology for the analysis of phenobarbital in a
substrate as intractable as animal chow which contains a broad spectrum of interfering coextractives could not be found in the literature. The following procedure was therefore developed to meet the
requirements of our experiments. The formula of phenobarbital is
shown in Figure 3.50.

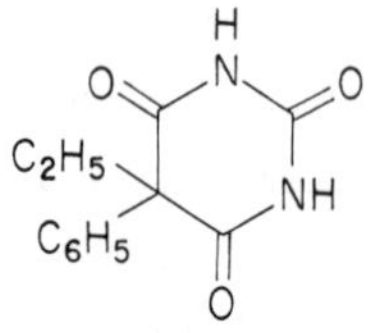

Figure 3.50. Formula of phenobarbital.
(From Bowman and Rushing [135].)

3. Experimental

a. *Materials*   The sodium phenobarbital (No. 56497, Merck and Co.,
Rahway, N.J.) was used as received since it contained no extraneous
peaks in assays by HPLC.

Silica gel (No. 3405, J. T. Baker Chemical Co., Phillipsburg,
N.J.) was heated overnight in an oven at 130°C and stored in a desiccator prior to use. The adsorbant was then partially deactivated
with water for use in the analytical procedure by adding 97 g of the
dry material to a glass-stoppered bottle containing 3.0 ml of water;
the contents were mixed well and allowed to stand for 24 hr with
occasional shaking prior to use.

All solvents were pesticide grade and all reagents were CP grade.
The animal chow was type 5010C (Ralston Purina Co., St. Louis, Mo.).

b. *Preparation of silica gel cleanup columns*   Columns (12 mm i.d.,
No. 420,000, Kontes Glass Co., Vineland, N.J.) equipped with a 50-ml
reservoir were prepared by successively adding a plug of glass wool
(ca. 3 mm i.d.), 0.25 g of sodium sulfate, 4 g of silica gel (3%
water), and 10 g of sodium sulfate. The columns were prepared immediately prior to use and washed with 20 ml of dichloromethane which
was discarded. [Note: The silica gel must be evaluated prior to
use to provide assurance that the phenobarbital (acid form) elutes
as indicated in the analytical procedure.]

c. *Extraction and cleanup of animal chow*   A 5-g portion of the
animal chow was weighed into a 100-ml glass-stoppered flask, 50 ml
of methanol was added, and the sample was mechanically extracted for
16 hr on a reciprocating shaker at a rate of 200 excursions per
minute. The extract was percolated through a plug of sodium sulfate
(ca. 25 mm diameter x 15 mm thick) and a 25-ml portion (2.5 g equivalents of chow) was transferred to a 100-ml round-bottom flask containing a glass bead and evaporated to dryness by using a 60°C water
bath and water pump vacuum. The residue was transferred to a 15-ml
culture tube equipped with a Teflon-lined screw cap by using 2-, 2-,
and 1-ml portions each of 0.1 N NaOH and dichloromethane; then 0.3 g

of NaCl was added and the contents were vigorously shaken for 2 min.
The tube was then centrifuged for 15 min at 2000 rpm and the dichloromethane layer (bottom) was carefully removed using a syringe and
cannula and then discarded. One-half milliliter of 2 N HCl and 5 ml
of dichloromethane were added to the aqueous layer, the contents were
vigorously shaken for 5 min to convert the sodium phenobarbital to
the acid form, and the tube was centrifuged as required to separate
the layers. The dichloromethane layer was carefully withdrawn and
added to a silica gel cleanup column prepared as described. The
aqueous acid phase in the tube was extracted with two additional 5-ml
portions of dichloromethane which were also successively added to the
column. Next, the column was eluted with 85 ml of dichloromethane
followed by 20 ml of dichloromethane-1% methanol and the eluate
discarded. Finally, the phenobarbital was eluted with 35 ml of
dichloromethane-1% methanol which was collected in a 100-ml round-
bottom flask and evaporated to dryness as described. In order to
remove the last traces of dichloromethane, the joint and walls of
the flask were rinsed with a 2-ml portion of methanol and the contents again taken to dryness as described. The residue was dissolved
in an appropriate volume (1 ml or more) of methanol for analysis by
HPLC.

d. High-pressure liquid chromatography   A Waters Associates, Inc.
(Milford, Mass.) liquid chromatograph equipped with a Model 6000
solvent delivery system, a Model U6K septumless injector, a Model 970
variable wavelength detector (Tracor, Inc., Austin, Tex.) operated at
210 nm, and a 30 cm x 4 mm i.d. μ-Bondapak C_{18} (reverse phase) column
(Waters, No. 27324) was used. The mobile phase (water-40% methanol)
flowed at a rate of 1 ml/min with a pressure of about 1600 psi.
Under these conditions the t_R values of both phenobarbital and sodium
phenobarbital were identical (6.80 min); with equal weights of the
compounds the response of sodium phenobarbital was 0.914 times that
of phenobarbital. All injections were made in 5 μl of methanol and
samples were quantified by relating their peak height to those of
known amounts of sodium phenobarbital.

e. *Extraction and recovery experiments*   In preliminary tests to
determine the most efficient means of extracting residues of sodium
phenobarbital from chow, samples (5 g) were spiked with 1 ml of
methanol containing 500 μg (100 ppm) of the chemical and the open
container was allowed to stand for 16 hr prior to extraction unless
otherwise specified. The spiked samples were then extracted for
various periods of time by using different procedures and a variety
of solvents.

Once the appropriate extraction procedure was selected, triplicate 5-g samples of chow in 100-ml glass-stoppered flasks were spiked
with 0, 2, 10, 100, and 1000 ppm of sodium phenobarbital by adding an
appropriate amount of the chemical in 1 ml of methanol. The open
flasks were allowed to stand overnight (16 hr), then the samples were
extracted, cleaned up, and analyzed by HPLC to determine the accuracy
and precision of the procedure.

f. *Stability experiments*   Tests were performed to determine the
stability of sodium phenobarbital in animal chow at the proposed dose
levels under simulated animal test conditions (i.e., open container,
0-16 days) and under storage conditions (i.e., closed container, 0-16
weeks). Batches of chow (1 kg) containing dose levels of 0, 100, or
1000 ppm of sodium phenobarbital were prepared by using a Model LV
Twin-Shell Lab Blender (Patterson-Kelley Co., Inc., East Stroudsburg,
Pa.). The appropriate amount of chemical dissolved in 50 ml of 95%
ethyl alcohol was added to the chow and an additional 25-ml portion
of the solvent was used as a rinse. The shell of the mixer was operated at 20 rpm during the 25-min mixing process and the intensifier
bar was operated at 3300 rpm during the first 5 min of mixing then
turned off. Each batch was transferred to a stainless steel pan and
dried in an autoclave at ambient temperature for 18 hr under reduced
pressure (ca. 0.11 atm). Each batch of chow was then divided into
two 500-g portions.

One portion of each dose level was placed in a crystallizing
dish (ca. 10 cm x 19 cm diameter) and allowed to stand in the open
vessel in a fume hood for 16 days. Duplicate samples for sodium

Table 3.55. Residues recovered from animal chow (5 g) spiked with sodium phenobarbital (100 ppm) by using various extraction systems[a]

Solvent	Volume of solvent (ml)	Extraction period (hr)	Recovery (%)
Methanol	20	1	73.7
Methanol	20	1	97.4[b]
Methanol	30	2	90.5
Methanol	50	4	85.6
Methanol	50	16	88.9
Methanol	110	16	59.7[c]
Methanol	20	2	87.0[d]
Methanol (1 N with NaOH)	20	1	0
Methanol (1 N with HCl)	20	1	17.8
Aqueous NaOH (0.01 N)	30	1	48.7
Aqueous NaOH (0.01 N)	60	2	69.4
Chloroform	30	1	74.8[e]
Chloroform	30	2	75.6[e]
Chloroform-10% methanol	30	2	89.1[e]
Chloroform-10% methanol	50	4	80.0[e]

Source: Bowman and Rushing [135].

[a]All extractions were by mechanical shaking (200 excursions per minute) except as indicated.

[b]Extracted immediately after chow was spiked.

[c]Extracted with Soxhlet at about 3 exchanges per hour.

[d]Vessel immersed in ultrasonic bath.

[e]Hydrochloric acid (5 ml, 0.1 N) added to chow prior to extraction.

phenobarbital assays and for dry matter determinations (material not
volatile at 110°C overnight) were taken immediately and 1, 2, 4, 8,
12, and 16 days later. The chow, which was initially about 3 cm deep
in the dish, was thoroughly mixed just prior to the removal of each
sample. The other 500-g portion of each dose level was transferred
to a sealed glass container and placed in a light-free cabinet at
ambient temperature. Duplicate samples for sodium phenobarbital
assays and for dry matter content were taken immediately and 1, 2,
4, 8, 12, and 16 weeks later.

4. Results and Discussion

Preliminary tests to determine an efficient means of extracting residues of sodium phenobarbital from the chow indicated that the chemical
is much more difficult to extract after the solvent used for spiking
has evaporated and the compound is sorbed by the substrate. For
example, a sample containing 100 ppm of the chemical, extracted with
methanol for 1 hr immediately after being spiked, yielded a recovery
of 97.4%, whereas a similar sample allowed to stand for 16 hr in an
open vessel prior to extraction yielded only 73.7%. Results obtained
with the various extraction procedures are presented in Table 3.55.
Extractions employing NaOH yielded low recoveries as did a Soxhlet
extraction with methanol, probably due to decomposition of the chemical. Also, attempts to extract the compound in the acid form after
addition of HCl failed to improve recovery or resulted in low recoveries; ultrasonication of a sample with methanol for 2 hr also failed
to significantly improve recovery. Although lesser periods of extraction with methanol appeared adequate, an overnight extraction (16 hr)
using a mechanical shaker operated at 200 excursions per minute was
arbitrarily selected for convenience and to provide a thorough extraction that yielded reproducible recoveries in excess of 85% at levels
of 2-1000 ppm.

Results from triplicate samples spiked at 0, 2.0, 10, 100, and
1000 ppm are presented in Table 3.56. All recoveries were within the
range of 85.1 to 91.8% and precision was excellent. The background
of unspiked chow was 0.07 ppm. Typical liquid chromatograms of an

Table 3.56. High-pressure liquid chromatographic analysis of animal chow spiked at various levels with sodium phenobarbital

Sodium phenobarbital added[a]		Milligram equivalents of chow used per analysis	Sodium phenobarbital recovered ($\overline{x} \pm SE$)[b]		
μg	ppm		μg	ppm	%
0	0	12.5	0.35 ± 0.05	0.07 ± 0.01	--
10	2	12.5	8.51 ± 0.18	1.70 ± 0.04	85.1 ± 1.8
50	10	6.25	44.6 ± 0.7	8.93 ± 0.14	89.3 ± 1.4
500	100	6.25	444 ± 4	88.9 ± 0.8	88.9 ± 0.8
5000	1000	0.625	4590 ± 10	918 ± 2	91.8 ± 0.2

Source: Bowman and Rushing [135].

[a]Per 5 g of chow.

[b]Per 5 g of chow. Mean and standard error from triplicate assays; spiked samples are corrected for background of unspiked chow.

analytical standard of sodium phenobarbital and of cleaned-up chow extracts unspiked and spiked with 2.0 or 100 ppm of the compound analyzed in the acid form are presented in Figure 3.51.

Complete results from the stability studies of chow spiked with sodium phenobarbital are presented in Table 3.57. Little degradation occurred at either 100 or 1000 ppm during the 16-day exposure in an open container or during the 16-week storage in a sealed container. The compound was therefore considered sufficiently stable in the chow for use in our toxicological test; although a few slightly erratic results were obtained, uniformity of the mixture was also considered to be acceptable.

In determining the appropriate wavelength for operating the liquid chromatographic detector, it was found that sodium phenobarbital (or its acid form) exhibits no pronounced ultraviolet absorption maximum but continually increases in absorbance from 280 nm to the ultraviolet cut-off of methanol near 205 nm. The variable wavelength detector allowed us to compare the response for

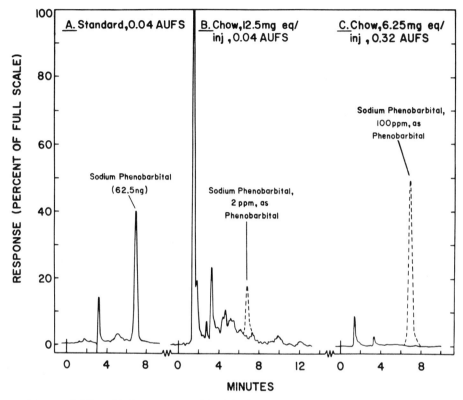

Figure 3.51. High-pressure liquid chromatograms.
A, analytical standard containing 62.5 ng of sodium
phenobarbital; in B and C solid lines are cleaned-
up extracts of unspiked chow, and broken lines
(superimposed) represent 2 and 100 ppm, respectively, of sodium phenobarbital analyzed in the
acid form. All injections were in 5 μl of methanol.
(From Bowman and Rushing [135].)

sodium phenobarbital and the background obtained with cleaned-up
extracts of untreated chow at 210 nm versus 254 nm which is generally
used with detectors having a fixed wavelength. Assays at 210 nm
instead of 254 nm enhanced the response of sodium phenobarbital
about 20-fold and decreased the background of the cleaned-up untreated chow from about 0.30 to 0.07 ppm; based on these data, we
used the 210 nm setting for all analyses.

Table 3.57. Results from stability studies with sodium phenobarbital in animal chow spiked at two levels

| | Percent of sodium phenobarbital recovered and dry matter content (%) for concentration indicated[a] | | | |
| | 100 ppm | | 1000 ppm | |
Sampling interval	Dry matter	Recovered	Dry matter	Recovered
Short-term Study[b]				
(days)				
0	95.6	103	96.1	987
1	93.8	101	94.0	966
2	92.1	102	93.0	979
4	92.5	104	92.8	968
8	92.8	104	92.8	957
12	92.3	98.1	92.4	969
16	92.3	100	92.1	933
Long-term Study[c]				
(weeks)				
0	95.6	103	96.1	987
1	95.7	105	96.0	980
2	95.8	105	95.7	1010
4	95.7	107	96.5	983
8	96.1	105	96.7	1040
12	96.4	102	96.0	963
16	96.0	104	95.9	964

Source: Bowman and Rushing [135].

[a] Average of duplicate assays, corrected for recovery and adjusted on basis of the dry matter of the 0-day sample.

[b] Open container, incandescent lighting, ambient temperature.

[c] Sealed container, light-tight cabinet, ambient temperature.

Table 3.58. Partition values for sodium phenobarbital in
benzene and dichloromethane.

| Aqueous system[a] | Partition value | |
	Benzene	Dichloromethane
NaOH (0.1 N)	0.01	0.00
pH 10	0.01	0.07
pH 9	0.02	0.42
pH 7	0.16	0.89
pH 5	0.25	0.87
pH 3	0.42	0.90
HCl (4 N)	0.48	0.90

[a]Solutions of various pH values were prepared by using small amounts
of aqueous NaOH and/or HCl.

Although assays can be accomplished without including the
liquid-liquid cleanup step (extraction of the alkaline sodium
phenobarbital phase with organic solvent), the cleanup is considered
beneficial especially at levels of 2 ppm or less. Partition-value
determinations were therefore performed for use in selecting an
appropriate solvent and pH for minimum loss of sodium phenobarbital
from the alkaline phase and for maximum recovery of the compound in
its acid form after acidification of the alkaline phase. Results
of these tests are given in Table 3.58.

Dichloromethane was the solvent of choice for the liquid-
liquid partitioning cleanup; based on the p-value data, the conditions selected for the liquid-liquid partitioning cleanup resulted
in minimal loss of the residue from the aqueous NaOH (0.1 N, pH 13)
by extraction with dichloromethane and essentially complete recovery
of the acid form from the acidified alkaline phase (ca. pH 1). The
addition of a small amount of NaCl (0.3 g) was required to help
break the emulsion formed by shaking the alkaline chow extract with
dichloromethane. Under these conditions, 98% of the sodium phenobarbital residue remained in the aqueous phase; however, if the

amount of NaCl was doubled or tripled only 90 and 59%, respectively, of the residue remained in the aqueous layer. Therefore, care must be taken to add exactly the recommended amount of NaCl (0.3 g). The cleanup on silica gel was required for assays of the drug in chow at levels below 1000 ppm.

It is recognized that only those engaged in toxicological research may be required to assay for residues of sodium phenobarbital in animal chow; however, the analytical chemical information and techniquew described should be useful in assaying other substrates not currently described in the literature.

VI THE *SALMONELLA TYPHIMURIUM* TEST FOR MUTAGENICITY (AMES TEST)[*]

A. General Description of Method

Especially constructed strains of *Salmonella typhimurium* are exposed to potential mutagens in the presence of a mammalian microsomal preparation and plated on a minimal agar medium. After incubation at 37°C for 48 hr, the mutated organisms grow into visible colonies. The stronger mutagens produce greater numbers of visible colonies. Nonmutagens will not alter the spontaneous mutation rates of the bacterial strains.

This test will not replace the need for animal carcinogenicity tests, but it is a valuable tool to be used in predictive estimation of potential risk.

B. Introduction

It has been estimated that 85% of all human cancer is caused by exposure to environmental toxicants. Since the number of these toxicants appears to be almost unlimited, assay systems that are rapid, sensitive, inexpensive, and reliable must be developed to identify and eliminate these agents from the environment. The Salmonella/microsome mutagenicity test as described by Ames et al. [151-153]

---

[*]The author is grateful to Dr. E. J. Lazear, National Center for Toxicological Research, Jefferson, Ark., for contributing this procedure.

has been sufficiently developed and validated in a number of laboratories to be considered as a valuable analytical tool for that purpose. Although long-term animal tests are expensive, they cannot be
eliminated as the ultimate safety test; however, the Salmonella assay
technique does show good correlation between mutagenicity in bacteria
and carcinogenicity in animals and therefore can be used as a predictive tool.

The chemicals to be tested for mutagenicity are spread on a lawn
of specially selected mutant strains of *Salmonella typhimurium*.
Direct-acting mutagens will penetrate the bacterial cells and cause
the organism to grow into a visible colony.

Homogenates of rodent (usually) livers may be added directly to
the petri plates to convert promutagens to the active state.

The appearance of a visible colony after a 48-hr incubation at
37°C is evidence that a mutation took place in a bacterial cell and
the daughter cells were able to grow on a minimal medium.

This relatively simple pour plate procedure is very flexible
and many modifications can be incorporated into the test procedure.
The chemicals to be tested can be dissolved in any nongermicidal
solvent and incorporated into a top agar and then spread evenly over
the surface of a minimal agar plate. [Note: DMSO is usually the
solvent of choice for preparing solutions of the test chemical.]

The chemical can also be applied to a filter paper disk which
is placed onto the surface of a preseeded agar plate. Another technique is to place a crystal of the compound directly onto the surface
of the plate. Each one of these techniques has its own advantages
and disadvantages.

C. Experimental

1. *Materials*

a. *Vogel-Bonner E minimal agar plates*   Prepare a 50-fold concentrate of minimal salt solution by dissolving 10 g of $MgSO_4 \cdot 7H_2O$,
100 g of citric acid ($H_3C_6H_5O_7 \cdot H_2O$), 500 g of K_2HPO_4, and 175 g of
$NaNH_4HPO_4$ in distilled water and adjusting the volume to 1 liter.

Dilute the minimal salt concentrate 50-fold with distilled water and add Bacto-agar to a final concentration of 1.5%. Sterilize the mixture at 120°C for 15 min. Add presterilized 20% glucose solution to a final concentration of 2% and dispense into sterile petri plates. (Caution: The plates must be level and free from bubbles.)

b. *Top agar*   The preparation, usually made in 100-ml amounts, contains 0.6% Bacto-agar and 0.6% NaCl. Autoclave this mixture at 120°C for 15 min.

c. *Reduced triphosphopyridine nucleotide (TPNH)*   The mammalian liver enzyme fraction (S-9 mix) is prepared to contain 8 mM of $MgCl_2$, 33 mM of KCl, 5 mM of glucose-6-phosphate, 4 mM of triphosphopyridine nucleotide and 100 mM of sodium phosphate (pH 7.4).

d. *Liver homogenate fraction (S-9 mix)*   Liver tissue is rich in enzyme activity and the investigator can select the species of choice; however, male rats are usually the preferred species. Enzyme activity may be increased by pretreating the rats with phenobarbital, 3-methylcholanthrene, or Aroclor 1254. Procedures for pretreatment are exceedingly variable from laboratory to laboratory and should be developed for each laboratory.

   The rats are anesthetized with diethyl ether and killed by cervical dislocation, then the livers are removed aseptically to a previously tared container and placed in an ice bath. The livers are washed with an equal amount (w/v) of sterile 0.15 M KCl and then homogenized in three volumes of sterile 0.15 M KCl by using a tissue grinder (Brinkman Polytron). The homogenate is centrifuged at 4°C at 9000 x G for 10 min, then the supernatant is decanted, pooled, dispensed into usable aliquots, and frozen at -70°C prior to use.

   For the plate test, three volumes of S-9 fraction are mixed with seven volumes of TPNH generating solution for addition to the reaction mixture.

e. *Bacterial strains*   The bacterial strains, *Salmonella typhimurium* LT-2 mutants designated as TA-1535, TA-1537, TA-1538, TA-98, and TA-100, are those constructed by Ames and his associates [151,153]. The

stock cultures are maintained on nutrient agar slants and are transferred to nutrient agar broth 24 hr prior to use in the mutagenesis
test. An 18 to 24-hr nutrient broth culture grown at 37°C with
shaking sould have 1-3 x 10^9 bacteria per milliliter.

f. *Histidine-biotin solution*   A trace amount of histidine is
required to allow for several cell divisions; this growth is necessary in many cases for mutagenesis to occur. This requirement is
met by using a solution containing histidine•HCl (0.5 mM) and biotin
(0.5 mM). The solution is sterilized by filtration through a 0.45-
µm membrane filter and stored at 4°C prior to use.

   2. Mutagenesis Assay on Plates
The Vogel-Bonner plates are removed from the refrigerator the day
preceding the test and allowed to equilibrate at room temperature
(in an inverted position).

   A flask containing 100 ml of top agar is liquified by heating,
allowed to cool slightly, then 10 ml of histidine-biotin solution is
added to the melted agar and uniformly mixed. Sterile test tubes
(12 x 75 mm) are placed in a constant-temperature bath (hot block)
at 45°C and the following ingredients are sequentially added: 2.5 ml
of molten top agar, 0.1 ml of the broth culture of the bacteria,
0.1 ml of the compound to be tested, and 0.5 ml of the S-9 mix.
After thorough mixing by vortex action, the contents of the tube
are poured onto the surface of a Vogel-Bonner plate. The plate is
rotated gently to assure even distribution over the entire surface
then placed on a level surface and allowed to harden. The total
elapsed time between the addition of the bacterial culture and the
pouring onto the minimal agar plate should be less than 1 min.
After the top agar has solidified, the plates are inverted and
incubated at 37°C in the dark for 48 hr.

   The colonies which develop on the minimal medium have mutated
to histidine prototrophy. The mutagenic potency is then estimated
by comparing the number of mutant colonies induced by the test
chemical to the number of spontaneous mutants on the control plates.
For screening compounds a wide dose range (e.g., 4 decades of

concentration) should be tested with and without the addition of the S-9 mix. The actual concentrations will be determined by factors such as solubility and toxicity. The investigator must decide on the number of replicate plates to be used for the various concentrations in each test. Fewer replicates may be used in range-finding assays than in the construction of dose-response curves where greater confidence levels are required.

D. Discussion

The Salmonella/mammalian microsome test is a very sensitive and simple bacterial test for the detection of carcinogens as mutagens and it has been used in laboratories all over the world to screen for potentially mutagenic environmental chemicals [154]. McCann et al. [155] summarized results of mutagenicity tests with 300 chemicals; a high correlation between carcinogenicity in animals and mutagenicity of the chemicals was demonstrated. Of the 174 recognized carcinogens, 156 (89%) were mutagenic in the Salmonella system. The number of compounds generally recognized as noncarcinogens which gave false positive reactions in the bacterial test was estimated to be approximately 10-13%. Many of these compounds have a chemical structure which is quite similar to known carcinogens and in many instances the carcinogenicity data are scant or lacking.

There are two large classes of chemical compounds which are generally considered to be nonreactive to the bacterial test as it is routinely performed. They are the heavy metals such as the lead and mercury compounds and the cocarcinogens such as the hormones.

The test as it was originally developed combined the test organisms and the suspected chemicals in a controlled medium. This procedure detected only the direct-acting mutagens. The test was later modified to include a mammalian microsomal preparation, usually from rat liver tissue, and this improvement allowed for the metabolic activation of promutagens which produced mutant colonies in the test organisms.

Another modification of the test procedure permits the detection of mutagenic metabolites in the urine of treated animals [156]. Urine is collected from animals which have been given the test chemical by the oral route, sterilized by filtration or by the addition of a germicide, and then tested for the presence of excreted metabolites which are mutagenic. For this test, glucuronidase from an external source is added to the other mammalian enzymes so that metabolites excreted as the glucuronides can be detected as mutagens.

E. Interpretation of Results

It is essential that adequate controls be performed with each test since a great deal of information can be attained by careful examination of the control plates. These plates should show that none of the individual components of the test were contaminated with extraneous organisms. Some contaminants could develop colonies and be mistaken for mutant colonies, thereby giving a false positive result. Good aseptic technique will minimize external contamination; however, some S-9 fractions may be contaminated due to an infection in the donor animals.

The spontaneous mutation rate for each strain is remarkably consistent from passage to passage. The spontaneous mutations in the control plates (with all ingredients except the test chemical) show that the indicator strain is capable of detecting induced mutations. Abnormally high background frequencies indicate that the test culture is not satisfactory. On the other hand, low background frequencies indicate that a toxic condition exists in the test. In either case, the reason for the deviation from the normal rates must be determined before the test can be evaluated.

A known positive control compound shows that the bacterial culture and the S-9 fraction are responding in a controlled manner. Variations in S-9 activity may result in fewer mutations than expected and an excessive S-9 fraction can add sufficient histidine to the test mixture to allow excessive growth of nonmutated organisms.

Dose-response curves that result from testing multiple dose levels are usually linear, but in most instances the curves will level off or even decrease at the higher concentrations.

A test is usually considered to be negative if the induced mutation frequency in the highest nontoxic concentration is less than twice that of the background frequency rate. A high mutation frequency in the bacterial culture does not necessarily mean that the test compound is a highly potent carcinogen in tests with a susceptible animal. Extensive research is currently being conducted in an attempt to correlate mutagenic potency with carcinogenic potency.

REFERENCES

1. M. C. Bowman and J. R. King. Analysis of 2-acetylaminofluorene: Residues in laboratory chow and microbiological media. *Biochem. Med. 9*, 390-401 (1974).

2. E. K. Weisburger and J. H. Weisburger. Chemistry, carcinogenicity and metabolism of 2-fluorenamine and related compounds. *Advan. Cancer Res. 5*, 331-431 (1958).

3. J. H. Weisburger and E. K. Weisburger. Biochemical formation and pharmacological, toxicological, and pathological properties of hydroxylamines and hydroxamic acids. *Pharmacol. Rev. 25*, 1-60 (1973).

4. B. B. Westfall. Estimation of 2-aminofluorene and related compounds in biologic material. *J. Nat. Cancer Inst. 6*, 23-29 (1945).

5. B. B. Westfall and H. P. Morris. Photometric estimation of N-acetyl-2-aminofluorene. *J. Nat. Cancer Inst. 8*, 17-21 (1947).

6. R. B. Sandin, R. Melby, A. S. Hay, R. N. Jones, E. C. Miller, and J. H. Miller. Ultraviolet spectra and carcinogenic activities of some fluorene and biphenyl derivatives. *J. Amer. Chem. Soc. 74*, 5073-5075 (1952).

7. C. C. Irving. N-hydroxylation of 2-acetylaminofluorene in the rabbit. *Cancer Res. 22*, 867-873 (1962).

8. J. H. Weisburger, E. K. Weisburger, H. P. Morris, and H. A. Sober. Chromatographic separation of some metabolites of the carcinogen N-2-fluorenylacetamide. *J. Nat. Cancer Inst. 17*, 363-374 (1956).

9. H. R. Gutmann and R. R. Erickson. The conversion of the car- cinogen N-hydroxy-2-fluorenylacetamide to o-amidophenols by rat liver in vitro (an inducible enzymatic reaction). *J. Biol. Chem.* 244, 1729-1740 (1969).

10. F. R. Fullerton, National Center for Toxicological Research, Jefferson, Ark., Personal communication.

11. M. Beroza and M. C. Bowman. Identification of pesticides at nanogram level by extraction p-values. *Anal. Chem.* 37, 291- 292 (1965).

12. M. C. Bowman and M. Beroza. Extraction p-values of pesticides and related materials in six binary solvent systems. *J. Ass. Offic. Anal. Chem.* 48, 943-952 (1965).

13. M. C. Bowman and M. Beroza. Identification of compounds by extraction p-values using gas chromatography. *Anal. Chem.* 38, 1544-1549 (1966).

14. M. Beroza, M. N. Inscoe, and M. C. Bowman. Distribution of pesticides in immiscible binary solvent systems for cleanup and identification and the extraction of pesticides from milk. *Res. Rev.* 30, 1-61 (1969).

15. M. C. Bowman, J. R. King, and C. L. Holder. Benzidine and congeners: Analytical chemical properties and trace analysis in five substrates. *Int. J. Environ. Anal. Chem.* 4, 205-223 (1976).

16. L. Rehn. Blasingeschwulste bei anilinarbeitern. *Arch. Klin. Chirurgie* 50, 588-600 (1895).

17. *Federal Register.* Carcinogens: Occupational health and safety standards. 39, 3756-3797 (January 29, 1974).

18. T. J. Haley. Benzidine revisited: A review of the literature and problems associated with the use of benzidine and its con- geners. *Clin. Toxicol.* 8, 13-42 (1975).

19. L. J. Sciarini and J. W. Meigs. Biotransformation of the ben- zidines. *Arch. Environ. Health* 2, 108-112 (1961).

20. R. K. Baker and J. G. Deighton. The metabolism of benzidine in the rat. *Cancer Res.* 13, 529-531 (1953).

21. M. A. El-Dib. Colorimetric determination of aniline derivatives in natural waters. *J. Ass. Offic. Anal. Chem.* 54, 1383-1387 (1971),

22. J. M. Glassman and J. W. Meigs. Benzidine (4,4'-diaminobiphenyl) and substituted benzidines. *AMA Arch. Ind. Hyg. Occup. Med.* 4, 519-532 (1951).

23. T. Akiyama. The investigation of the manufacturing plant of organic pigment. *Jikei Med. J.* 17, 1-9 (1970).

24. D. B. Clayson, E. Ward, and L. Ward. The fate of benzidine in various species. *Acta Unio. Intl. Contra. Cancerum. 15*, 581-586 (1959).

25. E. Rinde. Thesis. New York University, 1974.

26. M. C. Bowman and L. G. Rushing. Trace analysis of 3,3'-dichloro-benzidine in animal chow, wastewater and human urine by three gas chromatographic procedures. *Arch. Environ. Contam. Toxicol. 6*, 471-482 (1977).

27. T. Gadian. Carcinogens in industry, with special reference to dichlorobenzidine. *Chem. Ind.* (London) *19*, 821-831 (1975).

28. E. Sawicki, H. Johnson, and K. Kosinski. Chromatographic separation and spectral analysis of polynuclear aromatic amines and heterocyclic imines. *Microchem. J. 10*, 72-102 (1966).

29. C. L. Holder, J. R. King, and M. C. Bowman. 4-Aminobiphenyl, 2-naphthylamine, and analogs: Analytical properties and trace analysis in five substrates. *J. Toxicol. Environ. Health 2*, 111-129 (1976).

30. T. Walle and H. Ehrsson. Quantitative gas chromatographic determination of picogram quantities of amino and alcoholic compounds by electron capture detection: Part I, Preparation and properties of the heptafluorobutyryl derivatives. *Acta Pharm. Suecica 7*, 389-406 (1970).

31. H. Ehrsson, T. Walle, and H. Brotell. Quantitative gas chromato-graphic determination of picogram quantities of phenols. *Acta Pharm. Suecica 8*, 319-328 (1971).

32. E. A. Lugg. Stabilized diazonium salts as analytical reagents for the determinations of air-borne phenols and amines. *Anal. Chem. 35*, 899-904 (1968).

33. J. W. Bridges, P. J. Creaven, and R. T. Williams. The fluorescence of some biphenyl derivatives. *Biochem. J. 96*, 872-878 (1965).

34. K. Shimomura and J. F. Walton. Thin-layer chromatography of amines by ligand exchange. *Separation Sci. 3*, 493-499 (1968).

35. Y. Masuda and D. Hoffmann. Quantitative determination of 1-naphthylamine and 2-naphthylamine in cigarette smoke. *Anal. Chem. 41*, 650-652 (1969).

36. J. A. Knight. Gas chromatographic analysis of γ-irradiated aniline for aminoaromatic products. *J. Chromatogr. 56*, 201-208 (1971).

37. R. C. Gupta and S. P. Srivastava. Oxidation of aromatic amines by preoxodisulphate ion. *Z. Anal. Chem. 257*, 275-277 (1971).

38. I. M. Jakovljevic, J. Zynger, and R. H. Bishara. Thin layer chromatographic separation and fluorometric determination of 4-aminobiphenyl in 2-aminobiphenyl. *Anal. Chem. 47*, 2045-2046 (1975).

39. J. R. King, C. R. Nony, and M. C. Bowman. Trace analysis of diethylstilbestrol (DES) in animal chow by parallel high-speed liquid chromatography, electron-capture gas chromatography and radioassays. *J. Chromatogr. Sci. 15*, 14-21 (1977).

40. W. G. Smith and E. E. McNeil. Simple method for routine detection of residues of diethylstilbestrol (DES) in meat contaminated at levels as low as one part per billion. *Anal. Chem. 44*, 1084-1087 (1972).

41. D. E. Coffin and J. Pilon. Gas chromatographic determination of diethylstilbestrol residues in animal tissues. *J. Ass. Offic. Anal. Chem. 56*, 352-357 (1973).

42. A. L. Donoho, W. S. Johnson, R. F. Sieck, and W. L. Sullivan. Gas chromatographic determination of diethylstilbestrol and its glucuronide in cattle tissue. *J. Ass. Offic. Anal. Chem. 56*, 785-792 (1973).

43. G. H. Gass, N. Coast, and N. Graham. Carcinogenic does-response curve to oral DES. *J. Nat. Cancer Inst. 33*, 971-977 (1964).

44. A. L. Donoho, O. D. Decker, J. Koester, and J. R. Koons. A sensitive gas chromatographic determination of diethylstilbestrol in animal feeds. *J. Ass. Offic. Anal. Chem. 54*, 75-79 (1971).

45. E. W. Cheng and W. Burroughs. Determination of small amounts of diethylstilbestrol in feeds. *J. Ass. Offic. Agr. Chem. 38*, 146-150 (1955).

46. M. T. Jeffus and C. T. Kenner. Quantitative determination and confirmation of low levels of diethylstilbestrol in feeds. *J. Ass. Offic. Anal. Chem. 55*, 1345-1353 (1972).

47. L. Stoloff. Analytical methods for mycotoxins. *Clin. Toxicol. 5*, 465-494 (1972).

48. W. A. White and N. H. Ludwig. Isomerization of α,α'-diethylstilbestrol, isolation and characterization of the cis isomer. *J. Agr. Food Chem. 19*, 388-390 (1971).

49. M. C. Bowman and C. R. Nony. Trace analysis of estradiol by electron-capture gas chromatography. *J. Chromatogr. Sci. 15*, 160-163 (1977).

50. J. B. Brown. Some observations on the Kober colour and fluorescence reactions of the natural oestrogens. *J. Endocrinol. 8*, 196-210 (1952).

51. W. S. Bauld. Separation of oestrogens in urinary extracts by partition chromatography. *Biochem. J. 59*, 294-300 (1955).

52. J. B. Brown. A chemical method for the determination of oestriol, oestrone and oestradiol in human urine. *Biochem. J. 60*, 185-193 (1955).

53. J. W. Goldzieher. The measurement of estrogen mixtures by differential fluorometry. *Endrocrinology 53*, 527-535 (1953).

54. K. Matsumoto and T. Seki. A chemical method for the quantita-
    tive determination of estriol, 16-epi estriol, estradiol-17β
    and estrone in human male and non-pregnancy urine. *Endocrinol.*
    Japon. *10*, 183-189 (1963).

55. S. Fishman. Determination of estrogens in dosage forms by
    fluorescence using dansyl chloride. *J. Pharm. Sci. 64*, 674-
    680 (1975).

56. R. H. Bishara and I. M. Jakovljevic. The separation of some
    estrogens by thin layer chromatography. *J. Chromatogr. 41*,
    136-138 (1969).

57. I. Schoreder, G. Lopez-Sanchez, J. C. Medina-Acevedo, and Ma.
    del Carmen Espinosa. Quantitative determination of conjugated
    or esterified estrogens in tablets by thin layer chromatography.
    J. Chromatogr. Sci. 13, 35-40 (1975).

58. S. Siggia and R. A. Dishman. Analysis of steroid hormones
    using high resolution liquid chromatography. *Anal. Chem. 42*,
    1223-1229 (1970).

59. E. Gurpide, M. C. Giebenhain, L. Tseng, and W. G. Kelly.
    Radioimmunoassay of estrogens in human pregnancy urine, plasma,
    and amniotic fluid. *Amer. J. Obstet. Gynecol. 109*, 897-906
    (1971).

60. H. A. Robertson, T. C. Smeaton, and R. Durnford. A method for
    the extraction, separation and estimation of unconjugated
    estrone, estradiol-17α and estradiol-17β in plasma. *Steroids*
    20, 651-667 (1972).

61. E. Cerceo and C. Elloso. Rapid method for the estimation of
    total free estrogens in plasma. *Anal. Chem. 46*, 1578-1580
    (1974).

62. S. Sybulski and G. B. Maughan. A rapid method for the measure-
    ment of estradiol and hydrocortisone levels in maternal and
    fetal blood and amniotic fluid. *Amer. J. Obstet. Gynecol. 121*,
    32-36 (1975).

63. J. C. Touchstone, T. Murawec, O. Brual, and M. Breckwoldt.
    Improved method for quantitation of urinary estrogens. *Steroids*
    17, 285-304 (1971).

64. H. Adlercreutz, C. J. Johannson, and T. Luukkainen. Gas chromato-
    graphic and mass spectrometric studies in the influence of metabo-
    lites of bis(p-acetoxyphenyl)cyclohexylidenemethane on the esti-
    mation of estrogens in urine. *Ann. Med. Exp. Fenniae. 45*, 269-
    276 (1967).

65. H. Adlercreutz. Evaluation of gas-liquid chromatographic tech-
    niques for the estimation of oestrogens. *Clin. Chim. Acta 34*,
    231-240 (1971).

66. R. A. Mead, G. C. Holtmeyer, and K. B. Eik-Nes. A method for
    the determination of free estradiol in peripheral plasma by
    gas-phase chromatography. *J. Chromatogr. Sci. 7*, 554-560 (1969).

67. J. R. G. Challis and R. B. Heap. The estimation of steroids by using gas-liquid chromatography with an electron-capture detector: Preparation of heptafluorobutyrate esters and their purification on Sephadex LH-20. *Biochem. J. 112*, 36p (1969).

68. K. Honda and S. Kushinsky. Gas chromatographic analysis of estrogens. *Mickrochim. Acta* (Wien) *6*, 1182-1187 (1969).

69. D. W. R. Knorr, M. A. Kirschner, and J. P. Taylor. Estimation of estrone and estradiol in low level urines using electron-capture gas-liquid chromatography. *J. Clin. Endocrinol. 31*, 409-416 (1970).

70. S. Kushinsky, J. Coyotupa, K. Honda, M. Hiroi, K. Kinoshita, M. Foote, C. Chan, R. Y. Ho, W. Paul, and W. J. Dignam. Gas chromatographic determination of estrone, estradiol and estriol in non-pregnancy plasma. *Mikrochim. Acta* (Wien) *3*, 491-503 (1970).

71. F. L. Rigby, H. J. Karavolas, D. W. Norgard, and R. C. Wolf. Preparation of steroid heptafluorobutyrates for gas liquid chromatography utilizing vapor phase derivatization. *Steroids 16*, 703-706 (1970).

72. G. Adessi, D. Eichenberger, T. Q. Nhuan, and M. F. Jayle. Determination by gas chromatography of seven urinary oestrogens at the end of gestation. *Clin. Chem. Acta 55*, 323-331 (1974).

73. J. J. Ryan. Chromatographic analysis of hormone residues in food. *J. Chromatogr. 127*, 53-89 (1976).

74. C. L. Holder, C. R. Nony, and M. C. Bowman. Trace analysis of zearalenone and/or zearalanol in animal chow by high-pressure liquid chromatography and gas-liquid chromatography. *J. Ass. Offic. Anal. Cham. 60*, 272-278 (1977).

75. C. J. Mirocha, C. M. Christensen, and G. H. Nelson. Physiologic activity of some fungal estrogens produced by fusarium. *Cancer Res. 28*, 2319-2322 (1968).

76. R. A. Meronuck, K. H. Garren, C. M. Christensen, G. H. Nelson, and F. Bates. Effects on turkey poults and chicks of rations containing corn invaded by penicillium and fusarium species. *Amer. J. Vet. Res. 31*, 551-556 (1970).

77. C. M. Christensen, C. J. Mirocha, G. H. Nelson, and J. F. Quast. Effect on young swine of consumption of rations containing corn invaded by *Fusarium roseum. Appl. Microbiol. 23*, 202 (1972).

78. G. H. Nelson, C. M. Christensen, and C. J. Mirocha. Fusarium and estrogenism in swine. *J. Amer. Vet. Med. Ass. 163*, 1276-1277 (1973).

79. J. C. Wolf and C. J. Mirocha. Regulation of sexual reproduction in *Gibberella zeae* (*Fusarium roseum* graminearum) by F-2 (zeara-lenone). *Can. J. Microbiol. 19*, 725-734 (1973).

266 CHAPTER 3

80. R. W. Caldwell, J. Tuite, M, Stob, and R. Baldwin. Zearalenone production by Fusarium species, *Appl. Microbiol. 20,* 31-34 (1970).

81. C. J. Mirocha, C. M. Christensen, and G. H. Nelson. *Microbial Toxins* Vol. 7 (S. Kadis, A. Ciegler, and J. Ajl, eds.). Academic Press, New York, 1971, pp. 107-138.

82. H. Rothenbacker, J. P. Wiggins, and L. L. Wilson. Pathologic changes in endocrine glands and certain other tissues of lambs implanted with the synthetic growth promotant zeranol. *Amer. J. Vet. Res. 36,* 1313-1317 (1975).

83. G. D. Sharp and I. A. Dyer. Zearalanol metabolism in steers. *J. Anim. Sci. 34,* 176-179 (1972).

84. R. M. Eppley. Screening method for zearalenone, aflatoxin, and ochratoxin. *J. Ass. Offic. Anal. Chem. 51,* 74-78 (1968).

85. L. Stoloff, S. Nesheim, L. Yin, J. V. Rodricks, M. Stack, and A. D. Campbell. A multimycotoxin detection method. *J. Ass. Offic. Anal. Chem. 54,* 91-97 (1971).

86. C. J. Mirocha, B. Schauerhamer, and S. V. Pathre. Isolation, detection and quantitation of zearalenone in maize and barley. *J. Ass. Offic. Anal. Chem. 57,* 1104-1110 (1974).

87. J. A. Steele, C. J. Mirocha, and S. V. Pathre. Metabolism of zearalenone by *Fusarium roseum* graminearum. *J. Agr. Food Chem. 24,* 89-97 (1976).

88. L. Stoloff. Analytical methods for mycotoxins. *Clin. Toxicol. 5,* 465-494 (1976).

89. C. R. Nony, M. C. Bowman, C. L. Holder, J. F. Young, and W. L. Oller. Trace analysis of 2,4,5-trichlorophenoxyacetic acid, its glycineamide, and their alkaline hydrolyzable conjugates in mouse blood, urine and feces. *J. Pharm. Sci. 65,* 1810-1816 (1976).

90. *Report on 2,4,5-T: A Report of the Panel on Herbicides of the President's Advisory Committee.* Executive Office of the President, Office of Science and Technology, Washington, D.C., March, 1971.

91. W. N. Piper, J. Q. Rose, M. L. Leng, and P. J. Gehring. The fate of 2,4,5-trichlorophenoxyacetic acid (2,4,5-T) following oral administration to rats and dogs. *Toxicol. Appl. Pharmacol. 26,* 339-351 (1973).

92. P. J. Gehring, C. G. Kramer, B. A. Schwetz, J. Q. Rose, and V. K. Rowe. The fate of 2,4,5-trichlorophenoxyacetic acid (2,4,5-T) following oral administration to man. *Toxicol. Appl. Pharmacol. 26,* 352-361 (1973).

93. K. Erne. Distribution and elimination of chlorinated phenoxyacetic acids in animals. *Acta Vet. Scand. 7,* 240-256 (1966).

94. K. Erne. Animal metabolism of phenoxyacetic acid herbicides. *Acta Vet. Scand.* 7, 264-271 (1966).

95. M. T. Shafik, H. C. Sullivan, and H. F. Enos. A method for determination of low levels of exposure to 2,4-D and 2,4,5-T. *Int. J. Environ. Anal. Chem. 1*, 23-33 (1971).

96. I. H. Suffet. The p-value approach to quantitative liquid-liquid extraction of pesticides and herbicides from water: 3, Liquid-liquid extraction of phenoxy acid herbicides from water. *J. Agr. Food Chem. 21*, 591-598 (1973).

97. M. C. Bowman, C. L. Holder, and L. I. Bone. Roetnone and degradation products: Analysis in animal chow and tissues by high-pressure liquid chromatography. *J. Ass. Offic. Anal. Chem. 61*, 1445-1455 (1978).

98. E. Geoffrey. Contribution to l'etude du Robinia Nicou Aublet, as point de vue botanique, chimique et physiologique. *Ann. Inst. Colon. Marseille 2*, 1-7 (1895).

99. F. B. LaForge, H. L. Haller, and L. E. Smith. The determination of the structure of rotenone. *Chem. Rev. 12*, 181-213 (1933).

100. Environmental Protection Agency. *EPA Compendium of Registered Pesticides* Vol. III. III-R-3.1, 1972.

101. M. Gosalvez and J. Merchan. Induction of rat adenomas with the respiratory inhibitor rotenone. *Cancer Res. 33*, 3047-3050 (1973).

102. T. J. Haley. A review of the literature of rotenone. *J. Environ. Path. Toxicol. 1*, 315-337 (1978).

103. Anonymous. EPA lists pesticides that may be too dangerous to use. *Chem. Eng. News*, June 14, 1976, p. 18.

104. C. R. Gross and C. M. Smith. Colorimetric method for determination of rotenone. *J. Ass. Offic. Anal. Chem. 17*, 336-339 (1934).

105. L. D. Goodhue. An improvement on the Gross and Smith colorimetric method for the determination of rotenone and deguelin. *J. Ass. Offic. Anal. Chem. 19*, 118-120 (1936).

106. A. T. Frases. Reactions of quinine and rotenone with vanadium. *Biol. Soc. Quim. Peru 3*, 219-220 (1937).

107. M. Jacobson, I. Hornstein, and R. T. Murphy. The analysis of milk for rotenoids. *J. Ass. Offic. Anal. Chem. 42*, 174-176 (1959).

108. H. L. Cupples and I. Hornstein. Infrared spectra of rotenone and dehydrorotenone. *J. Amer. Chem. Soc. 73*, 4023-4024 (1951).

109. G. Vigneron. Infrared spectrum of rotenone. *Ann. Soc. Sci. Bruxelles Ser. I. 65*, 41-48 (1951).

110. R. G. Knoerlein. The infrared analysis of rotenone. *J. Ass. Offic. Anal. Chem. 44*, 577-579 (1961).

111. H. Begue. The chemical analysis of rotenone powders. *Ann. Agron. 9*, 121-132 (1939).

112. H. Matsumoto. Qualitative analysis of rotenone (derris root) by paper partition chromatography. *Kagaku To Sosa 11*, 19-21 (1958).

113. Y. Doi. Microdetection of rotenone. *Kagaku To Sosa 12*, 492-511 (1959).

114. T. Shishido. Chromatography of organic insecticides: III, Paper chromatography of rotenone and its derivatives. *Nippon Nogei Kagaku Kaishi 36*, 780-784 (1962).

115. N. E. Delfel. Hydriodic acid as a new selective reagent for detection of rotenone in chromatography. *J. Agr. Food Chem. 13*, 56-57 (1965).

116. N. E. Delfel. Thin-layer chromatography of rotenone and related compounds. *J. Agr. Food Chem. 14*, 130-132 (1966).

117. N. E. Delfel and W. H. Tallent. Thin-layer densitometric determination of rotenone and deguelin. *J. Ass. Offic. Anal. Chem. 52*, 182-187 (1969).

118. V. Mallet and D. P. Surette. Fluorescence of pesticides by treatment with heat, acid or base. *J. Chromatogr. 95*, 243-246 (1974).

119. G. W. Ivie and J. E. Casida. Sensitized photodecomposition and photosensitizer activity of pesticide chemicals exposed to sunlight on silica gel chromatoplates. *J. Agr. Food Chem. 19*, 405-409 (1971).

120. H. M. Cheng, I. Yamamoto, and J. E. Casida. Rotenone photodecomposition. *J. Agr. Food Chem. 20*, 850-856 (1972).

121. N. E. Delfel. Gas-liquid chromatographic determination of rotenone and deguelin in plant extracts and commercial insecticides. *J. Ass. Offic. Anal. Chem. 56*, 1343-1349 (1973).

122. N. E. Delfel. Ultraviolet and infrared analysis of rotenone: Effect of other rotenoids. *J. Ass. Offic. Anal. Chem. 59*, 703-707 (1976).

123. R. J. Bushway, B. S. Engdahl, B. M. Colvin, and A. R. Hanks. Separation of rotenoids and the determination of rotenone in pesticide formulations by high-performance liquid chromatography. *J. Ass. Offic. Anal. Chem. 58*, 965-970 (1975).

124. R. I. Freudenthal, D. C. Emmerling, and R. L. Baron. Separation of rotenoids by high-pressure liquid chromatography. *J. Chromatogr. 134*, 207-209 (1977).

125. R. Bushway and A. Hanks, Determination of rotenone in pesticide formulations and separation of six rotenoids by reversed-
phase high-performance liquid chromatography. *J. Chromatogr.*
134, 210-215 (1977).

126. J. R. King and M. C. Bowman. 4-Ethylsulfonylnaphthalene-1-
sulfonamide (ENS): Analytical chemical behavior and trace
analysis in five substrates. *Biochem. Med. 12*, 313-330 (1975).

127. G. M. Bonser and D. B. Clayson. A sulphonamide derivative
which induces urinary tract epithelial hyperplasia and car-
cinomas of the bladder epithelium in the mouse. *Brit. J.*
Urol. 36, 26-34 (1964).

128. D. B. Clayson and G. M. Bonser. The induction of tumours of
the mouse bladder epithelium by 4-ethylsulphonylnaphthalene-
1-sulphonamide. *Brit. J. Cancer 19*, 311-316 (1965).

129. D. B. Clayson, J. A. S. Pringle, and G. M. Bonser. 4-Ethyl-
sulphonylnaphthalene-1-sulphonamide: A new chemical for the
study of bladder cancer in the mouse. *Biochem. Pharmacol. 16*,
619-626 (1967).

130. P. E. Levi, J. C. Knowles, D. M. Cowen, M. Wood, and E. H.
Cooper. Disorganization of mouse bladder epithelium induced
by 2-acetylaminofluorene and 4-ethylsulfonylnaphthalene-1-
sulfonamide. *J. Nat. Cancer Inst. 46*, 337-343 (1971)

131. A. Flaks, J. M. Hamilton, and D. B. Clayson. Effect of ammonium
chloride on incidence of bladder tumors induced by 4-ethyl-
sulfonylnaphthalene-1-sulfonamide. *J. Nat. Cancer Inst. 51*,
2007-2008 (1973).

132. W. J. Moore. *Physical Chemistry* 4th Ed. Prentice-Hall,
Englewood Cliffs, N.J., 1972, 977 pp.

133. M. C. Bowman and M. Beroza. Gas chromatographic detector for
simultaneous sensing of phosphorus- and sulfur-containing compounds by flame photometry. *Anal. Chem. 40*, 1448-1452 (1968).

134. J. W. Stanley. National Center for Toxicological Research,
Jefferson, Ark. Personal communication.

135. M. C. Bowman and L. G. Rushing. Determination of sodium
phenobarbital in animal chow by high-pressure liquid chromatography. *J. Chromatogr. Sci. 18*, 23-27 (1978).

136. W. A. Joern. Gas chromatography of anticonvulsant drugs,
with no solvent evaporation. *Clin. Chem. 21*, 1548-1550 (1975).

137. A. Kumps and Y. Mardens. Rapid gas-liquid chromatographic
determination of serum levels of phenobarbital and diphenylhydantoin. *Clin. Chim. Acta 62*, 371-376 (1975).

138. P. Friel and A. S. Troupin. Flash-heater ethylation of some
anti epileptic drugs. *Clin. Chem. 21*, 751-754 (1975).

139. H. L. Davis, K. J. Falk, and D. G. Bailey. Improved method
     for the simultaneous determination of phenobarbital, primidone
     and diphenylhydantoin in patients' serum by gas-liquid chroma-
     tography. *J. Chromatogr. 107*, 61-66 (1975).

140. A. Brachet-Liermain and L. Ferrus. Use of the thermoionic
     detector for determining nitrogen-containing drugs in bio-
     logical fluids. *Ann. Falsif. Expert. Chim. 67*, 351-363 (1974).

141. P. A. Pranitis, J. R. Milzoff, and A. Stolman. Extraction of
     drugs from biofluids and tissues with Amberlite XAD-2 resin.
     J. Forensic Sci. 19, 917-926 (1974).

142. K. K. Kaistha, R. Tadrus, and R. Janda. Simultaneous detec-
     tion of a wide variety of commonly abused drugs in a urine
     screening program using thin-layer identification techniques.
     J. Chromatogr. 107, 359-379 (1975).

143. M. Kohsaka. Determination of phenobarbital and phenytoin in
     serum by thin-layer chromatography. *No To Hattatsu 6*, 441-
     443 (1974).

144. S. Hishida, M. Ueda, T. Tanabe, and Y. Mizoi. Experimental
     studies on the detection of hypnotics using thin layer chroma-
     tography. *Kobe J. Med. Sci. 18*, 1-10 (1972).

145. H. E. Booker and B. A. Darcey. Enzymatic immunoassay versus
     gas/liquid chromatography for determination of phenobarbital
     and diphenylhydantoin in serum. *Clin. Chem. 21*, 1766-1768
     (1975).

146. M. G. Horning, W. G. Stillwell, J. Nowlin, K. Lertratanangkoon,
     R. N. Stillwell, and R. M. Hill. Identification and quantifi-
     cation of drugs and drug metabolites in human breast milk using
     gas chromatography-mass spectrometry-computer methods. *Mod.
     Probl. Paediatr. 15*, 73-79 (1975).

147. I. L. Honigberg, J. T. Stewart, A. P. Smith, R. D. Plunkett,
     and E. L. Justice. Liquid chromatography in pharmaceutical
     analysis: IV, Determination of antispasmodic mixtures. *J.
     Pharm. Sci. 64*, 1389-1393 (1975).

148. S. H. Atwell, V. A. Green, and W. G. Haney. Development and
     evaluation of method for simultaneous determination of pheno-
     barbital and diphenylhydantoin in plasma by high-pressure
     liquid chromatography. *J. Pharm. Sci. 64*, 806-809 (1975).

149. V. Quercia. B. Tucci Bucci, and F. Rosmini. Determination of
     trace amounts of barbituates by liquid-phase chromatography.
     Boll. Chim. Farm. 113, 628-632 (1974).

150. J. E. Evans. Simultaneous measurement of diphenylhydantoin
     and phenobarbital in serum by high pressure liquid chroma-
     tography. *Anal. Chem. 45*, 2428-2429 (1973).

151. B. N. Ames, W. E. Durston, E. Yamaski, and F. D. Lee. Carcinogens are mutagens: A simple test system combining liver homogenates for activation and bacteria for detection. *Proc. Nat. Acad. Sci. U.S. 70*, 2281-2285 (1973).

152. B. N. Ames, F. D. Lee, and W. D. Durston. An improved bacterial test system for the detection and classification of mutagens and carcinogens. *Proc. Nat. Acad. Sci. U.S. 70*, 782-786 (1973).

153. J. McCann, N. E. Springarn, J. Kobori, and B. N. Ames. Detection of carcinogens as mutagens: Bacterial tester strains with R factor plasmids. *Proc. Nat. Acad. Sci. U.S. 72*, 979-983 (1975).

154. J. L. Fox. Ames test success paves way for short-term cancer testing. *Chem. Eng. News,* December 12, 1977, p. 34.

155. J. McCann, E. Choi, E. Yamaski, and B. N. Ames. Detection of carcinogens as mutagens in the Salmonella microsome test: Assay of 300 chemicals. *Proc. Nat. Acad. Sci. U.S. 72*, 5135-5139 (1975).

156. W. E. Durston and B. N. Ames. A simple method for the detection of mutagens in urine studies with the carcinogen 2-acetylaminofluorene. *Proc. Nat. Acad. Sci. U.S. 71*, 737-741 (1974).

4

A PROCEDURE FOR THE TRACE ANALYSIS OF THIRTEEN CARCINOGENS
AND ANALOGS IN ADMIXTURE IN HUMAN URINE AND WASTEWATER

I   INTRODUCTION

Two important factors relating to the control of test substances in nonclinical laboratory studies as proposed by the U. S.
Department of Health, Education, and Welfare, Food and Drug Administration [1] are (1) to provide assurance that personnel and work
areas remain free of contamination by the substances and (2) to
accomplish the safe disposal of contaminated experimental material.
Since long-term, low-dose toxicological studies with large numbers
of mice at our laboratory include tests with several chemicals known
to cause, or suspected of causing, cancer in humans by occupational
exposure [2-4], every effort must be made to ensure zero exposure of
personnel to carcinogens by periodically monitoring samples of urine
by the most sensitive and specific analytical methods available [5-
8]. In a similar manner, these methods are also used to routinely
monitor wastewater that has been treated for the removal of all test
chemicals [9] prior to sewage treatment and eventual discharge into
the environment. Methods based on spectrophotofluorescence (SPF),
high-pressure liquid chromatography (HPLC), or electron-capture gas
chromatography (EC-GC), have served us well in determining traces
[low or sub parts per billion (ppb; ng/ml)] of a few chemicals
analyzed separately. However, as the number of test compounds
increases, such methods fail to detect, identify, and quantify all
of the substances when they are present in admixture [10]. It
therefore became necessary to devise a procedure capable of simul-
taneously analyzing for traces of all of the substances of current

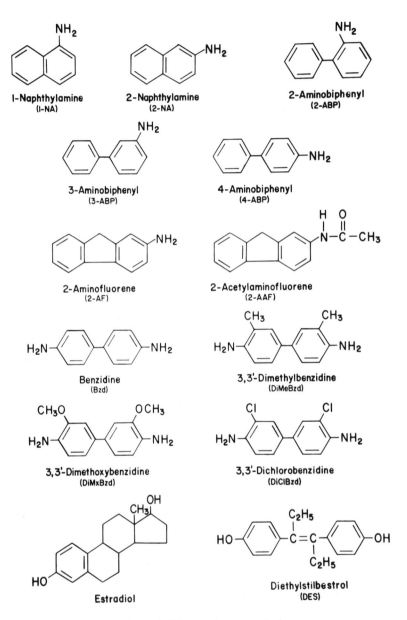

Figure 4.1. Formulas of 13 carcinogens and
related compounds. [From Nony and Bowman [15].)

interest at our laboratory. Formulas of these compounds and some
of their analogs, and the abbreviations used for them in this chapter,
are presented in Figure 4.1.

The 13 compounds shown in the figure may be classified according
to their chemical properties as follows: there are 10 primary amines
(basic), one secondary amine (neutral), and two estrogens (phenolic).
This provided the basis for separating them into groups via acidification, alkalinization, and solvent extraction. Because of the free
hydrogen atoms present in all compounds, including the secondary
amine (2-AAF) after acid hydrolysis and conversion to 2-AF, these
compounds can be reacted with fluorinating agents [8,11-14] to produce derivatives that exhibit high sensitivity in assays using EC-GC.

This chapter gives details for extraction, separation, detection, identification, and quantification of trace amounts of all 13
of these chemical carcinogens and analogs in admixture in wastewater
and human urine by EC-GC of their pentafluoropropionyl derivatives
[15,16].

II   EXPERIMENTAL

A.   Test Chemicals and Reagents

The chemicals shown in Figure 4.1 were obtained from several
suppliers as previously reported by Bowman and coworkers [5-8,13,14],
who also described their properties and purity. (See Chapter 3 for
details.)

All solvents were pesticide grade and all reagents were CP
(chemically pure) grade. Sodium sulfate and glass wool were extracted
with benzene for 40 hr in a Soxhlet apparatus and dried in an oven
overnight at 130°C prior to use. All culture tubes were borosilicate
glass and equipped with Teflon-lined screw caps. The 170-ml and 35-
ml culture tubes were fabricated by Shamrock Scientific Glassware
Co., Little Rock, Ark.

Pentafluoropropionic anhydride (PFPA) and heptafluorobutyric
anhydride (HFBA) were obtained from Pierce Chemical Co., Rockford,
Ill. (No. 65193), and Regis Chemical Co., Morton Grove, Ill.

(No. 270085), respectively. A 100-μl Hamilton syringe, fitted with Chaney adapter, was used to withdraw the derivatizing agent from the vial and deliver it into the reaction vessel. A fresh vial (1 g) was used for each group of samples. The trimethylamine (TMA) reagents (0.05 and 0.1 M in benzene), buffer solution (potassium monobasic phosphate, pH-6), sodium hydroxide (1 N), and sodium bicarbonate (1 M) were described by King et al. [13] and Bowman and Rushing [8]. The "keeper" solution was paraffin oil (20 mg/ml) in pentane. (See procedures for DES, estradiol, and DiClBzd in Chapter 3 for details.)

    B.   Extraction and Preparation of Samples for Analysis

    1. Wastewater

The sample (100 ml) and 10 ml of concentrated HCl were added to a 170-ml culture tube, shaken, and allowed to stand for 5 min. Benzene (20 ml) was then added, the contents were shaken for 1 min, then the tube was centrifuged at 550 revolutions per minute (rpm) for 10 min. The benzene layer was carefully withdrawn by using a syringe and cannula, percolated through a plug of sodium sulfate (25 mm diameter x 25 mm thick), and collected in a 100-ml round-bottom flask containing a glass bead and 0.5 ml of keeper solution. The extraction was repeated by using two additional 20-ml portions of benzene and the combined extracts, containing the phenolic and neutral compounds, were evaporated just to dryness by using water pump vacuum and a 60°C water bath. The acidified aqueous phase was reserved for subsequent extraction of the basic compounds.

    The flask containing the phenolic and neutral compounds was treated as described by Bowman and Nony [14], viz. 5 ml of benzene was used to transfer the residue to a 20-ml culture tube containing 4 ml of 1 N NaOH. The contents of the tube were shaken, centrifuged for 5 min at 1200 rpm, and the benzene layer was transferred to a 35-ml culture tube also containing 4 ml of 1 N NaOH. The contents of the second tube were shaken and centrifuged as described and the benzene layer was carefully withdrawn, percolated through a plug of sodium sulfate (18 mm diameter x 20 mm thick), and collected in a

50-ml round-bottom flask containing a glass bead and 0.5 ml of keeper solution. The flask and aqueous NaOH phases in both tubes were again sequentially washed and extracted in the same manner by using two additional 5-ml portions of benzene which were also percolated through a plug of sodium sulfate. The combined extracts containing the neutral fraction (2-AAF) were reserved for subsequent treatment. The contents of the 20-ml tube were transferred to the 35-ml tube and 10 ml of 1 M sodium bicarbonate, used to wash the 20-ml tube, was also added to the mixture. The mixture was then extracted three times with 15-ml portions of benzene; each extract was successively percolated through a plug of sodium sulfate (25 mm diameter x 25 mm thick) and collected in a 100-ml round-bottom flask containing a boiling bead and 0.5 ml of keeper solution. The combined extracts containing the phenolic fraction were evaporated to dryness by using water pump vacuum and a 60°C water bath. The residue was reserved for subsequent derivatization with PFPA and assay by EC-GC.

The neutral fraction was evaporated to dryness as described and the residue transferred to a 20-ml culture tube by using three 1-ml portions of chloroform. The solvent in the tube was then evaporated to dryness in a tube heater (No. 720,000, Kontes Glass Co., Vineland, N.J.) set at 40°C by using a gentle stream of dry nitrogen. The dry residue was hydrolyzed, as described by Bowman and King [5], by heating the sealed tube containing 4 ml of methanol and 2 ml of concentrated HCl in a tube heater set at 85°C for 2 hr. After the tube had cooled, 3 ml of water was added and the contents were extracted three times with 7-ml portions of benzene. Each extract was carefully withdrawn and discarded by using a 10-ml syringe and cannula. Next, 4 ml of 10 N NaOH was added and the contents were extracted three times with 7-ml portions of benzene. Each extract was successively percolated through a plug of sodium sulfate (18 mm diameter x 20 mm thick) and collected in a 50-ml round-bottom flask containing a boiling bead and 0.5 ml of keeper solution. The contents were evaporated just to dryness at 60°C by using water pump vacuum as described; the residue was transferred to an 8-ml culture tube by using three 1-ml portions of benzene which were also evaporated to dryness in a tube heater at 50°C by using a stream of dry nitrogen. The residue, containing 2-AF, was reserved for subsequent derivatization with PFPA and assay by EC-GC.

The acidified aqueous phase (basic fraction), previously reserved for later treatment, was made strongly alkaline by adding 15 ml of 10 N NaOH and extracted three times with 20-ml portions of benzene. Each extract was percolated successively through a plug of sodium sulfate (25 mm diameter x 25 mm thick) and collected in a 100-ml round-bottom flask containing a boiling bead and 0.5 ml of keeper solution. The combined extracts were evaporated to dryness by using water pump vacuum and a 60°C water bath. The residue was transferred to an 8-ml culture tube by using three 1-ml portions of benzene and evaporated to dryness in a tube heater at 50°C with a stream of dry nitrogen. The residue was reserved for subsequent derivatization with PFPA and assay by EC-GC.

2. Human Urine

Two 50-ml portions of the sample were added to two separate 75-ml culture tubes, each containing 5 g of NaCl; 5 ml of concentrated HCl was added to one tube (phenolic and neutral fractions) and 5 ml of 10 N NaOH was added to the other tube (basic fraction). After the tubes were shaken and allowed to stand for 5 min the contents were extracted three times with 15-ml portions of benzene which were successively percolated through plugs of sodium sulfate (25 mm diameter x 25 mm thick) and collected in 100-ml round-bottom flasks containing a boiling bead and 0.5 ml of keeper solution. Each of these combined extracts was then treated exactly as described for wastewater.

3. Recovery Experiments

a. Wastewater Triplicate samples (100 g) of wastewater in 170-ml culture tubes were separately spiked with 1 ml of methanol containing the appropriate amount of 10 selected carcinogens and analogs (i.e.,

2-NA, 4-ABP, 2-AF, 2-AAF, Bzd, DiClBzd, DiMeBzd, DiMxBzd, DES, and estradiol) to produce residues of 0, 0.10, 1.0, and 10 ppb. The tubes were sealed, mixed, and allowed to stand overnight at 5°C prior to analysis.

b. *Human urine*   Two sets of triplicate 50-g samples of urine in 75-ml culture tubes were separately spiked with 0.5 ml of methanol containing the appropriate amounts of the 10 compounds used for wastewater to produce residues of 0, 2.0, and 20 ppb. The tubes were sealed, mixed, and allowed to stand overnight at 5°C prior to analysis.

C. Preparation of Derivatives

Pentafluoropropionyl (PFP) and heptafluorobutyryl (HFB) derivatives of all compounds shown in Figure 4.1, except 2-AAF, were prepared by our modification of the procedures reported by Walle and Ehrsson [11] and Ehrsson et al. [12]. For derivatization of amines, TMA solution (0.5 ml, 0.05 M) was added to an 8-ml culture tube containing the compounds (10 µg or less) dissolved in exactly 1.5 ml of benzene (total benzene = 2.0 ml), then 50 µl of either PFPA or HFPA reagent was added. The tube was immediately sealed, shaken, heated in a 50°C water bath for 20 min, cooled, and the reaction was terminated by adding 2 ml of phosphate buffer (pH 6.0). The tube was shaken for 1 min, and after the phases had separated, the aqueous layer (bottom) was discarded. The extraction was repeated with an additional 2-ml portion of buffer; the tube was centrifuged for 1 min at 1000 rpm and the benzene layer (top) was either analyzed directly or appropriately diluted with benzene prior to analysis.

For derivatization of phenolic compounds, TMA solution (0.5 ml, 0.1 M) was added to a 50-ml round-bottom flask containing the compounds (10 µg or less) dissolved in exactly 0.5 ml of benzene (total benzene = 1.0 ml), then 50 µl of either PFPA or HFBA reagent was added. The flask was immediately sealed with a glass stopper, the contents mixed by gentle swirling, and allowed to stand at ambient temperature for 20 min. The reaction was terminated by adding 1 ml

of phosphate buffer (pH 6.0) and gently swirling the contents. A
1-ml portion of benzene was then added (total benzene = 2.0 ml),
mixed with gentle swirling, and the mixture was transferred to an
8-ml culture tube to allow the phases to separate. The aqueous
layer (bottom) was discarded, and the benzene phase was extracted
with an additional 2-ml portion of buffer, centrifuged, and analyzed
as described for the amines.

Final residues from the extraction and cleanup procedures of
the basic, neutral, and phenolic fractions from wastewater or urine
were dissolved in benzene (1.5 ml for amines; 0.5 ml for phenols)
and derivatized by using TMA solution and PFPA reagents as described.
For assays of wastewater containing amine or phenolic residues in
the order of 0.10, 1.0, and 10 ppb, the entire extract (100 g equivalents) of the cleaned-up sample was derivatized and 5-µl injections
containing 250, 25, and 2.5 mg equivalents, respectively, were assayed
by EC-GC. Likewise, for assays of urine containing residues in the
order of 2 or 20 ppb, the entire extract (50 g equivalents) was derivatized and 12.5 and 1.25 mg equivalents, respectively, were
analyzed.

D. Gas Chromatographic Assays

A Hewlett-Packard (Palo Alto, Calif.) Model 5750B instrument
equipped with a ^{63}Ni EC detector (Tracor, Inc., Austin, Tex.) and
125-cm glass columns (4 mm i.d.) containing 5% Dexsil 300, 5% OV-101,
or 5% OV-17, all on Gas Chrom Q (80-100 mesh) conditioned at 270°C
overnight prior to use, was operated isothermally at the various
temperatures (see Table 4.1, Section III) with a nitrogen carrier
flow of 160 ml/min. The detector, operated in the DC mode, was at
300°C and the injection port was 20°C higher than the column oven.
Lindane and heptachlor epoxide were used as reference standards to
monitor the performance of the EC-GC system; all injections were
made in 5 µl of benzene. Assays of the three fractions from wastewater or urine were performed on a column of Dexsil 300. Because
of the wide differences in retention time (t_R) for the various PFP

derivatives, the basic fraction was first analyzed at 165°C to
quantify 2-NA and 4-ABP then at 220°C for the other amines. The
neutral fraction was also assayed at 220°C and the phenolic fraction
was assayed at 190°C for DES then at 220°C for estradiol. Derivatized samples of unknown residue content (except DES) were quantified
by relating their peak heights to known amounts of the corresponding
PFP derivatives. The DES residue content was quantified as described
by King et al. [13] by relating the sum of the heights of the cis and
trans peaks expressed as the trans isomer (cis x 0.722 = trans) to
known amounts of PFP derivatives of DES calculated in the same manner.
Derivatized samples of unknown 2-AAF content were quantified by relating the peak height of the resulting PFP-2-AF to a known amount
of PFP-2-AF and then expressing the results as 2-AAF (2-AF x 1.23 =
2-AAF).

III   RESULTS AND DISCUSSION

A periodic analysis of the urine is one of the most convenient
means of determining human exposure to test chemicals. Although
metabolism of these substances is known to occur prior to excretion
in the urine, the unaltered parent compound is also believed to be
excreted in sufficient amounts to signal any appreciable exposure
in the event that highly sensitive analytical procedures are employed.
Therefore, in the absence of rapid and sensitive detection methods
for a wide variety of metabolites of each of the test compounds shown
in Figure 4.1, surveillance of personnel to detect accidental exposure to the test substance is based on periodic assays of the urine
for traces of the parent compounds.

Recent development of methodology at our laboratory for assaying
traces of DiClBzd [8], DES [13], and estradiol [14] based on derivatization with fluorinated acid anhydrides led us to investigate the
possibility of analyzing all of the compounds in the same manner.
Indeed, it was found that all of these compounds, with the exception
of 2-AAF, could be derivatized and analyzed with high sensitivity;

Table 4.1. Retention times of two EC derivatives of carcinogens
and analogs on three chromatographic columns

		Retention time and oven temperature for column indicated[a]					
		Dexsil 300		OV-101		OV-17	
Compound	Derivative	Temp. (°C)	t_R (min)	Temp. (°C)	t_R (min)	Temp. (°C)	t_R (min)
2-ABP	PFP	165	1.65	155	2.20	165	1.90
	HFB	165	1.70	155	2.40	165	1.90
1-NA	PFP	165	1.80	155	2.00	165	2.00
	HFB	165	1.95	155	2.25	165	1.95
2-NA	PFP	165	2.30	155	2.45	165	2.50
	HFB	165	2.50	155	2.75	165	2.50
3-ABP	PFP	165	4.50	155	4.80	165	4.90
	HFB	165	4.85	155	5.50	165	4.90
4-ABP	PFP	165	5.05	155	5.40	165	6.10
	HFB	165	5.55	155	6.30	165	6.10
2-AF	PFP	220	1.70	210	1.60	220	1.75
	HFB	220	1.80	210	1.80	220	1.70
Bzd	PFP	220	3.20	210	3.00	220	2.75
	HFB	220	3.55	210	3.60	220	2.65
DiClBzd	Underivatized	220	6.60	210	4.80	220	11.85
	PFP	220	4.30	210	4.10	220	3.00
	HFB	220	4.70	210	5.20	220	2.90
DiMeBzd	PFP	220	4.90	210	4.10	220	3.75
	HFB	220	5.50	210	5.20	220	3.60
DiMxBzd	PFP	220	8.25	210	6.90	220	6.00
	HFB	220	8.70	210	8.30	220	5.70
DES	PFP-cis	190	1.60	195	1.55	175	2.10
	HFB-cis	190	1.90	195	2.00	175	2.35
	PFP-trans	190	2.55	195	2.30	175	2.95
	HFB-trans	190	3.15	195	3.10	175	3.40
Estradiol	PFP	220	4.35	210	4.20	220	2.80
	HFB	220	5.15	210	5.45	220	2.95
Lindane	--	165	4.15	155	3.70	165	6.40
(reference standard)	--	190	1.65	195	1.05	175	4.25
	--	220	0.85	210	0.85	220	1.00
Heptachlor epoxide	--	165	11.50	155	11.90	165	--
(reference standard)	--	190	4.00	195	2.55	175	10.50
	--	220	1.75	210	1.75	220	2.20

Source: Nony and Bowman [15].

[a]All columns were 125-cm glass (4 mm i.d.) packed with 5% liquid phase on
Gas Chrom Q (80-100 mesh);

2-AAF, after hydrolysis to 2-AF [5] and subsequent derivatization could also be analyzed.

Both PFP and HFB derivatives of all of the compounds were prepared and subjected to GC analysis on columns of Dexsil 300, OV-101, and OV-17 by using a variety of isothermal operating conditions. Data concerning GC operations and retention times for all of these compounds as well as underivatized DiClBzd and reference standards of lindane and heptachlor epoxide are presented in Table 4.1. 3,3'-Dichlorobenzidine was the only test substance that demonstrated appreciable EC properties without being subjected to derivatization; nevertheless, conversion of the compound to the PFP derivative enhanced its response about 300-fold, which agrees with the value reported by Bowman and Rushing [8]. Although the PFP and HFB derivatives of the various compounds yielded about the same response, the use of PFP derivatives was adopted because the reagent was easier to use and generally produced fewer interference peaks. Data concerning the retention times of the PFP derivatives (Table 4.1) indicate that Dexsil 300 is the column of choice for the analytical procedure because better separation is obtained. Although the present procedure for wastewater and urine employs PFP derivatives on a column of Dexsil 300, the data concerning both the PFP and HFB derivatives on all three column packings may be useful in confirmatory tests. Typical gas chromatograms of PFP derivatives of all of the compounds, underivatized DiClBzd, and the reference standards assayed on a column of Dexsil 300 using various isothermal operating conditions are presented in Figures 4.2 and 4.3. Excellent responses are obtained from injections of picogram amounts of the PFP derivatives.

The partition values (p-values; fraction of solute partitioning into the nonpolar phase of an equivolume immiscible binary solvent system) are useful for confirming the identity of unknown GC peaks where insufficient amounts of substance are available for test by other means. Therefore, such values for all of the PFP derivatives in five solvent systems, determined as described by Bowman and Beroza [17,18], are reported in Table 4.2. Additional p-values were determined for all of the PFP derivatives in benzene versus the phosphate

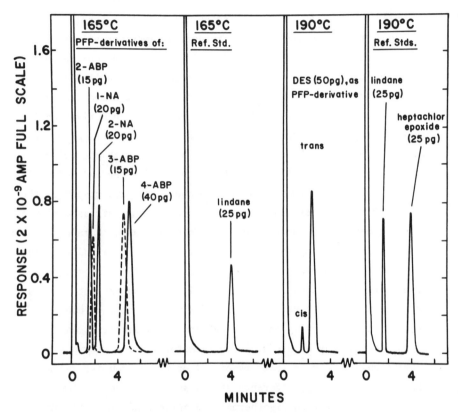

Figure 4.2. Electron-capture gas chromatograms of standards of PFP derivatives of carcinogens and their analogs, and reference standards of lindane and heptachlor epoxide. All injections were in 5 µl of benzene. (From Nony and Bowman [15].)

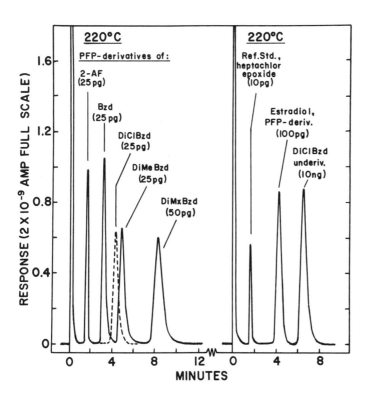

Figure 4.3. Electron-capture gas chromatograms
of standards of PFP derivatives of carcinogens
and their analogs, a reference standard of
heptachlor epoxide, and underivatized DiClBzd.
All injections were in 5 µl of benzene.
(From Nony and Bowman [15].)

Table 4.2. Partition values and GC-mass spectrometric verification of PFP derivatives of carcinogens and analogs

Compounds	Number of PFP groups per molecule	Hexane-acetonitrile	Heptane-40% acetonitrile (60% water)	Heptane-90% ethanol (10% water)	Isooctane-90% acetone (10% water)	Isooctane-80% acetone (20% water)
1-NA	1	0.038	0.63	0.11	0.46	0.62
2-NA	1	0.052	0.77	0.12	0.45	0.70
2-ABP	1	0.090	0.91	0.27	0.42	0.70
3-ABP	1	0.050	0.88	0.13	0.48	0.76
4-ABP	1	0.044	0.85	0.13	0.44	0.74
2-AF	1	0.046	0.86	0.14	0.56	0.73
Bzd	2	0.016	0.45	0.020	0.48	0.66
DiClBzd	2	0.042	1.00	0.14	0.59	0.78
DiMeBzd	2	0.031	0.52	0.046	0.50	0.66
DiMxBzd	2	0.044	0.98	0.22	0.69	0.86
DES-cis	2	0.40	0.97	--[a]	0.91	0.98
DES-trans	2	0.44	0.96	--[a]	0.91	0.99
Estradiol	1	0.50	0.99	0.88	0.90	0.97

Source: Nony and Bowman [15].
[a]Instability of derivative in solvent system precluded analysis.

buffer (pH 6) used to terminate the derivatization reaction; all of
the values were found to be 1.0, which indicated that no loss of the
derivatives occurred during the process. Results from GC-mass spectrometric tests of the individual derivatives to determine the number
of PFP groups added to each compound during derivatization are also
presented in Table 4.2. Benzidine, its analogs, and DES each contained two PFP groups while all of the other compounds contained one
PFP group.

Stability studies employing periodic assays of benzene solutions
(5 ng/ml) of the PFP derivatives stored in sealed tubes at 5°C indicated that all of the compounds were essentially stable during a
10-month period.

The chemical properties of the test substances provided a convenient means of separating them into basic, phenolic, and neutral
fractions. The analytical scheme used for the extraction, separation, and analysis of all 13 compounds in admixture in wastewater
is illustrated in Figure 4.4. Salient elements of the procedure,
after separation of the sample into three fractions, are extraction
of the phenolic residues with benzene (pH 10.2), hydrolysis of 2-AAF
in the neutral fraction and extraction of the product (2-AF) as the
free amine, extraction of the free amines from the basic fraction
(pH 12), conversion of all residues to the PFP derivatives, and
analysis via EC-GC by using three isothermal operating conditions.

Typical gas chromatograms of derivatized fractions from untreated wastewater along with 1-ppb amounts of 10 of the compounds
as PFP derivatives (superimposed) are presented in Figure 4.5.
Resolution was excellent for 8 of the 10 derivatives. Although
baseline resolution was not achieved for DiClBzd and DiMeBzd, no
problem was experienced in using peak height measurement to quantify
residues as low as 0.1 ppb.

Results from triplicate assays of wastewater unspiked and
spiked with 0.10, 1.0, and 10 ppb of 10 of the compounds in admixture are presented in Table 4.3. Recoveries were generally good
at the 10-ppb level but tended to drop significantly at 1 ppb. At

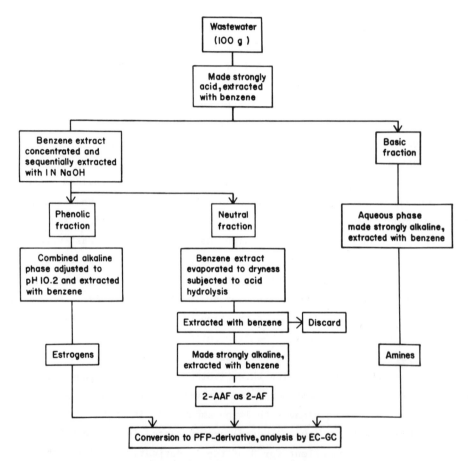

Figure 4.4.   Scheme for extraction, separation, and analysis of 13 carcinogens and related compounds in admixture in wastewater.   (From Nony and Bowman [15] and Bowman [16].)

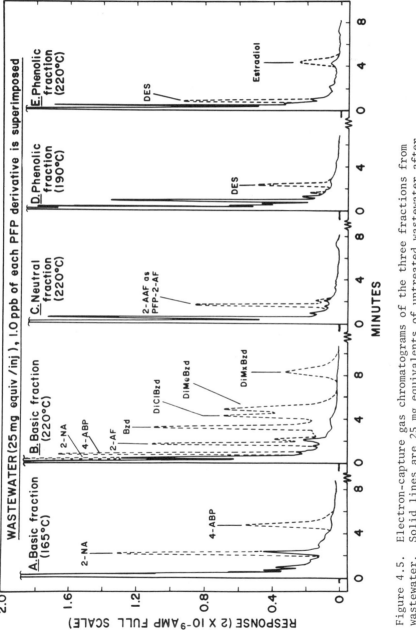

Figure 4.5. Electron-capture gas chromatograms of the three fractions from wastewater. Solid lines are 25 mg equivalents of untreated wastewater after derivatization; broken lines (superimposed) illustrate responses from 1-ppb amounts of the compounds assayed as PFP derivatives. All injections were in 5 μl of benzene. (From Nony and Bowman [15] and Bowman [16].)

Table 4.3. Analysis of wastewater unspiked and spiked with 0.10, 1.0, and 10 ppb of 10 carcinogens and analogs in admixture

		Recovery ($\bar{x} \pm SE$)[a]					
Compounds	Unspiked ppb	Spiked with 0.10 ppb		Spiked with 1.0 ppb		Spiked with 10 ppb	
		ppb	%	ppb	%	ppb	%
2-NA	0.123 ± 0.025	0.011 ± 0.004	11 ± 4	0.443 ± 0.039	44.3 ± 3.9	7.64 ± 0.60	76.4 ± 6.0
4-ABP	0.002 ± 0.001	0.040 ± 0.003	40 ± 3	0.657 ± 0.036	65.7 ± 3.6	8.52 ± 0.30	85.2 ± 3.0
2-AF	0.002 ± 0.000	0.022 ± 0.000	22 ± 0	0.555 ± 0.048	55.5 ± 4.8	8.17 ± 0.10	81.7 ± 1.0
2-AAF	0.002 ± 0.001	0.056 ± 0.006	56 ± 6	0.650 ± 0.042	65.0 ± 4.2	7.52 ± 0.06	75.2 ± 0.6
Bzd	0.002 ± 0.001	0.004 ± 0.003	4 ± 3	0.208 ± 0.009	20.8 ± 0.9	7.05 ± 0.33	70.5 ± 3.3
DiClBzd	0.003 ± 0.001	0.055 ± 0.004	55 ± 4	0.580 ± 0.064	58.0 ± 6.4	7.47 ± 0.08	74.7 ± 0.8
DiMeBzd	0.005 ± 0.002	0.028 ± 0.001	28 ± 1	0.583 ± 0.037	58.3 ± 3.7	8.39 ± 0.14	83.9 ± 1.4
DiMxBzd	0.003 ± 0.001	0.009 ± 0.001	9 ± 1	0.465 ± 0.048	46.5 ± 4.8	7.25 ± 0.10	72.5 ± 1.0
DES	0.016 ± 0.003	0.041 ± 0.005	41 ± 5	0.441 ± 0.060	44.1 ± 0.6	4.99 ± 0.24	49.9 ± 2.4
Estradiol	0.018 ± 0.006	0.078 ± 0.001	79 ± 1	0.839 ± 0.018	83.9 ± 1.8	8.91 ± 0.30	89.1 ± 3.0

Source: Nony and Bowman [15].

[a]Mean and standard error from triplicate assays; spiked samples are corrected for background of unspiked samples

0.10 ppb, recoveries of 2-NA, Bzd, and DiMxBzd were 11% or less; however, the fact that the compounds were detectable indicated that the procedure is useful even at this low level.

Urine is assayed by using the same scheme as for wastewater, except that the sample is initially divided into two 50-ml portions. One of the portions is made strongly alkaline for extraction and analysis of the basic fraction (amines), and the other is made strongly acid for extraction and analysis of the phenolic (estrogens) and neutral (2-AAF) fractions. Typical EC-GC curves of the derivatized fractions from untreated urine along with 10-ppb amounts of 10 of the compounds as PFP derivatives (superimposed) are presented in Figure 4.6. Results from triplicate assays of urine unspiked and spiked with 2.0 and 20 ppb of the 10 compounds are presented in Table 4.4. Recoveries at the 20-ppb level were good; however, a marked decrease in recovery was found at the 2-ppb level. Also, background interferences from untreated urine as high as 2 ppb were observed in the case of DiMxBzd. Nevertheless, the procedure does serve as an excellent means of monitoring for residues of the compounds at levels of 1-2 ppb in the urine of our personnel.

Recently, tests with the monoacetyl analog of benzidine (AcBzd), a metabolite of benzidine found in urine, have indicated that it also responds to the analytical procedure. The retention time (t_R) of PFP-AcBzd on the Dexsil 300 column operated at 200°C was about 12.6 min. Quantitation of AcBzd, as the PFP derivative, is best accomplished with the Dexsil 300 column operated at 260°C (t_R = 2.85 min). Under these conditions a 5-μl injection of benzene containing 250 pg of PFP-AcBzd yields a response of about 6×10^{-10} amp, which is about 10 times less than that of PFP-Bzd; nevertheless, this sensitivity is adequate for the measurement of AcBzd in urine at the low ppb level.

It should be noted that no cleanup steps are used in the procedure for wastewater and urine, although, some cleanup was achieved by our method as a result of the extraction, separation, and derivatization steps. Bowen [19] was also able to assay for certain

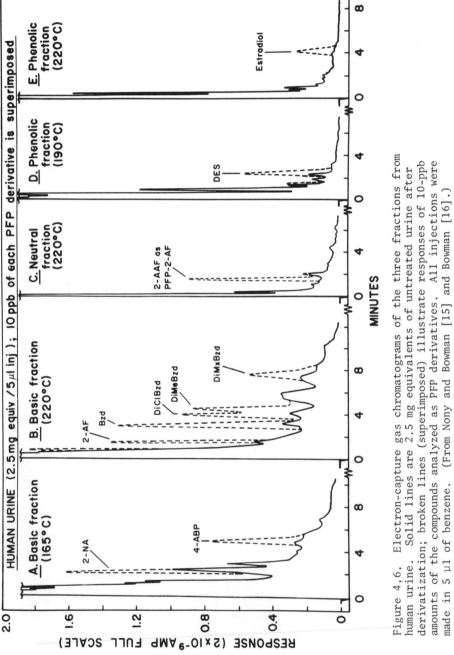

Figure 4.6. Electron-capture gas chromatograms of the three fractions from human urine. Solid lines are 2.5 mg equivalents of untreated urine after derivatization; broken lines (superimposed) illustrate responses of 10-ppb amounts of the compounds analyzed as PFP derivatives. All injections were made in 5 μl of benzene. (From Nony and Bowman [15] and Bowman [16].)

Table 4.4. Analysis of human urine unspiked and spiked with 2.0 and 20 ppb of 10 carcinogens and analogs in admixture

Compounds	Unspiked ppb	Recovered ($\bar{x} \pm SE$)[a]					
		Spiked with 2.0 ppb		Spiked with 20 ppb			
		ppb	%	ppb	%		
2-NA	0.788 ± 0.038	0.637 ± 0.172	31.9 ± 8.6	13.3 ± 0.7	66.6 ± 3.3		
4-ABP	1.06 ± 0.08	1.03 ± 0.08	51.3 ± 4.0	17.3 ± 0.2	86.5 ± 1.1		
2-AF	0.515 ± 0.031	0.480 ± 0.040	24.1 ± 2.0	14.9 ± 0.2	74.2 ± 1.0		
2-AAF	0.023 ± 0.005	1.16 ± 0.12	57.7 ± 5.9	15.9 ± 0.8	79.2 ± 3.8		
Bzd	0.213 ± 0.023	0.907 ± 0.023	45.1 ± 1.2	14.1 ± 0.2	70.4 ± 0.9		
DiClBzd	0.830 ± 0.038	1.41 ± 0.06	70.7 ± 2.8	19.9 ± 0.3	99.3 ± 1.4		
DiMeBzd	0.215 ± 0.037	0.973 ± 0.012	48.6 ± 0.4	17.3 ± 0.3	86.4 ± 1.3		
DiMxBzd	2.13 ± 0.00	0.953 ± 0.021	47.5 ± 1.0	18.6 ± 0.3	92.6 ± 1.6		
DES	0.543 ± 0.014	0.876 ± 0.006	43.8 ± 0.3	11.1 ± 0.7	55.3 ± 3.5		
Estradiol	0.730 ± 0.014	1.22 ± 0.02	60.8 ± 0.8	17.6 ± 0.1	88.0 ± 0.5		

Source: Nony and Bowman [15].
[a]Mean and standard error from triplicate assays; spiked samples are corrected for background of unspiked samples

aromatic amines at ppb levels in aqueous waste streams via flame ionization GC without sample treatment in many cases. Although extensive studies of cleanup procedures were conducted at our laboratory employing XAD-2 resin and Sephadex LH-20 prior to derivatization and alumina and silica gel before and after derivatization, no system could be devised that allowed good recoveries of all compounds at the levels tested. Therefore, it appears that further refinement of the present procedure to improve sensitivity and recovery should be directed toward the individual compound and substrate.

This method may easily be adapted to the monitoring of work areas (animal cages, floors, apparatus, air filters, etc.) suspected of being contaminated with the test chemicals. The procedure currently used at our laboratory [6] for sampling surfaces employs a kit consisting of a cotton applicator and a 5-ml culture tube containing a known volume of a suitable solvent. The applicator is saturated with the solvent and used to swab a specific area then the applicator is vigorously stirred in the solvent after each of several swabbings of the same area. In a similar manner fiberglass filters used to trap particulate matter from the air may be cut into small pieces and extracted with a suitable solvent. These extracts may then be screened for contaminants by slightly modifying the procedure described.

IV   SUMMARY

A GC method has been described for determining traces of 13 carcinogens and related compounds (aromatic amines and estrogens) in admixture in wastewater and human urine. This method was developed for use in toxicological research for monitoring the safe disposal of wastewater and to signal any accidental exposure of personnel to hazardous test substances. Salient elements of the procedure are extraction of phenolic and neutral residues from the acidified sample, liquid-liquid partitioning cleanup and separation of neutral from phenolic residues at pH 14 and 10.2, acid hydrolysis of the neutral component, subsequent alkalinization of the sample

and extraction of the basic residues as the free amines, conversion
of all residues to the corresponding PFP derivatives, and quantification by EC-GC. Residues were detectable in wastewater and urine
at the 0.1 and 1 ppb levels, respectively. Additional information
has been provided concerning partition values for all PFP derivatives
in five solvent systems, structure verification of the derivatives by
mass spectrometry, and the adaptation of this method to the monitoring
of surfaces and air in potentially contaminated work areas.

REFERENCES

1. *Federal Register.* Nonclinical laboratory studies: Proposed
    regulations for good laboratory practices. *41,* 51206-51230
    (November 19, 1976).

2. *Federal Register.* Carcinogens: Occupational health and safety
    standards. *39,* 3756-3797 (January 29, 1974).

3. T. J. Haley. Benzidine revisited: A review of the literature
    and problems associated with the use of benzidine and its con-
    geners. *Clin. Toxicol. 8,* 13-42 (1975).

4. L. M. Games and R. A. Hites. Composition, treatment efficiency
    and experimental significance of dye manufacturing plant efflu-
    ents. *Anal. Chem. 49,* 1433-1440 (1977).

5. M. C. Bowman and J. R. King. Analysis of 2-acetylaminofluorene:
    Residues in laboratory chow and microbiological media. *Biochem.
    Med. 9,* 390-401 (1974).

6. M. C. Bowman, J. R. King, and C. L. Holder. Benzidine and
    congeners: Analytical chemical properties and trace analysis
    in five substrates. *Int. J. Environ. Anal. Chem. 4,* 205-223
    (1976).

7. C. L. Holder, J. R. King, and M. C. Bowman. 4-Aminobiphenyl,
    2-naphthylamine and analogs: Analytical properties and trace
    analysis in five substrates. *J. Toxicol. Environ. Health 2,*
    111-129 (1976).

8. M. C. Bowman and L. G. Rushing. Trace analysis of 3,3'-dichloro-
    benzidine in animal chow, wastewater and human urine by three gas
    chromatographic procedures. *Arch. Environ. Contam. Toxicol. 6,*
    471-482 (1977).

9. C. R. Nony, E. J. Treglown, and M. C. Bowman. Removal of trace
    levels of 2-acetylaminofluorene (2-AAF) from wastewater. *Sci.
    Total Environ. 4,* 155-163 (1975).

10. M. C. Bowman, Control of test substances. *Clin. Toxicol.*, in
    press (1979).

11. T. Walle and H. Ehrsson. Quantitative gas chromatographic determination of picogram quantities of amino and alcoholic compounds by electron capture detection: Part I, Preparation and properties of the heptafluorobutyryl derivatives. *Acta Pharm. Suecica 7*, 893-406 (1970).

12. H. Ehrsson, T. Walle, and H. Brotell. Quantitative gas chromatographic determination of picogram quantities of phenols. *Acta Pharm. Suecica 8*, 319-328 (1971).

13. J. R. King, C. R. Nony, and M. C. Bowman. Trace analysis of diethylstilbestrol (DES) in animal chow by parallel high-speed liquid chromatography, electron-capture gas chromatography and radioassays. *J. Chromatogr. Sci. 15*, 14-21 (1977).

14. M. C. Bowman and C. R. Nony. Trace analysis of estradiol in animal chow by electron-capture gas chromatography. *J. Chromatogr. Sci. 15*, 160-163 (1977).

15. C. R. Nony and M. C. Bowman. Carcinogens and analogs: Trace analysis of thirteen compounds in admixture in wastewater and human urine. *Int. J. Environ. Anal. Chem. 5*, 203-220 (1978).

16. M. C. Bowman. Trace analysis: A requirement for toxicological research with carcinogens and hazardous substances. *J. Ass. Offic. Anal. Chem. 61*, 1253-1262 (1978).

17. M. C. Bowman and M. Beroza. Identification of compounds by extraction p-values using gas chromatography. *Anal. Chem. 38*, 1544-1549 (1966).

18. M. Beroza and M. C. Bowman. Identification of pesticides at nanogram level by extraction p-values. *Anal. Chem. 37*, 291-292 (1965).

19. B. E. Bowen. Determination of aromatic amines by an adsorption technique with flame ionization gas chromatography. *Anal. Chem. 48*, 1584-1587 (1976).

5

REMOVAL OF TEST SUBSTANCES FROM WASTEWATER

I INTRODUCTION

It has been reported that the national goal for the control of water pollution in the United States is the elimination of pollutant discharge into navigable waters by the year 1985 [1]. In complying with the Federal Water Pollution Control Act Amendments of 1972 (Public Law 92-500), industry often finds that it is more economical to treat wastewater for reuse than for discharge into the environment. Of the various processes available for the treatment of wastewater, the most promising are chemical treatment, filtration, activated carbon, and microscreening [2]. Peacock [3] concluded that physico-chemical processes consisting of chemical flocculation, filtration, and granular activated carbon could replace conventional biological processes, especially when upsets from toxic chemicals could be anticipated.

The National Center for Toxicological Research (NCTR) is engaged in long-term, low-dose feeding studies of known carcinogens [2-acetyl-aminofluorene (2-AAF) was our first test substance] and potential carcinogens in mice and other experimental animals. In such studies residues of the carcinogens are introduced into our wastewater primarily through the cleaning procedures used for decontaminating the animal cages, feeders, and containers used to prepare and store the toxicant-treated diets. Therefore, the objective of our wastewater cleanup can be no less than total removal of any deleterious residues, thereby rendering the water safe for recycle or direct discharge into the environment.

The size of the complex of laboratories and ancillary functions places the NCTR in the small to medium category with regard to the magnitude of its wastewater program. When all of our programs become operational, about 500,000 gallons of wastewater will be discharged daily. Prior to the development of our present wastewater treatment at NCTR, carcinogen-containing wastewater was isolated from other water and held in tanks pending the development of an acceptable means of removing the residues (2-AAF). However, in order to evaluate the effectiveness of any proposed cleanup system for wastewater, it was first necessary to develop a highly sensitive chemical procedure for the analysis of traces of the contaminant in wastewater. Since sub parts-per-billion (ppb; ng/g) sensitivity was sought, special emphasis was also placed on the confirmation of the identity of trace amounts of the carcinogen. This chapter describes the experiments that ultimately led to a workable means of cleaning up wastewater contaminated with traces of carcinogens [4].

II   EXPERIMENTAL

A.   Analysis of 2-Acetylaminofluorene in Wastewater

The following method for determining traces of 2-AAF was developed for use in evaluating the behavior of such residues in several experiments proposed for cleaning up contaminated wastewater.

Residues of 2-AAF and/or its hydrolysis product, 2-aminofluorene (2-AF), were assayed by a modification of the procedure of Bowman and King [5]. The sample (250 ml) in a 500-ml separatory funnel containing 2 g of NaCl and 1 ml of 10 N aqueous NaOH was extracted twice with 25-ml portions of chloroform, which were successively percolated through a plug of sodium sulfate (15 mm diameter x 10 mm thick) and collected in a 100-ml glass-stoppered flask containing a boiling bead and one drop of diethylene glycol as a "keeper" solution. The contents were evaporated to near dryness under water pump vacuum at 60°C and quantitatively transferred to a culture tube (20 x 150 mm, sealed with a Teflon-lined cap) by using three 2-ml portions of chloroform.

The contents were evaporated to near dryness with a jet of dry air
and finally to dryness with water pump vacuum and a 60°C water bath.
Hydrolysis of 2-AAF to 2-AF was then accomplished by adding 4 ml of
methanol and 2 ml of concentrated HCl to the dry residue and heating
it in the sealed tube at 80°C for 2 hr using a tube heater (No.
720,000, Kontes Glass Co., Vineland, N.J.). After the tube had
cooled, 3 ml of distilled water was added and the contents were
extracted twice with 7-ml portions of benzene; each portion of
benzene was carefully withdrawn and discarded by using a 10-ml
syringe and cannula. Next, 4 ml of 10 N NaOH was added and the contents were extracted three times with 7-ml portions of benzene. Each
portion was successively percolated through a plug of sodium sulfate
(15 mm diameter x 10 mm thick) and collected in a 50-ml glass-
stoppered flask containing a boiling bead and a drop of keeper solution. The contents were evaporated just to dryness under water pump
vacuum at 60°C as described and the residue was dissolved in 10 ml
of methanol for subsequent spectrophotofluorescent (SPF) analysis.

An Aminco-Bowman instrument (American Instrument Co., Silver
Spring, Md.) equipped with a xenon lamp and a 1P28 detector was used
with 1-cm cells and a 2-2-2-mm slit program to measure the fluorescence of the 2-AF [wavelength maxima for excitation (λ_{Ex}) and emission
(λ_{Em}) are 297 and 366 nm, respectively]. Samples of water known to
be free of carcinogens were carried through the entire procedure and
used for correcting the analytical results. Since residues of 2-AAF
are analyzed as 2-AF, the analytical results are multiplied by a
factor of 1.23 to express them as 2-AAF. Recoveries of 2-AAF from
water spiked at the 10-ppb level averaged about 80%; the analytical
data are corrected for both background and recovery. Based on twice
the background fluorescence, the sensitivity of the method to 2-AAF
(assayed as 2-AF) is 0.2 ppb. The identity of 2-AAF and/or 2-AF
residues in wastewater at levels as low as 0.2 ppb may be easily
confirmed by comparing the λ_{Ex} and λ_{Em} values of the unknown sample
with those for 2-AF. The analytical method detects combined residues
of 2-AF and 2-AAF; since no residues of 2-AF have been found in the

wastewater, all results are expressed as 2-AAF. The individual residues may be analyzed as described by Bowman and King [5].

B. Evaluation of Cleanup Procedures for Wastewater

Several possible approaches to cleaning up the wastewater were investigated in the laboratory; they included millipore filtration, distillation, organic solvent extraction, alkaline hydrolysis, and carbon and nonionic polymeric adsorption. In addition, information concerning the adsorption of 2-AAF from aqueous dispersions by the soil at the NCTR was also sought.

Two distillation experiments were performed to investigate the effectiveness of the process as a cleanup procedure and to approximate the vapor pressure of 2-AAF. In the first experiment, 200 ml of distilled water containing 2 mg of solid 2-AAF (10 µg/ml) was distilled a 1 atmosphere until 100 ml of distillate was collected; the distillate was assayed for 2-AAF content. The initial concentration of 2-AAF in the distilling flask (10 ppm) and subsequent levels were undoubtedly below the saturation level at 100°C. Secondly, 100 ml of distilled water and 200 mg of solid 2-AAF were distilled until 80 ml of distillate was collected. The distillate was analyzed for 2-AAF and the equation of Rassow and Schultzky [6] was used to approximate the vapor pressure. The water in the distilling flask was observed to be supersaturated with 2-AAF during the entire distillation.

In laboratory evaluations of adsorbents for removing traces of 2-AAF from water, glass columns containing activated carbon (Witco Grade 718, 50 g, 20 mm diameter x 280 mm thick) or a nonionic polymeric resin (Amberlite XAD-2, 70 g, 20 mm diameter x 240 mm thick) supported by a plug of glass wool and topped by a plug of glass wool were each prewashed with 2 liters of distilled water. Fifteen liters of an aqueous dispersion of 2-AAF (5.0 ppm) were then separately percolated by gravity through each column; 1-liter fractions from the columns were analyzed for residues of 2-AAF.

A sample of alluvial silt soil of the type found in the oxidation and equilization ponds of the sewage treatment system at the NCTR was used for laboratory tests to determine its ability to adsorb 2-AAF residues from aqueous dispersion. Duplicate 250-ml beakers were prepared by adding the appropriate amount of soil to provide a layer 6.5 cm in diameter and about 1.7 cm thick in the bottom of each container. Deionized water (150 ml) was added to one container to serve as a control and aqueous 2-AAF (150 ml, 5.0 ppm) was added to the other. The aqueous layers over the soil were about 4.1 cm deep. Another beaker (soil absent) containing 150 ml of the aqueous 2-AAF was also prepared to monitor any change in concentration due to settling or adsorption of the 2-AAF by the container. Aliquots (10 ml) of the aqueous phases were withdrawn from the geometrical center of the supernatants after they had stood at 25°C for 2 hr, then 3, 7, 14, 21, and 28 days later. The containers were tightly sealed with aluminum foil, except during the sampling process, to prevent evaporation of the water and possible "codistillation" of the 2-AAF. Evaporation of the water could also cause the 2-AAF residue to precipitate. Each aliquot was assayed for 2-AAF content.

C. Evaluation of a Pilot-scale Wastewater Cleanup System

A pilot-scale cleanup system for removing 2-AAF residues was implemented by modifying an existing system of stainless steel tanks. A flow diagram of the system is presented in Figure 5.1, in which the fifteen components are designated by the letters A through O. The carcinogen-containing wastewater, isolated from other wastewater, was stored in two 30,000 gallon tanks (A and B). The tanks were piped so as to allow the wastewater to flow into one (A) and be withdrawn from the other (B). Liquid levels in each tank were equalized through interconnecting pipes. Wastewater was forced through the filtration and adsorption system by a horizontal single-stage centrifugal pump (C) driven by a 3-horsepower motor; the pump was rated at 5 gallons/min against a 72-foot head. The water was pumped through

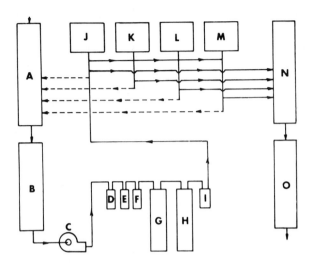

Figure 5.1. Flow diagram of pilot-scale system
for treating carcinogen-containing wastewater at
the NCTR. A and B, holding tanks for raw wastewater (30,000 gallons each); C, centrifugal pump;
D, E, and F, filters (40, 25, and 5 μm, respectively); G, granular carbon (Witco Grade 718,
25 pounds); H, polymeric resin (Amberlite XAD-2,
45 pounds); I, membrane filter (99% retention of
0.45-μm particles); J, K, L, and M, holding tanks
for cleaned-up wastewater (7,000 gallons each);
N and O, holding tanks for cleaned-up wastewater
(30,000 gallons each). (From Nony et al. [4].)

a series of coarse (D), medium (E), and fine (F) depth filtration
filter elements (40, 25, and 5 μm, respectively) for clarification
and then through the primary adsorber (G) which consisted of 25
pounds of Witco Grade 718 granular carbon contained in a conventional
water treatment tank. The secondary adsorber (H) was located immediately downstream from the primary adsorber. It consisted of 45
pounds of Amberlite XAD-2 nonionic polymer, also contained in a
conventional water treatment tank. This unit provided assurance
that any 2-AAF residues penetrating the carbon adsorber would still
be retained in the cleanup system. Finally, the water was passed
through a membrane filter (I). This filter (99% retention of 0.45-
μm particles) was to retain any fine particles of the two adsorbents

which might escape from their respective tanks and carry adsorbed
2-AAF along with them. Treated water was stored in 5000-gallon
batches in the 7000-gallon tanks (J, K, L, and M) pending the results
of chemical analysis concerning the presence or absence of 2-AAF.
These tanks were equipped with turbine mixers to allow representative
sampling. Treated water found to contain 2-AAF is returned to tanks
A and B for reprocessing. Water found to be free of 2-AAF is transferred to holding tanks (N and O) for reuse or discharge into the
environment. The operation of the cleanup system was monitored by
a series of gauges and valves located in a manner that permitted the
determination of pressure drop and 2-AAF concentration across any
component of the system.

III   RESULTS AND DISCUSSION

Preliminary experiments with millipore filtration (99% retention
of particles 0.45 μm or larger) of actual wastewater (32.6 ppb of
2-AAF, pH = 9.42) yielded a 40% cleanup, which presumably resulted
from the removal of sludge which has sorbed a portion of the 2-AAF
residue. Since the solubility of 2-AAF is about 7 ppm in water at
25°C [5], filtration would not be expected to effectively clean up
the water unless all of the residue had been irreversibly sorbed by
the sludge. Moreover, the millipore filtration concept proved unsatisfactory because the accumulation of sludge on the filter drastically
reduced the rate of filtration. The experiment was repeated after the
wastewater had been adjusted to a pH of 7.0 and essentially the same
results were obtained.

The possibility of removing 2-AAF residues from the wastewater
by organic solvent extraction was also investigated. After the wastewater was saturated with chloroform [ca. 1%, volume/volume (v/v)], a
single extraction of 100 ml of water by using 1 ml of chloroform removed 93% of the residue. The 1% solubility of chloroform in water
is a decided disadvantage and makes this procedure impractical. A
similar disadvantage would also be expected with other immiscible
solvents of sufficient polarity to extract the 2-AAF from water.

Hydrolysis procedures such as a 24-hr digestion (82°C) of waste-water previously adjusted to pH 11 with NaOH failed to destroy any of the 2-AAF. The carcinogen is very difficult to hydrolyze, as is evidenced by the analytical procedure; such processes are not amenable to the decontamination of wastewater.

Results from distillation tests indicated that 2-AAF distills with water. In one test, 200 ml of water containing 10 ppm of 2-AAF (presumably in solution) yielded 1.3 µg (13 ppb) in the first 100 ml of distillate; in another test, 100 ml of water containing 2000 ppm of 2-AAF (supersaturated) contained 297 µg (3.71 ppm) in the first 80 ml of distillate. Results of the latter were used to approximate the vapor pressure at 100°C for 2-AAF at about 2.3×10^{-4} mm [6]. Distillation, in addition to being inefficient, would be a slow process and its energy requirements are prohibitive.

In the laboratory tests, evaluating the effectiveness of adsorbents for removing 2-AAF residues from water by percolating 15 liters of aqueous 2-AAF (5.0 ppm) through them, residues (0.96 ppb) were found only in the 4- to 5-liter fraction from carbon. With XAD-2 resin, residues were detected only in the 3- to 5-liter and 12- to 14-liter fractions, which averaged 1.03 and 2.89 ppb, respectively. These few instances, where 2-AAF was found in the eluate, were believed to have resulted from small particles of the adsorbent being swept through channels in the column; such difficulties could be easily overcome by using appropriate filters for the column effluent. There was no evidence that the adsorption capacity of either column for 2-AAF had been depleted and both systems generally achieved a cleanup of 100,000-fold. Based on these data, a system consisting of filters and adsorption units was proposed for pilot-scale evaluation.

Results of tests to determine possible sorption of 2-AAF from aqueous dispersions by the alluvial silt soil at the NCTR are illustrated in Figure 5.2. The concentration of the aqueous 2-AAF in the presence of soil declined from 5.0 to 0.004 ppm during the 28-day test period, while a portion of the same dispersion (soil absent)

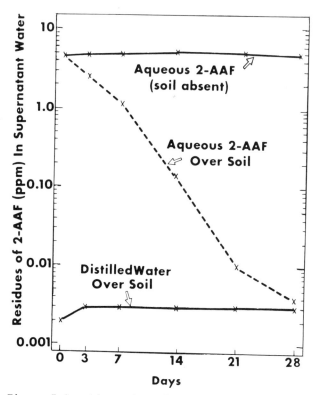

Figure 5.2. Adsorption of 2-AAF from an aqueous dispersion (5 ppm) by alluvial silt soil at the NCTR. (From Nony et al. [4].)

remained essentially unchanged. In the unlikely event that 2-AAF-containing wastewater accidently escaped from our cleanup system and entered the sewage treatment process, none of the residues would be expected to be discharged from the NCTR. The 30-day journey through the sewage processing system would probably allow complete sorption of the residues by the soil.

The pilot-scale cleanup system was evaluated using 59,000 gallons of 2-AAF-containing wastewater; results of these tests are presented in Table 5.1. Samples were collected across each major component of the system at 1000-gallon intervals during the processing of the first 5000 gallons. The depth filters were shown to have

Table 5.1. Residues of 2-AAF in wastewater at various stages of the pilot-scale cleanup process

Wastewater processed (gallons x 10³)	Raw wastewater (untreated)[a]	Residues of 2-AAF (ppb)		
		After filtration	After filtration and carbon adsorption[b]	After filtration and carbon and resin adsorption[c]
0[d]	3.3	2.0	<0.2	<0.2
1	7.0	6.7	<0.2	<0.2
3	8.3	5.9	<0.2	<0.2
4	7.1	6.4	<0.2	<0.2
5	2.6	3.4	<0.2	<0.2
10	7.8	--	0.6	<0.2
18	8.5	--	1.2	<0:2
20	6.7	6.9	0.8	<0.2
30	7.5	--	<0.2	<0.2
35	3.2	--	<0.2	<0.2
40	3.8	--	<0.2	<0.2
45	3.0	--	<0.2	<0.2
50	4.3	--	1.1	<0.2
55	4.4	--	<0.2	<0.2
59	55.9	--	44.3	<0.2

Source: Nony et al. [4].

[a]The pH ranged from 6.3 to 7.5; however, it was generally 7.0 ± 0.1.

[b]The carbon adsorber was replaced after 20,000, 30,000, and 50,000 gallons had been processed.

[c]No residues of 2-AAF were detected in any of the samples.

[d]Initial sample was taken after only a few gallons had been processed.

little or no effect on the residue levels of 2-AAF; therefore, routine monitoring of the water between the filters and the primary absorber was discontinued. Nevertheless, the filters are considered necessary for the removal of suspended material that could accumulate in the adsorbers and cause a reduction of flow rate and/or deactivation of the adsorbents. No residues of 2-AAF penetrated either adsorber during the purification of the first 5000 gallons. Slight penetration of 2-AAF residues through the carbon adsorber occurred during the processing of the next 5000-gallon batch; nevertheless, only the depth filters were replaced at this point, and an additional 10,000 gallons were processed in order to challenge the secondary adsorber. No residues penetrated the secondary adsorber during this treatment. The performance of the system indicated that the primary carbon adsorber should be changed after processing 10,000 gallons of water; however, its longevity is undoubtedly related directly to the concentration of extraneous contaminants in the water. Therefore, after 20,000 gallons of water had been processed, the carbon adsorber was replaced and another 10,000 gallons were processed. The effluents of both adsorbers were free of 2-AAF residues. At the 30,000-gallon interval, the depth filters, carbon adsorber, and membrane filter were replaced and the water treatment process continued. No residues were detected in the effluent of either adsorber after 40,000 gallons; the longevity of the carbon adsorber was again tested by subjecting it to an additional 10,000 gallons of wastewater. At the 50,000-gallon interval, 2-AAF residues had again penetrated the carbon but not the resin. The carbon adsorber was replaced and the treatment continued. As the holding tanks were being emptied (59,000 gallons processed) residual sludge containing high levels of 2-AAF (e.g., 55 ppb) was inadvertently picked up from the bottom of the tanks and introduced into the cleanup system. This caused high levels of 2-AAF (44 ppb) to penetrate the carbon adsorber; however, no residues passed the secondary adsorption unit. The pilot-scale evaluation was terminated when the supply of wastewater was essentially exhausted and sludge began to enter the system. Results of the evaluation are illustrated in Figure 5.3. No residues of 2-AAF (<0.2 ppb) were detected in the

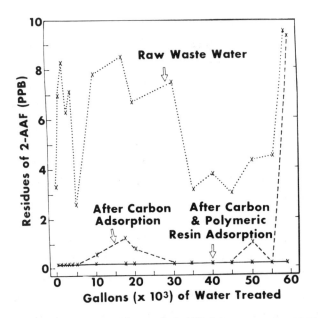

Figure 5.3. Residues of 2-AAF in raw wastewater (dotted line), after adsorption on activated carbon (broken line), and finally on polymeric resin (solid line). The carbon adsorber was replaced after 20,000, 30,000, and 40,000 gallons had been treated. (From Nony et al. [4].)

effluent of the secondary adsorber at any time during the tests. Flow rates of the wastewater through the cleanup system ranged from 0.8 to 1.7 gallons/min with the pressure drop being greatest across the primary adsorber. The spent carbon adsorbent and filters removed from the system were destroyed by incineration at 900°C. Contaminated XAD-2 resin may be incinerated or cleaned up by percolating acetone through it; the acetone effluent should be destroyed by incineration.

Future modifications of the cleanup system include the scaling-up of the components to provide a higher capacity. This could be accomplished with several complete systems consisting of larger filters and adsorbers arranged in parallel. Each system would include two carbon adsorbers in tandem to protect the more costly polymeric resin. Once the upstream carbon unit became depleted, the second unit would be brought upstream and a new unit installed

downstream   Fine-porosity depth filters should also be installed
downstream from each adsorber to prevent particles of adsorbent from
being carried from one unit to another and to protect the membrane
filter.

Consideration was given to the recycling of the treated wastewater for use in the boilers and cooling tower at the NCTR and chemical analyses indicated that its quality was acceptable. However,
microbiological assays of one of the treated samples revealed the
presence of a variety of microorganisms that prevented its immediate
reuse; chlorination would probably correct the deficiency.

In laboratory evaluations of the carbon and XAD-2 columns tested
with wastewater as previously described, traces of all compounds
tested thus far have been effectively removed by both adsorbents.
These include 4-aminobiphenyl, benzidine, 3,3'-dimethylbenzidine,
3,3'-dimethoxybenzidine, and 3,3'-dichlorobenzidine, all as free
amines or hydrochloride salts, and 2-AAF, 2-AF, diethylstilbestrol,
estradiol, lindane, and rotenone.

The pilot-scale cleanup system described above has functioned
well for decontaminating relatively small volumes of water. However,
a system capable of processing much larger volumes of wastewater is
required at the NCTR as toxicological testing is expanded. Such a
high-capacity system, based on the principles of the pilot-scale
cleanup, is currently being designed; the projected total cost of
the facility is about 1.5 million dollars.

Other researchers [7] who face cleanup problems with relatively
small volumes of contaminated wastewater are employing the basic
principles described in our pilot-scale system.

It should be noted that any appreciable amounts of organic solvents present in the wastewater could destroy the adsorptivity of
both the carbon and the XAD-2, therefore such solvents are collected
separately and destroyed by incineration. A possible alternative to
separate collection and disposal of organic solvents might be found
in the use of a new hydrophobic crystalline silica molecular sieve
[8]. Although this product has not yet been evaluated by the author,

the use of such a material is an attractive alternative for the removal of organic solvents of low molecular weights prior to treatment with other adsorbers.

REFERENCES

1. H. M. Malin Jr. Industry looks at wastewater reuse. *Environ. Sci. Technol. 7*, 500 (1973).

2. J. M. Cohen and I. J. Kugelman, Wastewater treatment: Physical and chemical methods. *J. Water Poll. Control Fed. 45*, 1027-1038 (1973).

3. C. E. Peacock. *Chem. Abs. 74*, 67408K (1971).

4. C. R. Nony, E. J. Treglown, and M. C. Bowman. Removal of trace levels of 2-acetylaminofluorene (2-AAF) from wastewater. *Sci. Total Environ. 4*, 155-163 (1975).

5. M. C. Bowman and J. R. King. Analysis of 2-acetylaminofluorene: Residues in laboratory chow and microbiological media. *Biochem. Med. 9*, 390-401 (1974).

6. B. Rassow and H. S. Schultzky. General principles of "codistillation." *Zeitscher. Agnew. Chem. 44*, 669-670 (1931).

7. J. N. Keith. How to design a building safe against hazards. *Occup. Health Safety 47*, 46-48 (1977).

8. E. M. Flanigen, J. M. Bennett, R. W. Grose, J. P. Cohen, R. L. Patton, R. M. Kirchner, and J. V. Smith. Silicalite, a new hydrophobic crystalline silica molecular sieve. *Nature 271*, 512-516 (1978).